# THINK
## AND GROW
# THIN

## Charles D'Angelo
### "THE WEIGHT-LOSS COACH"

RKP ROBERT KENNEDY PUBLISHING

Published by
Robert Kennedy Publishing
400 Matheson Blvd. West
Mississauga, ON
L5R 3M1 Canada
RKPubs.com
TAGTbook.com

Library and Archives Canada Cataloguing
in Publication

D'Angelo, Charles, 1985-
    Think and grow thin : the revolution-
    ary diet &
        weight-loss system that will
    change your life in
        88 days / Charles D'Angelo.

Includes index.

ISBN 978-1-55210-099-8
1. Reducing diets.  2. Weight loss--Psycho-
logical aspects.  I. Title.

RM222.2.D37 2012        613.2'5
C2011-905392-6

10 9 8 7 6 5 4 3 2 1

Distributed in Canada by
NBN (National Book Network)
67 Mowat Avenue, Suite 241
Toronto, ON
M6K 3E3

Distributed in USA by
NBN (National Book Network)
15200 NBN Way
Blue Ridge Summit, PA
17214

Printed in Canada

## Robert Kennedy Publishing
# BOOK DEPARTMENT

MANAGING DIRECTOR
**Wendy Morley**

SENIOR EDITOR
**Amy Land**

EDITOR, ONLINE AND PRINT
**Meredith Barrett**

ASSOCIATE EDITOR
**Rachel Corradetti**

ONLINE EDITOR
**Kiersten Corradetti**

EDITORIAL ASSISTANT
**Brittany Seki**

ADMINISTRATIVE ASSISTANT
**Jeannie Mahoney**

ART DIRECTOR
**Gabriella Caruso Marques**

ASSISTANT ART DIRECTOR
**Jessica Pensabene Hearn**

EDITORIAL DESIGNER
**Brian Ross**

ART ASSISTANT
**Kelsey-Lynn Corradetti**

SENIOR WEB DESIGNER
**Christopher Barnes**

MARKETING COORDINATOR
**Patricia D'Amato**

ONLINE ASSISTANT
**Chelsea Kennedy**

RECIPE PHOTOS
*Photographer—* **Donna Griffith**
**www.donnagriffith.com**
*Food Stylist—* **Marianne Wren**
*Props provided by* **Laura Branson,
The Prop Room, Robert Kennedy
Publishing, Donna Griffith**

INDEXING AND PROOFREADING
**James De Medeiros**

RECIPE WRITING & TESTING
**Ashif Tejani**

OTHER PHOTO CREDITS
**Paul Buceta:** *9, 17, 72, 137,
187 (Model: Fran Dennis), 194-218*
**Corbis Images:** *28*
**Vincent D'Angelo:** *52, 78*
**Tony Meoli:** *22, 74, 108, 193*

*All other photos of Charles provided by
Charles D'Angelo.*

*All Success Story photos provided by
each respective person.*

*Cover photography by* **Paul Buceta**

*All other photos* **istockphoto.com**

## IMPORTANT

The information in this book reflects the author's
experiences and opinions and is not intended to
replace medical advice.

Before beginning this or any nutritional or exercise
regimen, consult your physician to be sure it is
appropriate for you. Ask for a physical stress test.

To you who feel there is no hope left. You hold in your hands tangible evidence of Grace and divinity at work in your life! Make use of the tools within!

And to the great visionaries and teachers who have come before me, illustrating that all things are possible and inspiring me to use my gifts to serve others, particularly Walt Disney, Napoleon Hill, Anthony Robbins, Wayne Dyer, Richard Simmons, J.K. Rowling and Steven Spielberg, my unending gratitude.

# CONTENTS

## SECTION IV: Recipes    222

## Maintenance Recipes    252

# FOREWORD

I grew up in the Venezuelan tropics, where we had a healthy and plentiful mix of fresh fruits and vegetables, fish and meat along with some carbohydrate staples. Combine that with parents of Eastern European background, and I developed a passion for eating at an early age. But no matter how well we ate, thanks to our steady diet of Hollywood movies and television we were always envious of the American way of life. When I first came to the US to practice medicine, I could not believe the endless buffets, the incredible variety and the supersized meals. I arrived in the 1970s and there was plenty of obesity, but nothing like today's epidemic.

Unfortunately, as I adapted to this country, so did my eating and exercise habits. I suddenly found myself among the increasingly overweight population. As a physician I knew all the medical implications of being overweight, but that didn't change my habits. It took a chance encounter with a friend and client of weight-loss coach Charles D'Angelo to start the chain of events that put me on the path to a healthier life.

When I first met Charles, I was struck by his energy and enthusiasm. He's in excellent shape, and if you didn't know already, you would never dream that as a teenager he weighed 360 pounds. He found the strength to change and overcome what seemed like an inevitable family destiny. And he did this despite the fact that he was suffering from a crippling lack of self-confidence, and despite the fact that many of his family members suffered from severe obesity due to extremely unhealthy attitudes about food. It is this very personal story that will pull you in and inspire you to join Charles' successful team. By sheer will, determination and hard work he broke the cycle for himself and has now helped countless men, women and children lose thousands of pounds of excess weight.

As a kidney doctor dealing with hypertension, diabetes and dialysis, I am very familiar with the need for dietary health restrictions, which are often difficult to accomplish without the necessary drive. And we are all familiar with the roller-coaster effect of fad diets. In this book, Charles explains why those diets are often doomed to failure. In a clear, articulate and engaging way, he explains the importance of balance and how severe fat or carbohydrate restriction can lead to cravings followed by binges. He then provides you with an easy and understandable list of good, moderate and bad foods. There is no guesswork on the reader's part: This is a road map anyone can follow.

I had years of careless eating under my ever-growing belt and the pounds had piled up. Charles proved to me that being overweight begins in the mind. That's where his focus lies – in changing the way we think.

Throughout this book, Charles offers anecdotes and imagery to which we all can relate. His clear and knowledgeable guidance makes it possible – and even exhilarating – for someone to establish new patterns and habits, which is key to his program's success. His is a very simple approach – there are no magic tricks or gimmicks. Reinventing yourself takes effort, will and a true desire to change for the better.

Charles D'Angelo helped me find that motivation to incorporate a well-balanced, consistent diet and program of physical fitness into my life without any feelings of deprivation. I am confident that he can do the same for you.

**Marcos Rothstein, M.D.**
Professor of Medicine,
Washington University in St. Louis

Medical Director, Dialysis Services,
Barnes-Jewish Hospital

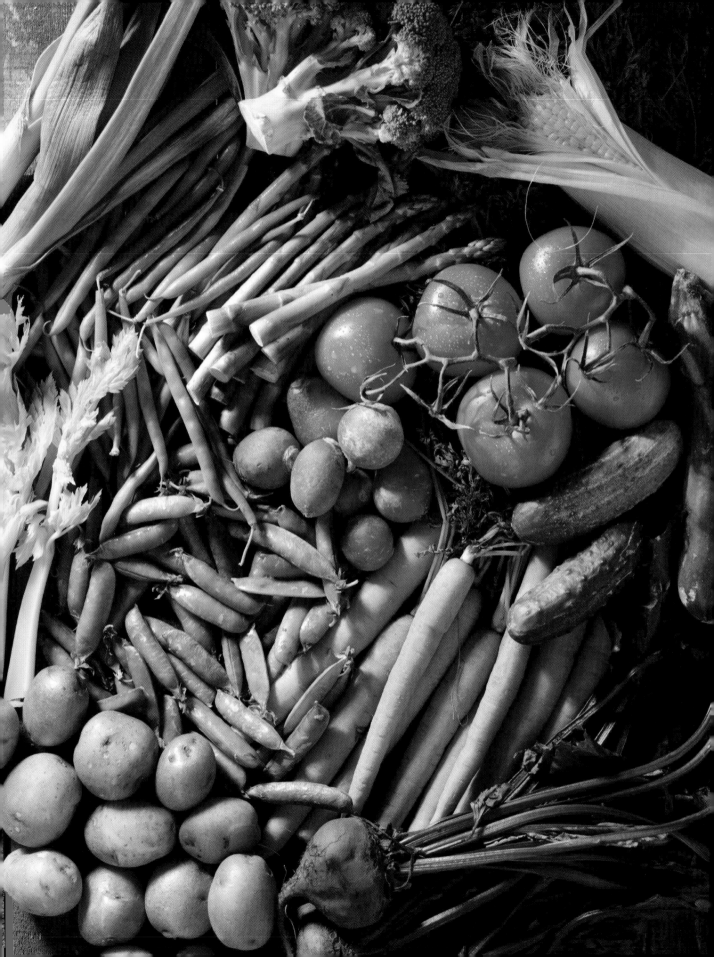

# INTRODUCTION

When you meet Charles, you know he has found what he was meant to do. His passion, enthusiasm, indefatigability and faith are clear as day. But he wasn't always this way. You'd never know meeting him now, but for the first 17 years of his life, Charles' obesity held him back from living the life he was meant to live. Being overweight is a significant barrier to fulfilling your greatest purpose and destiny. It was by losing his excess weight that Charles was able to find his. Charles' life mission is to serve others, inspiring and providing his strategies to as many people as he can, helping them realize their true potential by getting their health and habits in check. Now God has put this book in your hands so Charles can help you as he has helped so many others, including my son, a number of my friends and me, by reminding us of our potential. Your unique purpose is waiting for just you.

As a young man growing up in Clinton, Montana in the 50s and 60s, I could easily have followed the path of least resistance. Although I wasn't overweight, I faced tremendous adversity similar to the discrimination Charles experienced because of his obesity. Thankfully, God had blessed me with a mother and father who taught their eight children the value of faith and hard work when we were young. They stressed that nothing comes without the two. We learned from them that the world was ours for the taking despite the racism we faced.

During this time of civil rights upheaval, I was the only African-American boy to graduate from my high school. I realized that things had to change. A group of friends and I decided to make our own personal statement and desegregate the local swimming pool. One day we went to the pool and just jumped right in. I don't know what we expected, but we found no resistance. That brave first step brought about everlasting change. You can also realize everlasting change when you follow Charles' *Think and Grow Thin* program. Go ahead and take the plunge. Dive right in.

Real change happens only when you put yourself out there without reservation, resist the norms and risk it all. You must have faith that God will carry you through. This message is clear in Charles' book. I see a lot of myself in Charles. Tremendous faith in God, hard work, persistence, passion, empathy and a willingness to serve – an extraordinarily rare set of qualities that can make this world a better place.

In his book *Think and Grow Thin*, Charles can help free you from the shackles of adversity your weight has you chained to. I urge you to embrace the profoundly simple strategies and wisdom found inside these pages. Go at it with all of your heart and your life will be changed for the better, and forever. After you've read his book, you will understand that you do have a mission to fulfill. It is a mission that requires you to feel your best – physically, spiritually and emotionally. Don't allow your weight to stop you from reaching your full potential.

Let Charles be your guide – he may very well be the answer you've been praying for. God bless you on the journey you're about to embark on; Charles has certainly been a blessing to me and to so many others. I wish you success and much happiness.

**David Steward**
Chairman and founder, Worldwide Technology, Inc.

100 Most Influential Black Americans - *Ebony* magazine

America's 14th-Best Entrepreneur - *Success* magazine

Ernst & Young Technology Entrepreneur of the Year

National Society of Black Engineers Entrepreneur of the Year

Small Business Association Hall of Fame Inductee

*St. Louis Sentinel* Business Person of the Year

Author of *Doing Business by the Good Book*

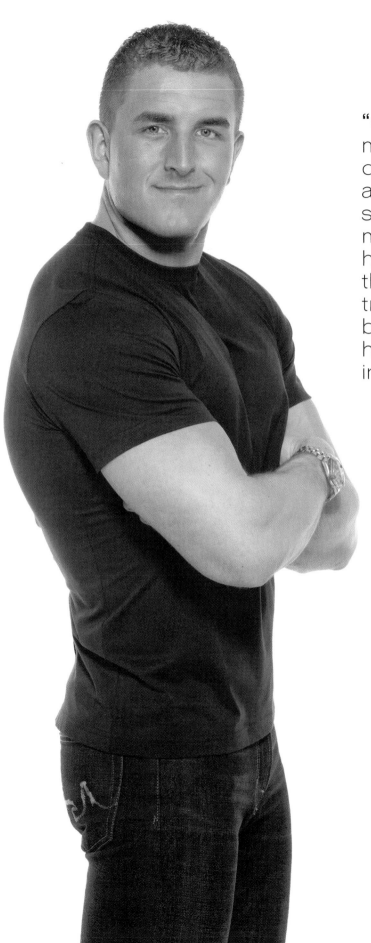

"Charles' life mission is to serve others, inspiring and providing his strategies to as many people as he can, helping them realize their true potential by getting their health and habits in check."

I

# section I

## You and I
## Are a Lot Alike

# CHAPTER ONE
## My Story: Facing Reality

"Most people condemn themselves to prison all their lives, despite the fact that they carry the keys to their prison without knowing they possess them. The prison consists in the self-imposed limitations they set up in their own minds, or permit others to set for them."

– Napoleon Hill, *You Can Work Your Own Miracles*

If you were to look at a photo of my extended family, you would probably guess that I'd end up fat – and you'd be right. Practically everyone in my family was fat, and I fit right in.

I started life as a large baby, and, as time passed, I only got larger, and larger, and larger still. I was a 200-pound fourth grader, if you can imagine that. By the time I was 17, my weight had ballooned to 360 pounds. Simple activities like tying my shoes felt like exercise to me. I had a hard time getting up the flight of only four stairs at my high school. I would break out in a cold sweat, just sitting at my desk in air-conditioned classes. I felt self-conscious everywhere I went, thinking all eyes were on me, and for all the wrong reasons.

The truth is, my life was miserable and even embarrassing. I had no self-esteem. I began to feel that life wasn't worth living. I saw my future in my relatives who suffered from obesity-related illnesses such as diabetes. One time, I saw the "future me" at a restaurant. This solitary, middle-aged man looked like he weighed around 400 pounds. I imagined his only friend was the big bowl of pasta in front of him, and that he would probably be going home to an empty house, feeling that nothing he did made a difference.

I was crossing to the dark side with all the negatives I was focused on. I had no friends – I had isolated myself from everyone because I feared their criticism. I was in such a negative place in my life. If I had kept on at the rate I was going, you wouldn't be reading this right now. Though many people had tried to tell me I was headed for an early grave, it didn't really sink in until one day when I was 17. On that frightening day, which I'll describe later in this chapter, I came to the grim realization that if I didn't make a change that very instant, I would not be alive to graduate from high school the next year. I would never have any true friends. I would never experience the love of a girl. I would never have my own family, nor would I ever be able to make a difference in anyone's life. I would have wasted the one chance I had to make a difference to others because of what my bad habits had done to my health.

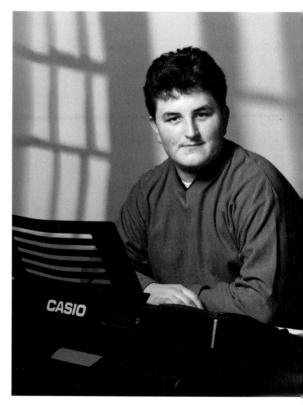

▶ MUSIC HELPED ME ESCAPE THE LONELINESS AND BULLYING DURING GRADE SCHOOL.

This realization made me finally change my ways forever. My life immediately began to transform that day, going from one of misery, loneliness, depression, ridicule and poor health to one of energy, excellent health, power, success and excitement. I went from weighing a sloppy, out-of-shape 360 pounds to building myself a chiseled, fit, muscular, jacked body. I went from being a kid who could only dream of one day having a date to being chosen as one of Cosmo's "Shirtless Sweethearts."

# I KNOW YOU CAN SUCCEED!

When I first made the decision to get healthy, I figured a gym was the place to start. I got a minimum wage job at my high school and saved money until I had enough to join a gym. I was terrified of walking through the doors. After all, wasn't the gym a place where all the attractive, popular, strong and assertive people hung out? I wasn't any of those things and I feared what lay ahead. Still, I knew I must do *something*, so I made my way in and talked to a salesperson. He looked young enough to be one of my classmates and didn't seem very emotionally invested in me, but I was desperate. I mustered up my courage and said, "Sign me up."

He took me to the front desk and started my paperwork. Standing there filling out the form, I thought of how great it would be to finally have the body I wanted and the confidence I yearned for. A manager had come over to talk to the salesperson, and it struck me something was wrong. I was right. Unfortunately, a credit card was needed to sign up, and I only had cash. I was turned away.

I left the gym more discouraged than ever. After psyching myself up for so long to have the courage to go in, I was rejected. It felt so familiar, like all those times I felt that magical butterflies-in-the-stomach feeling for a girl, but was turned down and not even given a

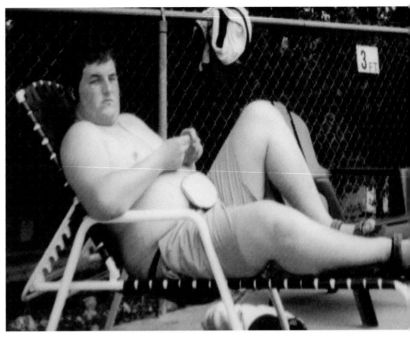

chance because I was fat. When I got home, I went up to my bedroom. I was lying on my back in bed and tears began to well up in my eyes. This is hopeless, I thought. I'm destined to be fat, miserable and alone.

Although my parents' house was air-conditioned and it had been an hour since I had been outside, I was still sweating profusely. I lay there and thought about the more than 150 pounds of pure fat I was carrying with me every day. I started to feel totally overwhelmed and depressed. I remember watching my gut rise up so high that it blocked my view of the TV. I looked up to the ceiling, and just started talking with God. I begged for His help, and promised that if he would help me to just be "normal" looking, I would do everything in my power to positively contribute to other people's lives in some way. After that short prayer, I went from hopeless to having a spark of hope.

Did I know then that a decade later I would not only have met all my goals, but also be helping thousands of other people transform their health and achieve the bodies they deserved? No! I would have never imagined such a thing. And yet, over the next two years, I lost more than 150 pounds of pure fat. I have kept my weight off, taken my body to a whole new level through weight training and kept my promise. It just goes to show you that you are part of this plan, too. God, Allah, Moses, Bhagwan, Buddha – whatever name you choose to call your higher power – has put this book into your hands at this moment. You are looking at these pages for a special reason.

It's my life's mission to help as many people as I can to break free from the prison they have eaten themselves into. I know how it feels to have people point and laugh at you. I know how it feels to hide in the bathroom until school begins, so you don't have to face kids in the schoolyard. I know how it feels to have TV and food as your only friends. To envy a couple you see at the mall, holding hands, totally in love, while you know you couldn't ever gather the courage to even approach a person you like. I've been where you are. I know how it feels to be scared to try because you feel like you've tried it all before and were shut down. I understand where you're coming from!

> ## "It's my life's mission to help as many people as I can to break free from the prison they have eaten themselves into."

You don't have to be as overweight as I was to be a prisoner to overeating. You might be only 20 or 30 pounds overweight, or you might have an extra 50, 100, 200 or more pounds to lose. Whatever the case, you are keeping yourself in that prison because of your mindset and the decisions you are making consistently. Know this: Today can be the day that you break free. I know you can break free, because I did it, and so have the thousands of others I've personally coached. You don't have to allow unhealthy food to use you anymore. After all, that's what it's doing. It's using you, controlling you and keeping you from the life you want and deserve.

So, if you are really willing to give it your all, then I am willing to offer you a plan that can turn your life upside down faster than anything you've tried before. Why am I so certain I can help you? I'm certain because everything has a pattern. Weight-loss success has a pattern. I've developed a pattern of eating and exercising that can cause your body to crank through fat at lightning-fast speeds while also helping you deal with the psychological and emotional sources that are at the root of your issue. If I can do it, you can do it. You deserve wellness. You deserve health and good looks. Now is the time to give yourself the permission to achieve it.

## WHAT'S YOUR EXCUSE?

I've worked with people from all walks of life – politicians, CEOs, lawyers, soccer moms and teens – which means I've heard practically every reason and rationalization for being overweight, including:

➡ "I was raised in a family that's overweight."

➡ "It's just part of my heritage."

➡ "I'm too busy to eat properly."

➡ "Food makes me happy."

➡ "I had a traumatic childhood."

Listen, I know you have your reasons for being overweight, just like I once had. The truth is, the only real reason you are overweight is because you have allowed yourself to believe your extra fat is something outside of your control.

I get it. I felt that way at one time, too. But here's the thing: If you really want to change your life – and I mean change it forever, not just for three months – then you need to start examining your beliefs about yourself. In the book *From Poverty to Power*, James Allen offers the following advice, "Cease your complaining and fretting; none of these things which you blame are the cause of your [problems]; the cause is within yourself, and where the cause is, there is the remedy." When being unhealthy becomes part of your identity, things can get dangerous. If you think of yourself as a "fat" person, if you *really believe* that's who you are, your behavior is going to reflect that belief. Wow!

Maybe you have never been in shape. Maybe you're like me and you've struggled with your weight as far back as you can remember. Today can be the day when you decide you're no longer a "fat" person. You can create a mental picture of yourself as a lean, fit, healthy, energetic and vibrant person who wants to be healthy not only for herself or himself, but also for others. Once you start to believe that you are a fit and healthy person who is simply carrying around extra fat, we can work at getting rid of that fat and sculpting the body you desire!

## GO BEYOND YOUR LIMITS

Being overweight limits the person you can be, doesn't it? It certainly limited me. All of my decisions, including where I would go, what I could wear, where I could shop, who I could talk to and where I sat, were affected by my weight. How I lived my life was not the way I would have chosen. I honestly believe that we are all here on this beautiful planet we call Earth to make everyone else's experience here as positive as possible. Yet I was so unhappy with myself that the last thing I could do was even *think* about helping others. As James Allen wrote in *As A Man Thinketh*, "A strong man cannot help a weaker unless that weaker is willing to be helped. And even then the weak man must become strong of himself. He must, by his own efforts, develop the strength which he admires in another. None but himself can alter his condition."

Now, maybe you are someone who thinks that all of that excess weight isn't really affecting your life. If so, let me ask you a few questions:

→ Are you the best parent you can be when you don't have energy?

→ Are you the most productive employee if you don't feel good while at work?

→ Are you able to function happily and efficiently when you are constantly worrying about what people are saying and thinking about you?

→ Are you able to give the most to your family if your mood is controlled by the diabetic medications you're forced to take because of your weight?

Of course not! You have so much potential, and the first step toward tapping into it is changing the beliefs you have about yourself.

You can be so much more.

"Cease your complaining and fretting; none of these things which you blame are the cause of your [problems]; the cause is within yourself, and where the cause is, there is the remedy."

– James Allen, *From Poverty to Power*

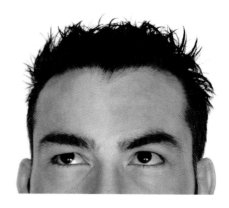

> "Remember, the brain is here to make you feel good, but some brains aren't the greatest long-term planners."

## REWIRING YOUR BRAIN

Our brains are unbelievably complex, useful and sometimes mysterious things. Whether you realize it or not, your brain is constantly at work trying to make you feel good. It wants you to be in a constant state of joy, elation and happiness. Somehow, though, you've got your wires crossed. My wires were once crossed, too. Your brain has connected a level of pain to exercise and eating healthy foods, and it has connected pleasure to things like junk food and laziness, which are actually (and ironically) keeping you in your state of misery.

Your brain's wires are crossed because it isn't looking at the long-term effects of your behavior. Remember, the brain is here to make you feel good, but some brains aren't the greatest long-term planners. When we start to feel bad, our brain goes to work trying to come up with ways to help us immediately feel better. If we feel sore and tired when trying to exercise, our brain says, "This doesn't feel good. Go watch some TV instead." It doesn't say, "This may be hard right now, but if you keep it up it will get easier and you'll feel good later." If you're used to eating foods filled with fats, sugars and salt, then when you eat healthy food, your brain says, "Where's that good feeling and taste? Go get a donut instead!" It doesn't say, "You'll soon love the taste of this healthy food and despise the taste of that donut," or "You're going to feel a lot better after a week without donuts!"

It may seem hard to believe now, but just as you can go from being a serious shopaholic to a super-frugal saver who gets pleasure from watching your savings grow and grow, you can rewire your brain to get pleasure from eating foods that fuel your health and fitness. You can get the same feelings of pleasure from an exercise session as from a piece of chocolate. In fact, you can get *more* pleasure once you become used to the exercise!

## UPGRADE YOUR LIFE

We can always find excuses to avoid doing the things we don't want to do. Think about it. If you want to find excuses for remaining overweight, isn't it easy? Just try to remember all the things you've told yourself up to this point. There are lots of reasons and rationalizations that can make those extra pounds on your frame seem acceptable, but I think something deep inside of you is whispering (or perhaps SHOUTING) that it's time to change. This book has been put into your hands at this moment for a very important reason. It's here with you because you are a person who *can* change. The circumstances that brought this book to fruition are almost magical. There is a far greater force at work here, and it wants you to benefit from the information contained within these pages.

You can have so much more in your life than you have right now. Imagine having so much energy that you could work out *twice* a day! Imagine leaving the office looking forward to being home with your family and having the energy to enjoy their company. Imagine feeling with absolute certainty that you are in control of your life and your decisions. Imagine knowing that you – not your friends, family or circumstances – are the one who will determine the quality of your life. Imagine finally having the confidence to reach for the things you once thought impossible – to approach the person you've longed to meet or go after that job you know you deserve. All of these things are waiting for you. Wayne Dyer has said, "What you want wants you, and is simply waiting for you to be on the same frequency to find it!" Know that anything you want, you can create, including the body of your dreams, *as soon as you decide this is true*.

Let's face it. It's time to upgrade your life. What you've done up to this point hasn't given you the results you deserve. And even if you've had short-term success but then gained all the weight back, you didn't fail. You simply got a result. The result you got was one that you don't want to get again. It's time to try something different, something that has given thousands of people a result so unique and exciting that it is now in this book. You've picked up this book because you're the type of person who wants more out of your life – and you deserve it. So don't be afraid, I am going to be right there beside you!

I am so excited for you!

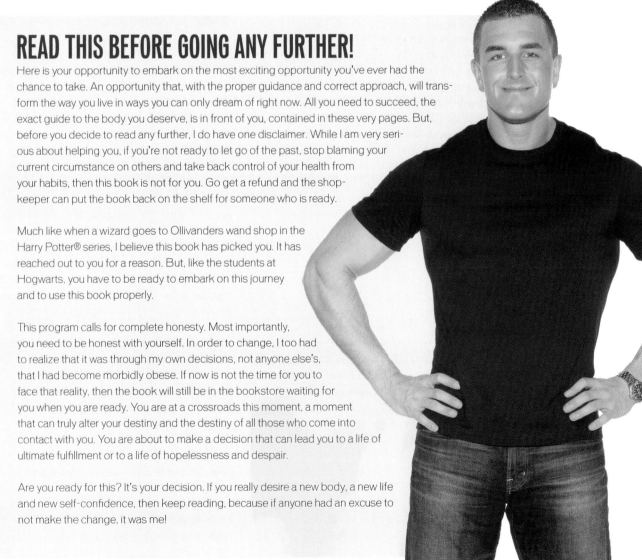

# READ THIS BEFORE GOING ANY FURTHER!

Here is your opportunity to embark on the most exciting opportunity you've ever had the chance to take. An opportunity that, with the proper guidance and correct approach, will transform the way you live in ways you can only dream of right now. All you need to succeed, the exact guide to the body you deserve, is in front of you, contained in these very pages. But, before you decide to read any further, I do have one disclaimer. While I am very serious about helping you, if you're not ready to let go of the past, stop blaming your current circumstance on others and take back control of your health from your habits, then this book is not for you. Go get a refund and the shopkeeper can put the book back on the shelf for someone who is ready.

Much like when a wizard goes to Ollivanders wand shop in the Harry Potter® series, I believe this book has picked you. It has reached out to you for a reason. But, like the students at Hogwarts, you have to be ready to embark on this journey and to use this book properly.

This program calls for complete honesty. Most importantly, you need to be honest with yourself. In order to change, I too had to realize that it was through my own decisions, not anyone else's, that I had become morbidly obese. If now is not the time for you to face that reality, then the book will still be in the bookstore waiting for you when you are ready. You are at a crossroads this moment, a moment that can truly alter your destiny and the destiny of all those who come into contact with you. You are about to make a decision that can lead you to a life of ultimate fulfillment or to a life of hopelessness and despair.

Are you ready for this? It's your decision. If you really desire a new body, a new life and new self-confidence, then keep reading, because if anyone had an excuse to not make the change, it was me!

# FAMILY MATTERS

I think I understand people and their reasons for rationalizing their problems so well because I could be the king of excuses if I chose to be. As I said earlier, I grew up in a family filled with overweight people. My grandparents, my father and his brothers were all overweight. Were we genetically predisposed to being fat? Maybe. Were we all brought up with terrible eating and exercise habits? Definitely. And those habits manifested themselves not only in a family of fat people, but a family of fat people filled with every preventable disease you can think of.

My great-grandfather died of a heart attack when my grandfather was only a young man, so my grandfather had to quit school at a young age to go to work in order to help support his family. You could say this was the genesis of my family's obesity: Since my grandfather had to quit school, he never learned how to read and therefore couldn't even consider learning about health and nutrition. Also because of his lack of education, he and his family were always poor. And when you're poor, food becomes a luxury.

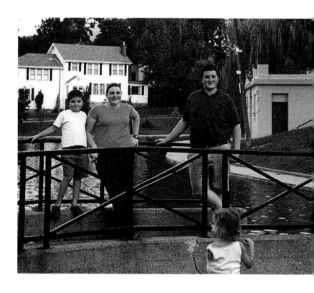

My grandfather and grandmother had four sons, including my father, and putting enough food on the table was never easy. Four growing boys want to eat – a lot – but feeding them healthy foods on a salary that was barely minimum wage was definitely a challenge. My grandparents, like many people affected by the economy today, filled their boys up the best way they knew how: with cheap, simple starches that tasted good. My dad remembers his daily breakfast consisting of stacks of white toast covered in butter and syrup. Lunch was white bread with jelly and maybe a little peanut butter. Dinner was pasta noodles with olive oil and butter. It's no surprise this diet resulted in four kids and two parents who were not only obese, but also suffered from heart disease, diabetes and even shortened lives.

## "Were we genetically predisposed to being fat? Maybe. Were we all brought up with terrible eating and exercise habits? Definitely."

And if you're thinking that these health risks apply only to the obese – they don't. According to the Centers for Disease Control, even slightly overweight adults (those carrying an extra 10 to 20 pounds) are at increased risk of premature death. They are also increasing their risk of developing a myriad of other serious health issues, including liver and gallbladder disease, certain types of cancer, pregnancy and fertility complications, musculoskeletal issues and emotional, social and psychological problems.

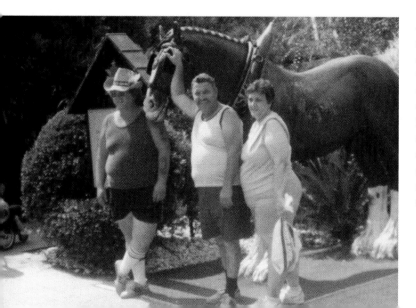

# FOOD AS CELEBRATION, PACIFICATION, JUSTIFICATION

Maybe it was because of our Italian heritage or maybe it was because food was scarce, but in my family no cause for celebration went without a sugary, salty mound of greasy food. For us, food was not just a form of sustenance. If any food was on the table, especially fast food or take out, it meant we were doing well. Food itself was an "event." Playing outside for an hour was rewarded with a night of take-out pizza and movies. So much for activity! Holing myself up on the couch with mountains of junk food was a surefire way to distract myself from the challenges I faced. Food never judged me – it just tasted good and it made me feel better.

One of the most primal needs we humans have is the need to provide food for our families, and in my house the colorful bags of potato chips, candy and chocolate meant that we were fed. By this standard, the fat that puffed out our bodies and muffin-topped over our pants did not mean poor health, it meant we could afford the most effectively marketed yet lowest-quality food. To a kid, that was fantastic. From my father's family, whether by genes or by environment, I inherited a feeling that I continually had to put more and more unhealthy food in my mouth. It was incessant. I have memories of sitting at my grandparents' table, eating one cherry pie after another while sipping on coffee with three tablespoons of sugar in cup after cup. I was slowly and steadily committing caloric suicide alongside my most-loved family members.

The flip side of that coin was my mother's family. Although individually they were not as much of an influence in my life as my dad's parents, the legacy they left me was. My mother's entire family was made up of alcoholics. They may not have been overweight, but their idea of dealing with a situation was the same as my dad's family. They used this other drug, alcohol, to distract themselves and hide from their problems. I have never yet had a sip of alcohol, but I too once was an addict, and my drug of choice was food. I used food as a pacifier when I was upset. I used it to lift me up when I was down. I used it as a distraction when I was worried. It was my state changer. Ironically, I used food, the very thing that was at the source of my problems, to help me get through my days of torment at school.

My day would start off with four or five Pop Tarts and a liter of regular soda. On the way to school, I would stop at 7-Eleven and pick up a bag of Chex Mix, a candy bar and a Big Gulp to "enjoy" in the car as I prepared myself for a miserable day of bullying. As the day wore on, I was far more likely to be stuffing my mouth with butter noodles, candy or nachos than anything that gave me any nutrition. My school had a lunch program in which you paid very little for second servings, and I remember going back for four plates of noodles to eat alongside my pizza, which had small ponds of grease floating on top of each slice. I didn't have much certainty in my life, but I knew that unhealthy food was the one thing that would make me feel better. Recipe for disaster? You'd better believe it! At the time I didn't know any better and neither did my family, but now I do. I've conquered it, and I can help you conquer it as well.

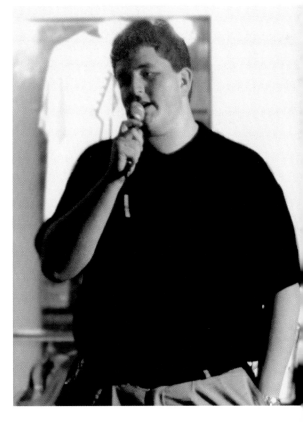

▼ NEAR THE BEGINNING OF MY JUNIOR YEAR.

## BACK TO YOU

Why did I tell you these intimate details of my personal life? I want you to know these things because you need to realize that we're not that different from each other. I once had a ton in common with you – pardon the pun. I'm sure you have your own "reasons" for being overweight. I did too. That's why, when I hear people say things like, "My whole family is overweight, therefore I will always be," I don't let them get away with it. I call "bull" right there. As you now know, my whole family was overweight. Our lifestyles and habits were a vicious breeding ground for obesity and ultimately life-ending disease.

As we near the end of this chapter, I can almost hear those negative voices in the back of your head (Remember, I've been right where you are now.) Right now you are thinking that you can't change because you've always been overweight, or because your family doesn't encourage you to, or because it's too hard. Well, have I got exciting news for you! You CAN change. It doesn't matter what shape you're in, how much money you make, what job you have, who your parents are or what education you have. None of that is as important as tapping into your desire to change now.

## MY MOTIVATION

By now you might be wondering, after 17 years of lonely nights, gym-class humiliations, and constantly being referred to as "the fat kid" – what finally made me change?

Over the years, countless people had told me that I should change my ways for the good of my health. Sometimes, that's just too ambiguous and doesn't bring the level of urgency that it takes to move someone to action. Being a smart kid, I knew that what they said was true logically and cognitively, but it didn't matter because emotionally I just didn't make the connection. I had strongly conditioned myself to associate positive emotions with bad foods for so long that these feelings outweighed the short-lived negative criticism I often received. After all, I had long given up on dating or even approaching a girl. I was in a terrible mental state in which I really didn't care. Even though it made me deeply unhappy, I had come to accept myself as obese. Like a smoker or alcoholic being lectured to quit, I just let their words go in one ear and out the other. I would nod gravely as they spoke, but I was really thinking about whether I would have McDonald's or Burger King that night. I figured I'd get around to changing sooner or later but, as it turned out, sooner came much more quickly than I thought it would. God often has a way of nudging us in the right direction and giving us a chance to see what the future holds if we choose not to do what's right. Over a couple of days in my junior year of high school, I suddenly understood the reality of what I was doing to my body.

One night, as usual, I was lying on the couch watching TV alone. To fill the void of loneliness, I had consumed a huge box of salty, greasy breadsticks, a large pepperoni and cheese pizza and a two-liter bottle of sugary soda. I fell asleep, likely due to the crash after the sugar high. When I awoke, my eyesight had disappeared. I couldn't see anything. I panicked, but at the same time I kind of pretended it wasn't happening. I kept waiting for my vision to come back, but it didn't. I went back to sleep, hoping that this was just a strange temporary occurrence. Thoughts of my grandma raced into my head. She had type 2 diabetes. I knew that diabetes was caused by a poor diet, and I also knew that it could cause blindness. This was not news to me, but the reality of these facts had never really sunk in. When my eyesight disappeared, the reality struck me in the head like a brick. This was to be my future. When I realized what was in store for me should I continue with my unhealthy habits, I was terrified. Luckily my eyesight returned, and I never found out the reason for its disappearance,

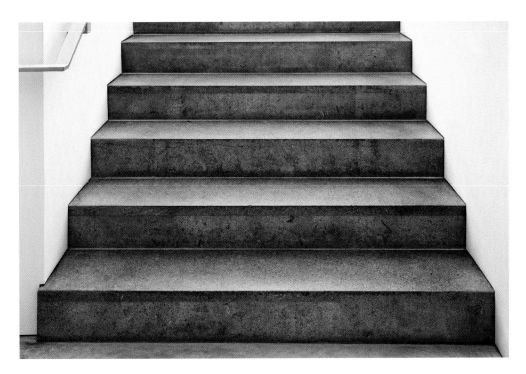

but that was one of the first emotional steps toward my transformation.

The next day at school, climbing up four stairs – not four *flights* of stairs, just four *stairs* – caused me so much difficulty that my heart was racing when I reached the top. Later on in class, I suddenly felt a sweaty chill. I was cold but sweating. My palms were sopping. I felt horrible. That moment also passed, but it has long remained seared in my mind.

I thought of my graduation the next year, and I just knew that if I kept doing what I had been doing, I would never live to see my graduation day. Although my life had been pretty horrible up until that point (as you will find out later in this book), I really did not want to end it.

That day when I got home, I called a gym. Less than a year later, I had lost 120 pounds, I felt great and I even had a date for the prom. By the winter of that same year, my first year in college, I had lost the last 40 pounds. While at college, I carved out my own niche, became a weight-loss coach and started weight train-

"The next day at school, climbing up four stairs – not four *flights* of stairs, just four *stairs* – caused me so much difficulty that my heart was racing when I reached the top."

ing with intensity. I poured myself into my passion, and within a very short time my story and reputation had attracted a lot of attention. I suddenly had clients flying in to St. Louis from out of state, seeking my advice and coaching. I've met and shared my story with two US presidents and countless celebrities. I've helped thousands of people from all walks of life reach their own goal weights, and I've helped dozens lose more than 100 pounds each. I've kept the weight off for nearly a decade, beating all the statistics, and now I'm ready to help you. Are you up for this?

Getting what you want out of life may not be easy. You may have failed in the past but you've

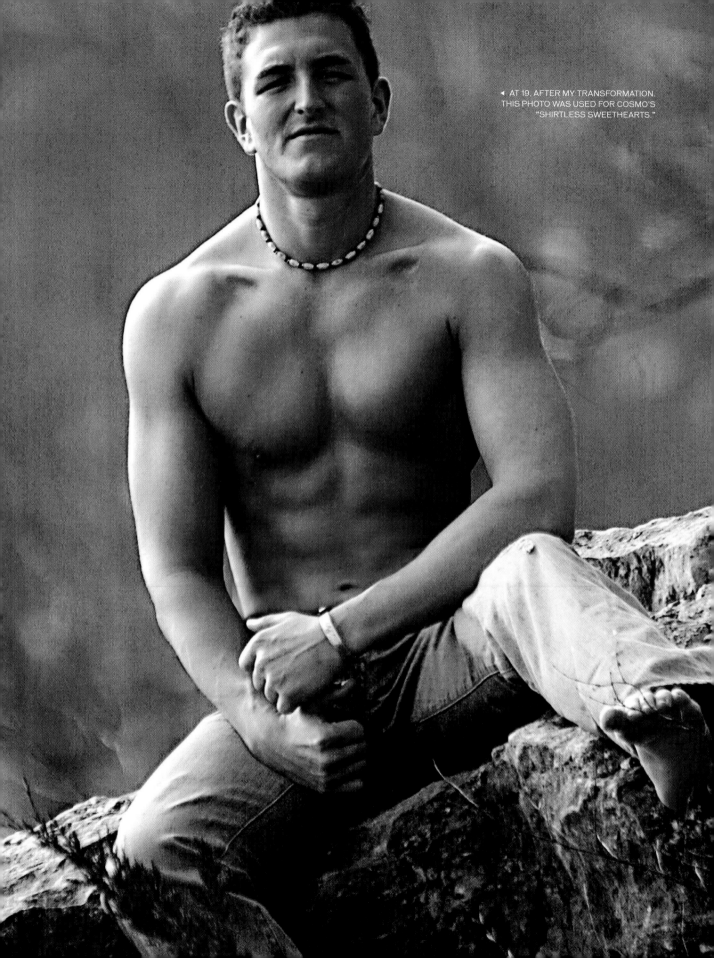

never worked with me. The majority of people give up at the first bump in the road (Remember my first attempt at joining a gym?). Since you're still reading, I know this isn't how you are! There may be some short-term pain, but you will change, and the long-term pleasure will make it all worth it. The time to change is now!

I want you to enlist the help of your higher power (I choose to call mine God). Send off prayers of gratitude, as well as requests for things you need help with, daily – or hourly – if needed. I know God has led you to this book for a miraculous reason. You may feel this is a lot to swallow. You may feel overwhelmed by the task ahead, but know that no matter how far beyond hope you feel, it's certainly not too late! Now is the time to take MASSIVE action. You are a very special person with an unbeliev-able destiny waiting for you to discover it. As Ralph Waldo Emerson said, "Once you make a decision, the universe conspires to make it happen." Forces you cannot even perceive are working to bring about positive changes in your life – if you choose to jump into the flow.

Sometimes life beats us down. We feel worn out, miserable and out of luck. We feel like we've tried it all. It's time to put that past behind you now. It's over. You are not the same person you were, and the experiences you're having now are not the same as before. Stop replaying the negative tapes and recordings. It's time to make a new recording, an achieve-ment that is not only going to change your life, but also inspire millions of others.

Everything gets better as you change what you're focused on. Thank God that you have the ability to even understand the words you're reading, that you can see them or hear them. We take completely for granted that which is familiar. That's one of the reasons your weight is out of control right now. Perhaps a health issue has scared you into doing this. Think of the years you ate whatever you wanted whenever you wanted

to without any perceived consequence. The truth is that *everything* we do has a conse-quence. Every food choice counts. Every rep and every minute on the treadmill counts. Make the most of the time you have and stop wasting your life focusing on perceived limitations. I don't say that judgmentally; I say it with the utmost respect for you. I almost fell victim to the belief that life is miserable. It's not! Wake up and see what's possible!

When you're grateful, you keep your mind in a positive state, focused on the good. You aren't the only one who will benefit immensely from following the recommendations I put forward in this book. Countless others will come to know your goodness because you will be con-tributing more to the world. Being overweight, unable to move, unhappy, down on yourself and on life doesn't allow for much contribu-tion to others. I know. I was once there. Sure, you may smile as people approach but believe me, many can see right through that façade.

The following pages contain a precise plan to take you to the place of your dreams, looking and feeling your best. I am thankful for the chance to be a part of your journey. Although I'm not sitting in the room with you, I hope you can sense how much I care about you and your success. I hope my personal trans-formation has more of an impact on you than anything else has. I have been blessed with so many opportunities and successes, not only for my own good, but so I could sow the seeds of possibility in your mind and heart.

I want to help you see just how much grace is available when you get yourself on track and start doing the good you're capable of doing. When you're living your mission and being your best, then miracles begin to occur in your life. Synchronicity kicks in, putting the right things in the right places at the right times. It is not an accident that you have this book in your hands right now. This is the time for you to take that step and become the person you were meant to be.

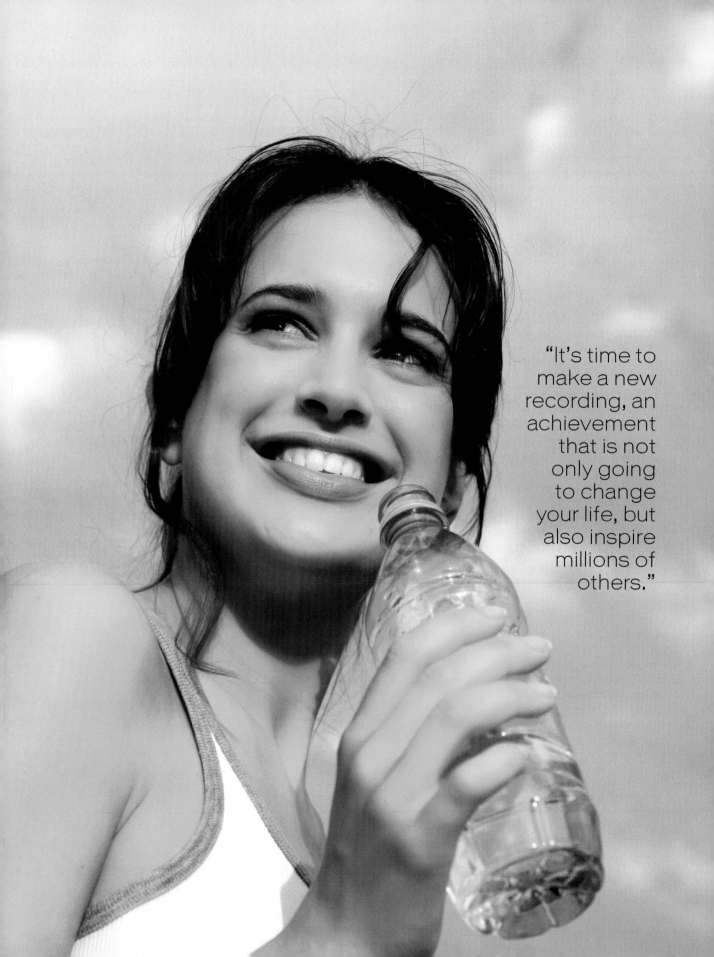

"It's time to make a new recording, an achievement that is not only going to change your life, but also inspire millions of others."

## "It never occurred to me that I was beginning to look not 'big,' but ridiculous."

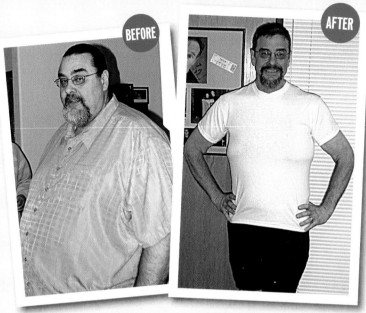

BEFORE

AFTER

**NAME:** Buzz Brown
**AGE:** 59
**HEIGHT:** 6'3"
**WEIGHT BEFORE:** 442 lbs
**WEIGHT AFTER:** 204 lbs
**WEIGHT LOSS:** 238 lbs

as Buzz calls it, was Charles, who helped Buzz lose an incredible 226 pounds within a year!

These days Buzz is constantly surprised at how he can now accomplish and even enjoy seemingly insignificant everyday tasks. He can sit in a normal-sized chair without worrying about breaking it. He can cross his legs comfortably. He can also ride a bike, climb stairs without getting winded and enjoy shopping. Best

**EVERY SATURDAY AT GRANDMA'S HOUSE WAS "BUZZIE" DAY. THIS MEANT THAT, AS THE ELDEST GRANDCHILD, BUZZ BROWN WAS ALLOWED TO EAT ANYTHING HE WANTED AND AS MUCH OF IT AS HE COULD HANDLE.** In his family, extra fat was considered healthy and, at a young age, Buzz learned that food was equivalent to love. He also learned that it could erase many unpleasant emotions. Eventually food became Buzz's addiction and main companion in good times and bad.

Sadly, both Buzz's grandmother and father died of heart complications related to obesity and diabetes. Buzz found himself heading down the same path – he was on medication for a heart condition and wound up in the hospital at least once a year – and felt powerless to do anything about it. His condition was also affecting his relationships, especially his marriage, not only because of the physical im-

plications of having extra weight, but also because of the cost of clothes and food. Buzz's turning point came when he weighed in at 442 pounds at the doctor's office. In Buzz's own words: "I guess it never occurred to me that I was beginning to look not 'big,' but ridiculous."

Although Buzz could list off a litany of weight-loss trials and errors over the years, none of them ever "stuck." As soon as he reached his goal weight, he would return to his emotional eating, which resulted in him gaining back all the weight and more.

At his lowest moment, Buzz found himself suicidal and eventually wound up in a 12-step program to help him cope with the emotional aspects of his obesity. After years of hard work, he formed a network of support to help him deal with his emotions. The final piece of the puzzle, though, or "the key that opened the lock"

legs comfortably. He can also ride a bike, climb stairs without getting winded and enjoy shopping. Best

## "He was on medication for a heart condition and wound up in the hospital at least once a year."

of all, he is completely off his heart medication and sees his cardiologist only on an as-needed basis.

Buzz stays motivated by maintaining contact with his support group, sticking to his 12-step program and following Charles' plan. According to Buzz, "'Thank you' seems so lame for someone who has saved my life."

# DIABETES DETOX
## Beating the Silent Killer

*More than 25 million Americans have an evil, debilitating disease, and roughly a third of them don't even know they have it until it's too late. For many of these people, their wake-up call comes in the form of significant health issues – vision problems, numbness in fingers and toes and impotence – that force them to confront just how much damage their poor eating and exercise habits have brought about.*

This silent killer is type 2 diabetes, and the International Diabetes Federation has called it the epidemic of the 21st century. The dramatic rise in cases of type 2 diabetes is directly related to the increase in the number of people who are overweight and obese. In fact, according to the Surgeon General, more than 80 percent of people with diabetes are overweight or obese.

When your body is unable to regulate blood sugar, as is the case with type 2 diabetes, it can lead to a variety of health complications including heart disease and stroke. Dr. Oz, Oprah's

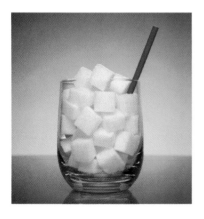

favorite doctor and a cardiac surgeon, has said that 25 percent of the patients he operates on have diabetes. He compares the extra sugar in the bloodstream to shards of glass scraping at the arterial walls, which can result in a clot buildup breaking free and causing a heart attack or stroke and ultimately death.

Still, there is hope for anyone who's suffering or at risk. "Most diabetes is preventable," Dr. Oz says. "It is treatable, even reversible. Ninety percent of type 2 diabetics can actually reverse their problem."[1]

When I was 17 and awoke after a huge sugar binge, I found my eyesight had disappeared. Thankfully it was temporary, but at the time I had thought I'd suddenly lost my sight to diabetes. That brief but terrifying experience helped motivate me to take action! Here are some simple and profound ways to help control your blood sugar and possibly prevent or even reverse diabetes if you've already fallen victim. *(See **NOTE** on following page.)

## 1 Eliminate ALL simple sugars!

As Dr. Oz says, if it's white or processed, get rid of it. This means foods containing everything from table sugar to white flour to high fructose corn syrup. When your body is insulin resistant, you need to recondition it to process carbs and sugars effectively again. It's been my experience that eliminating all simple sugars is a tremendously effective way of doing that.

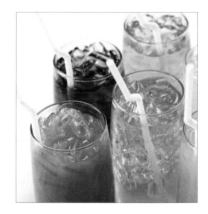

## 2 Eliminate all caloric drinks

Low-sugar and no-sugar-added beverages are not enough. You need to consume only zero-calorie drinks such as water (which is the best choice), mineral water, tea, etc. Don't drink juices, which are like glasses of pure liquid sugar with some vitamins thrown in.

## 3 Limit your starches

Starches break down into sugars. This means you will need to limit potatoes, sweet potatoes and bananas along with any product made with grains. Make sure the starches you do eat are unrefined (whole grains, brown rice, etc.), that you only eat small quantities of them and not at every meal.

## 4 Start doing at least 30 minutes of cardio every day!

Regular activity helps you control your blood sugar and it helps your body to become more sensitive to the insulin you do make.[2] Exercise also helps you lose excess fat, which further contributes to diabetes management.

**NOTE:** Before making any changes in diet and/or exercise, you should consult a physician. If you are on diabetes medication, it's even more critical that you consult your physician before making these changes. If you are taking medication that pulls sugar from your blood and there's not enough sugar, you can have a diabetic reaction, which can result in a coma or even death.

1. "Diabetes: America's Silent Killer," Feburary 1, 2010, www.oprah.com/oprahshow/Diabetes-101-with-Dr-Oz-Dr-Ian-Smith-and-Bob-Greene

2. "Top 10 Benefits of Being Active," American Diabetes Association, www.diabetes.org/food-and-fitness/fitness/fitness-management/top-10-benefits-of-being.html

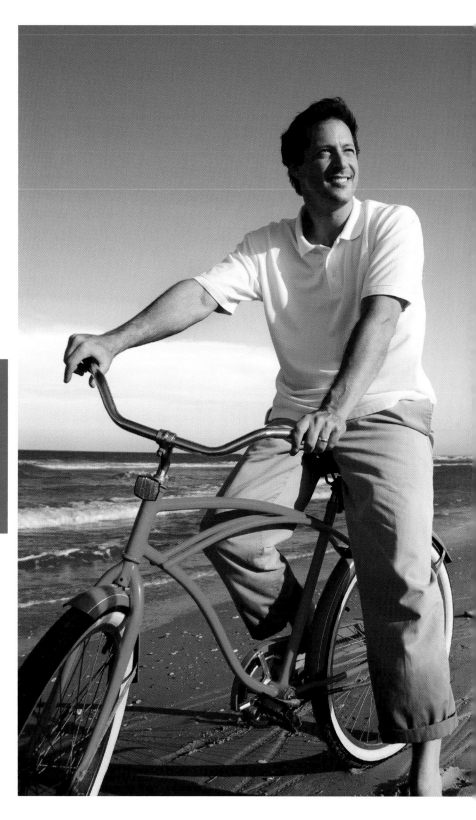

## CHAPTER TWO
## Growing Up As "The Fat Kid"

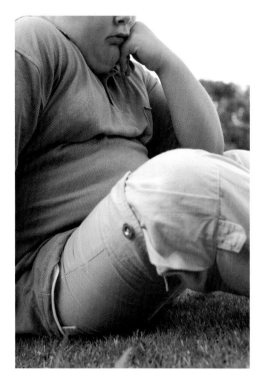

> "Change your thoughts, and you change your world."
>
> – Norman Vincent Peale

While a lot of people remember their first year of school as being fun filled – playing games, singing songs, making new friends and sharing lunch – I remember my kindergarten days as being terrifying. I'd sit there watching the minutes on the smiley face clock tick away until I could go home to my mom where I was safe. Even a seemingly harmless game of "Duck, Duck, Goose" would leave me panic-stricken because once I was "it" I was never fast enough to touch another person. I felt I had no control. I just had to endure the laughter.

And so began my long and miserable voyage through the school system. I always wondered how the kids could be so mean – after all, what had I done to them? But it didn't matter what I'd *done to* them. I was different from them, and kids don't like different. When it comes to outsiders, none are tormented as mercilessly as the fat kid. The fat kid is everyone's punching bag. No matter how short, nerdy, ugly, dumb or smart you are, you're "allowed" to laugh at the fat kid. The fat kid makes everyone else feel superior.

I wish I could say that things improved after grade school. However, as with many people, the most difficult stage of my life started right after I turned 12. I don't know what it is about kids of this age, but cruelty seems to reach a pinnacle during this time. I had just been invited over to a classmate's house to work on a speech for class. It was thrilling for me because I was never invited to anyone's house, ever. This classmate was part of the "in" crowd, which made it all the more exciting. My parents even took me to JC Penney to buy new clothes so I would fit in. What I didn't yet understand was that no matter what I was wearing, I was still different. And I was about to learn (the hard way) that different kids don't belong.

My classmate lived in a very large house, tucked into a wooded subdivision where the majority of the other kids lived too. That afternoon, we were working away on our speech in a room with floor-to-ceiling windows. Suddenly we heard loud voices coming from outside. I turned to see a huge group of kids from our class, boys and girls, looking in the windows and yelling out such hurtful and hateful things as: "Hey lard ass!" "You fat fag!" "You're a tub of lard!" "Get the f*** out of here!"

I didn't know how to react. As the adrenaline pumped through my body, the electrician in my brain was busy crossing wires and making some of those connections that I mentioned in the first chapter of this book. In my messed-up mind, engaging with others now equaled terrible pain and embarrassment. And since our brains try to keep us away from pain, I made certain to avoid any future circumstances where I would be alone with a classmate ever again. That afternoon was supposed to be happy and exciting – a big turnaround for me – but any happiness I had felt was utterly destroyed.

That event sent me into a deep depression. I didn't want to go to school and face those kids anymore. Unfortunately, my experiences are not unique. It seems we are often hearing about yet another young person who has tragically chosen to end his or her life because of bullying. If you're one of these people who is about to do the same, DO NOT. I'm living proof you don't need to end it. There is so much waiting for you in the future. The fact that you're reading this right now shows me that you are capable of loving yourself. Please know that you are not alone. I am there with you in spirit, and there are lots of great professionals out there who can help you on the path to feeling happy, strong and healthy.

In my case, the religion teacher, who also happened to be heavyset, was key to helping me cope. Just having someone who understood what I was going through really helped me to be strong and stay in school. Sticking it out did not mean living a normal school life, however. I would get my dad to drop me off at school before any of the other kids arrived so I could hide in the bathroom until class began. In seventh grade, I talked my way out of a class camping trip because I was so scared of those kids. It's pretty sad that I'd rather do a full week of extra schoolwork than go camping with them.

Lunch-hour recess, a time most kids look forward to, was just another anxiety-inducing segment in an already stressful day. But in my efforts to avoid the other kids, I stumbled across something that turned out to be a blessing. It was then that I discovered a gift that gave me enough self-confidence to make

friends and be a little more accepted in high school later on.

Our school had a wonderful music teacher named Valerie Fradkin. He was a Ukrainian who had come to the US shortly after the Chernobyl incident. He had been well known in his homeland and had one of the highest degrees, but because his credentials were obtained outside of the country, he had to start over. I would spend time with him at lunch recess so I could avoid the kids who tormented me. I would listen to him play piano and then play back exactly what I had heard. He compared me to Mozart, saying I had a great gift. I loved playing because it allowed me to escape from my daily hell, taking me to a magical world where I could express my emotions freely.

Looking back, I realize that music (and food) weren't my only forms of escape. When I was quite young, I was also lucky enough to discover that I had a passion for magic tricks. I went

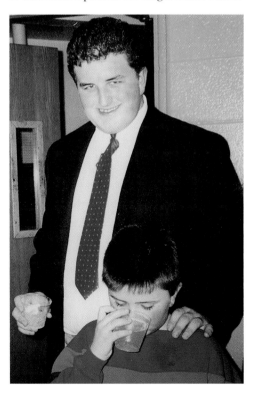

◀ WITH MY BROTHER VINCE.

to the library and borrowed a bunch of books on how to perform them, and I practiced and practiced. I would watch tapes of David Copperfield's TV programs over and over, trying to figure out his secrets. He has an energy that charges up his audience and I quickly fell in love with the art. All of this practicing had kept me busy, giving me something other than my unhappiness to focus on, and – bonus! – it had made me quite good at magic tricks. This ability helped me live through the awkwardness of being fat by taking the focus off of my appearance and putting the focus on the trick. Suddenly I was interesting, and people were interested in me. My "performances" even brought a little joy to people's lives.

I am extremely grateful to have discovered the gifts of music and magic. Although both were only a short-term fix, they did wonders for building my confidence and have given me great pleasure and many opportunities in life. I found things I could do that others couldn't.

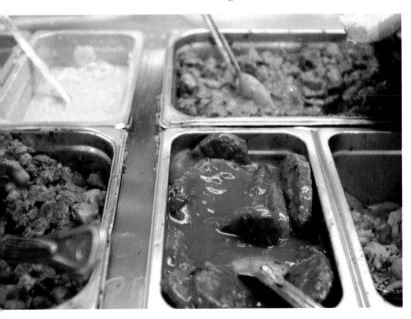

"I may have been an unusually fat kid, but my horrible eating habits were not that unusual."

I was unique and so are you! Whether your gift is singing, dancing, working with animals, writing poetry, gardening … whatever it is, it's in there somewhere! Now is the time to find it!

## THIS IS CALLED IRONY

I often came home from school in tears. My mom, who was there to comfort me, knew that I was having a terrible time. She knew how much I hated going to school, how I got picked on and how unhappy I was. She loved me so much and wanted to help. She had grown up on a diet of junk food and knew that it was the one thing that put a smile on my face, so she made sure I had plenty of it to make me feel better. If I came home after a bad day – and as you can probably guess, most days were bad days – then a trip to McDonald's was in order. She'd get me a Happy Meal complete with a new toy, to make my day sunny. Until recently I never thought about how ironic it was that she gave me foods that made me fat in order to help make up for the misery I felt because I was fat!

I may have been an unusually fat kid, but my horrible eating habits were not that unusual. I guess you could even say that I was on the cusp of a great American trend. According to the Centers for Disease Control, obesity rates in the US have been steadily increasing since 1985 (For a shocking and enlightening interactive year-by-year illustration, visit **www.cdc.gov/obesity/data/trends.html**). Statistically, over a third of those kids who made my life miserable are now obese themselves. In fact, some of those kids who bullied me are now my devoted clients! Go figure!

And it's no wonder. My school district, St. Louis, Missouri, recently won the prize as the school district with the worst health practices in the entire country[1]. We had a lunch program in our school whereby we would pay around four dollars for lunch and only 50 cents for each extra helping. And I'm not

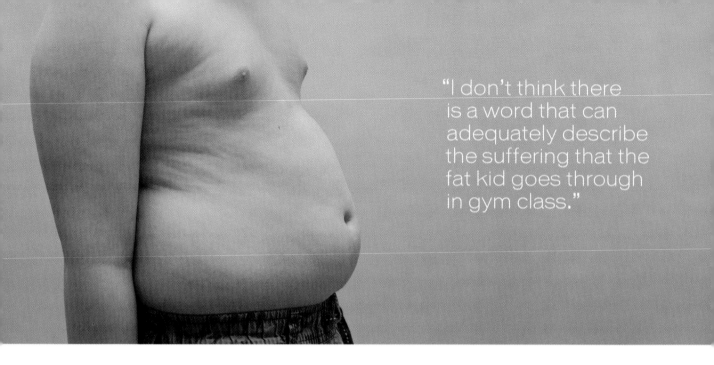

"I don't think there is a word that can adequately describe the suffering that the fat kid goes through in gym class."

talking about a healthy lunch here. No fruit. No vegetables. No healthy proteins or whole grains. We had butter noodles, pizza and other high-fat, simple-sugar lunches. And with each additional serving costing just 50 cents, I would go back again and again.

An argument has been raging in recent years about whether or not schools should be allowed to serve unhealthy foods or whether they should be held accountable for kids' health. I can see both sides of the argument. On the one hand, I do feel it is the parents' responsibility to teach kids about nutrition, and the best place to teach them is by example in the home. On the other hand, if, like me, they are not being taught about nutrition in the home and are being fed garbage at school, then where are they supposed to learn how to eat properly?

Many schools have argued that they rely on their food programs to support school activities, and if they remove unhealthy foods from the menu they will lose overall revenue because kids won't buy the healthy stuff. However, many of the schools across the country that have been bold enough to cut the worst foods and encourage kids to eat better report *increased* food revenue, so that argument is no longer valid.

## GYM CLASS

I don't think there is a word that can adequately describe the suffering that the fat kid goes through in gym class. Getting naked in front of the other boys was horrible. I knew my body didn't look like theirs, and they knew it too. Not only was my stomach extremely large, but my thighs also stuck together and I had stretch marks all over my gut. I tried to be as invisible as possible, but the other kids had a keen curiosity and wanted to get a good look at this "different" body. They wanted to see the freak, so they could laugh and feel even more superior.

Unfortunately, the situation was far from improved once gym class actually began. I simply couldn't do anything. I remember a time in sixth grade when we had to run a full mile for the Presidential Physical Fitness Test. This was actually a week of tests – things like pull-ups, sit-ups, long jump – activities we had no training or practice in, but were expected to do. The kids who played sports and were natural athletes looked forward to the opportunity to showcase their abilities. I, on the other hand, tried to fake being sick for a week so I wouldn't have to go at all. But that didn't work. I had to face the music. Even though I couldn't finish many of the tests, I ended up

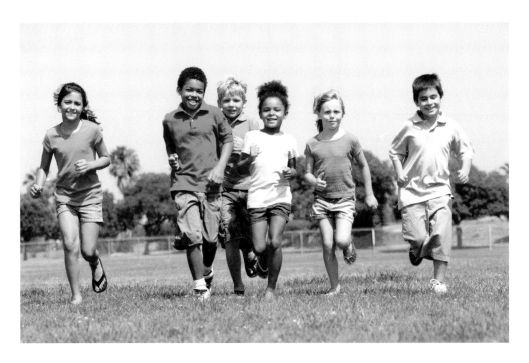

"completing" them, thanks to a kind partner who risked failing the class by lying for me, saying I had finished when I hadn't even done a third!

When the time came to do the mile run, it was a blistering hot day. We had to run a certain number of times around the asphalt parking lot as the sun beat down on us. All the fit kids finished really quickly, the average kids a minute or two after and then the slower kids a few minutes later. Me? I was determined to finish, but after every few steps I would have to rest and walk. My teacher even tried to get me to stop, but I wouldn't. I felt like I was going to throw up all over the steaming hot pavement, but something kept me going. By the time I finished that mile, the rest of the kids were dressed in their uniforms and ready to go back to class. They all stood there at the window, watching me as I rounded the last lap. In my opinion, giving a physical test without providing a conditioning program to help students prepare is like giving a calculus test to students who have been working on addition all semester – and then basing the majority of their grade on that calculus test. And not only

that, but also making them do the test publicly in front a group that is familiar with calculus. I feel that these types of experiences do not build self-confidence in the future leaders of society.

# FIND YOUR SENSE OF SELF

People often ask me how I turned my life around so radically. After all, I had spent my whole life as "The Fat Kid." I had also spent my whole life buying into several lies that were constantly being reinforced by those around me. *You were meant to be fat. Your family is fat; it is your destiny. There's nothing wrong with junk food if it makes you feel better.*

So, how *did* I turn my life around? I believe the answer lies in the way I was thinking. I changed my thoughts, and doing so changed my life. Food wasn't the only thing that was draining my energy and self esteem; my thoughts were. I was completely preoccupied with what others thought of me. I was in a constant state of panic, and the drug I used to calm me was food. If someone happened to look my way, I immediately assumed the worst. Did I have sweat stains? Was a flap of fat protruding from under my shirt? To me, the idea of someone just giving me a friendly glance was inconceivable. As you can probably see, I was not a positive thinker. I always assumed the worst because in my past that is typically what happened. I figured that if I expected the worst I'd never be hurt.

American writer and publisher Elbert Hubbard said, "To avoid criticism, do nothing, say nothing and be nothing." In other words, instead of trying and risking not hitting the target, you can just never try and therefore never risk failure. That was me. I never risked reaching out to another person because I didn't want to experience the pain that came from being rejected.

This way of thinking only furthered my isolation from others. In turn, as I felt more and more isolated, I filled the void with my oldest and best friend: junk food. As I grew more and more obese, my negative expectations eventually became a reality of my own making – a self-fulfilling prophecy. As Buddha said, "All that we are is a result of what we have thought."

My thoughts had fueled my overeating to the point where I was out of control. I ended up eating so much that, as fat as I was and as tall as I am, I became like a car crash – people couldn't help but look at me, whether they wanted to or not. Maybe they looked out of shock or fear, maybe out of sadness and pity – all I know is that people looked. And the more they looked the more isolated I felt. See the downward spiral here?

The way I changed was by first deciding to take control of my life and then by setting goals for myself. Things weren't just going to magically happen. If I wanted to feel better and look better, no wizard was going to come and wave his magic wand. I had to take action. I started by redefining who I was. I decided to

no longer buy into the lie that I was destined to be fat and unhealthy just because that was the way I had always been. I decided to transform my beliefs about myself.

Once I accepted that I was a lean, fit, attractive young man with a six-pack who just happened to be carrying an extra 160 pounds of fat around, my behavior changed. I no longer acted like a "fat" person. I started to seek out role models – people who looked the way I wanted to look and lived the type of life I wanted to live – and I got their advice. I spent countless months studying what made it all work for them. After all, if they could be fit and healthy, why couldn't I? And if they can and I can, then why can't you?

> "You can immediately change – this second – if you choose to redefine yourself and realign yourself with a new identity, one that is fulfilling and exciting, the true you!"

So let me ask you a question: How do you define yourself? Are you giving away your power by allowing others to define you? Do you wear certain clothes or dress a certain way to avoid criticism? Do you hide at home, or do you hide behind unattractive clothes or even behind your fat so you don't have to deal with other people?

You can immediately change – this second – if you choose to redefine yourself and realign yourself with a new identity, one that is fulfilling and exciting, the true you! If all you are allowing yourself to be is "the fat kid," "the fat lady," "the fat guy" or whatever other title you or others have bestowed upon you, then how will you ever get out? You will not escape the excess fat if that fat has become who you are. Change your identity. This will change how you live every day!

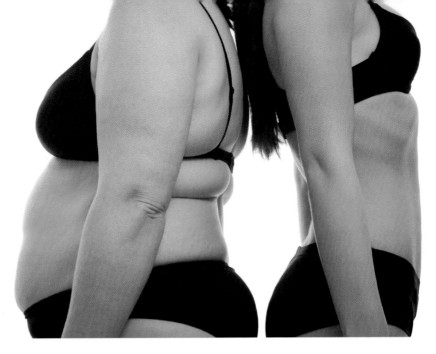

> **"You need to find the 'you' underneath those extra pounds."**

You need to find the "you" underneath those extra pounds. What are you good at? Think about the last time you felt incredible. Think about who you were with, what music was playing, whether it was during the day or night, if it was cool or warm. Close your eyes and get as associated with the memory as you can. Begin to feel the incredible feelings you felt. Was it a feeling of purpose that made you feel great? Was it a feeling of accomplishment? Was it your friend that made you feel special? The truth is that *you* were making yourself feel a certain way by the way you were processing the events that were happening to you.

You can make this present journey – and your life – just as exciting as that moment if you choose to give each feeling an empowering meaning. Instead of feeling tired, feel like you're recharging. Instead of feeling deprived, feel like you're rewarding your body for all the hard work it does for you by feeding it the best food. After you've defined yourself and where you want to be, you need to reaffirm the purpose of doing this. In the short term, it may be for your parents, spouse or kids, or it may be for a reunion or other special event, but ultimately you have to be doing it for yourself. You have to make this journey something that fulfills you. Otherwise you will enjoy only short-term happiness and results, and you'll soon return to the way you were.

What gives your life purpose? Having a sense of purpose will make losing your excess fat – which is not *you*, but just excess baggage you carry around all day – much easier. After all, you are a success. You have chosen to take initiative and read this book. You went to the store and picked it up. If this was given to you, you are a success because others love you enough to want you to be around for them.

Sometimes we get caught up in negative emotions and forget all the blessings we've been given. Think about your gift. It can be working with horses, building websites, learning mechanics, painting or doing magic tricks and playing the piano like me – anything you can dream up. Identify yourself with your passions, your abilities, the way you treat others, the way you live your life. Love these things about yourself. Abandon your incessant need for the approval of others. What they think doesn't matter. You will never be able to change from being the fat person if you believe the fat person is who you are. You must come to realize that you are a fit, healthy person with many gifts. Determine your strengths by deciding who it is you want to be. It's time to get curious and start discovering your unique God-given gifts today!

1. "PCRM Report Card Reveals School Lunch Disparities," Physicians Committee for Responsible Medicine Online, September 2007)

## *"Throw out your excuses."*

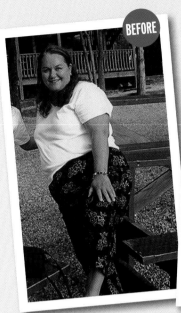

BEFORE

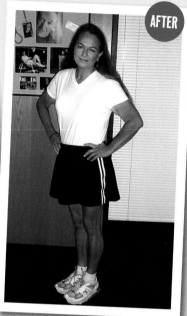

AFTER

**NAME: Kristine Kopczynski**
**AGE: 49**
**HEIGHT: 5'6"**
**WEIGHT BEFORE: 238 lbs**
**WEIGHT AFTER: 128 lbs**
**WEIGHT LOSS: 110 lbs**

**IMAGINE LOSING ALMOST HALF OF YOURSELF IN LESS THAN ONE YEAR!** That is exactly what Kristine Kopczynski was able to achieve with the help of Charles D'Angelo. After years of emotional eating combined with a lack of exercise, she found herself weighing 238 pounds. With this extensive weight gain came a series of health issues, namely, hypertension, anxiety, diabetes, restless leg syndrome and sleep apnea. Kristine was on expensive prescriptions for each of these conditions, including using a sleep-apnea (CPAP) machine on a nightly basis.

Tired of feeling miserable, both physically and mentally, Kristine finally decided to change because she wanted to enjoy quality time with her husband and two children. But before she went full steam ahead, Kristine needed to decide which plan was best for her. In the past she had tried Weight Watchers "at least 15 times"

and was successful only twice, at least until she gained the weight back after only a few months. Consistency was not Kristine's strong point. Luckily, this is where Charles shines.

Charles made Kristine face her weight problem out loud at their first meeting. He stressed the importance of proper diet and exercise, but he also made this way of life accessible by giving Kristine a narrow food plan. This meant she did not need to worry about choosing from too many options, which is where she had gone wrong in the past. Kristine also needed Charles' conviction that she could succeed at this. With his motivation and encouragement along with a strict eating and exercise plan, Kristine was able to shave off her excess weight in under a year! She was also able to ditch *all* of her medications and the CPAP machine. As Kristine continued to make improvements, she was soon able to tackle a ton of

new activities, including climbing to the top of Pikes Peak, Colorado, with her husband. Best of all, her confidence skyrocketed and she began to feel good all the time.

In order to avoid relapsing back to her old ways, Kristine relies heavily on her support system, including Charles and her family and friends. She also remembers how awful she felt when she was at her heaviest. This is enough to keep her on track on a daily basis. She continues to set goals for herself, such as celebrating one year at her goal weight.

## *"Charles is young and a little cocky, but he knows what he is talking about."*

If it wasn't for Charles and his no-nonsense approach, Kristine knows she would still be struggling with her weight. She says his encouragement and attitude are what motivated her to reach her goals. According to Kristine, "Charles is young and a little cocky, but he knows what he is talking about. Throw out your excuses and surrender yourself to what he says to do."

# BLAST YOUR PAST!
## 6 Ways to Let Go and Lose Weight

*I recently received a call from a woman who had heard about me helping people lose hundreds of pounds. After a brief conversation, I got the feeling she was very cynical about weight loss. Although we hadn't delved into her dieting history, I suspected she'd tried many plans before, always abandoning them before any real change could take effect. I called her back and was right on. She explained that she needed to lose about 150 pounds, but didn't know if she needed my program or therapy because she believed that her past was driving her to overeat.*

*As I said to her then, I don't think the options of therapy and my program need to be mutually exclusive. Understanding your past is an excellent tool in taking control of your life and succeeding on my program. Until you are able to use your past in an empowering way it will control you, whereas you should be in the driver's seat of your own life. Here are some simple ways to learn from and let go of the past, so you can take control of your weight loss and your life!*

### 1 Choose to forgive.

Are you letting the pain of the past cause you to feel angry and powerless? These feelings are both reactions to fear. You may subconsciously choose to feel this way because you are afraid of taking personal responsibility and dealing with difficult emotions. "The decision to forgive touches you to your very core, to who you are as a human being," says psychologist and founder of the International Forgiveness Institute Robert Enright, PhD. "It involves your sense of self-esteem, your personal worth, the worth of the person who's hurt you, and your relationship with that person and the larger world." Stop allowing the past to wield so much power. Acknowledge how you've designed your life up to this point and, more importantly, that you will be designing your life in the future.

One of the first steps to forgiveness is to realize its value in your life. Several studies, including many by Enright, Frederic Luskin (director of the Stanford Forgiveness Projects), Loren Toussaint and others, have shown that forgiveness can lead to lower blood pressure, reduced levels of anxiety, depression and chronic pain, healthier relationships and a lower risk of alcohol and substance abuse. It stands to reason that forgiveness

would improve your risk of becoming (or remaining) a junk-food addict as well.

### 2 Choose to own your life.

When you blame other people or circumstances for the way your life has turned out, you are handing over your personal power. When you are angry, vengeful or looking to cast responsibility on others, you are giving them –

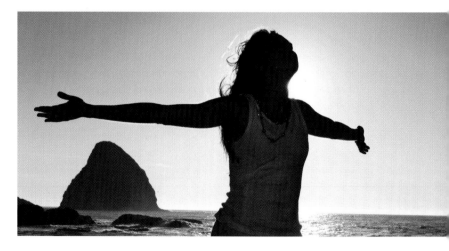

or more appropriately, your memory of them – control of your life. When you actively choose to no longer be a victim, you will release the power that your tormentor had. As Ann Landers said, "Hanging onto resentment is letting someone you despise live rent-free in your head." Don't relinquish your personal power by allowing the dark side of anger and negativity to grip you. In most cases, you are the only one being tormented by the hurtful events of the past. Those who've wronged you have likely moved on and have long since forgotten the incidents.

## 3 Put a new spin on old wounds.

Reinterpreting the painful memories that compel you to overeat can change the way you feel about past events and thus change how they continue to influence you. If this sounds easier said than done, think of the incident and ask yourself: "What else could this mean?" Famed motivational speaker Tony Robbins said that the moment he began asking himself this question about upsetting times, his life changed for the better. Asking it helps you realize that you aren't really upset because of something someone has done, you're upset because of the meaning you've attached to the person's actions. Instead of saying: "She did it because she hates me," you might say: "Maybe she did it because she's angry at the world and never learned how to express emotions in a healthy way." If you are used to looking at yourself and the world in a negative light it may be challenging to see the positive angles, but for each incident, try to come up with as many empowering meanings as disempowering ones.

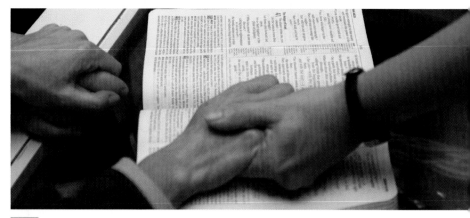

## 4 Replace pain with gratitude.

I know, I know, feeling grateful for your traumatic past may sound strange or even impossible, but several studies including many by Robert Emmons, a professor of psychology at the University of California and a pioneer in gratitude research, have shown that people who frequently feel grateful are happier, healthier, more energetic, earn more, and have more life satisfaction than those who do not. While you may have had difficult experiences at a time in your life when you didn't have a support system or control over your environment (when you were a child, for example), you need to recognize that you are no longer that person and those experiences don't need to affect you in the ways they once did. You can rise above these traumatic events by viewing them as opportunities for learning and growth. Be grateful that they shaped you into who you are and led you to the place you are now – building a better life by taking personal responsibility for yourself.

## 5 Find closure.

If you believe a particular relationship, person or event set you on the path to obesity, write a letter to the person at the core of the situation. Putting your emotions on paper will force you to face your demons head-on while giving you a sense of understanding, control and empowerment. Your letter may end up covered in tears, but force yourself to do it! If there is more than one specific person or event, write multiple letters in one evening – this task needs to be complete before you begin your transformation. Put the letters in envelopes and write the offending name on each one. Then go to a fireplace or barbecue pit and free yourself by placing each letter into the flames. As they burn, feel the chains of your past lifting as you relieve yourself of years of suffering. Go forward, knowing you are now officially the captain of your fate!

## 6 Embrace unconditional love for yourself and others.

Accept those around you as they are, and don't try to change them. There is no scarcity, so jump in the world of abundance. Give out that which you seek. Want support from others? Be supportive of others! Want to feel loved? Do loving things for others regularly and you will get it back tenfold. You cannot bring about that which you don't already possess mentally. Envision the body, health and life of your dreams and attract it by being loving in all of your actions in each and every moment of your life.

# CHAPTER THREE

## My Drug of Choice: Food!

> "Stop and think about it for a moment. Do you know of a single instance where any real achievement was made in your life, or in the life of any person in history, that was not due to a problem with which the individual was faced?"
>
> – Napoleon Hill and W. Clement Stone,
> *Success Through a Positive Mental Attitude*

I've never touched a drop of alcohol, taken an illicit drug or smoked a cigarette, and yet I am a recovered addict. Do you think that sounds crazy? It may, but addiction comes in many forms. We use substances or actions we are addicted to in order to distract us from our pain, to fill a void in our life or simply as a coping mechanism. I turned to junk food for all these reasons and more.

The fact is that as humans, we often turn to activities and substances outside of ourselves to give us a feeling of certainty or validity instead of looking inside for the answer. We tend to look for some sort of external stimulus when we feel we need help getting through the day or coping with a stressful situation,

or when we're feeling down, or when we're celebrating, or when we're bored. You can see how often some of us might turn to these external stimuli. It was at those times I turned to food. And more specifically, junk food.

Food did not mean the same thing to me that it does to most people. Food wasn't just something to fuel my day or fill me up; food was my closest friend. When I unwrapped a steaming, gooey McDonald's cheeseburger, ripped open a Little Debbie cake or reached out for my Dairy Queen ice cream from the drive-thru window, I would get a rush of endorphins. I got excited, as excited as you get when you walk down the stairs on Christmas morning to see if Santa came. I know it sounds messed up, but that's how it was for me.

You could almost say I had a love affair with junk food. The thought of having my favorite nachos smothered with "beef paste" and "cheese product" from 7-Eleven made me salivate. When I peeled back the wrapper of a Snickers or Hershey's bar, I felt a tingling sensation of love in my gut. I started the day, got through the day and ended the day with junk food. A typical breakfast was four or five Pop Tarts. Throughout the day I would munch on nachos, candy, chocolate bars, entire pizzas, boxes of breadsticks – and every morsel was washed down with Coke. The calories most people consumed throughout a week, I ate in a day. It's obvious now that this was not a normal or healthy relationship with food. Food is meant to fuel our lives; it is not meant to *be* our lives. Eating is meant to give us the energy to do the things we love to do; it is not meant to be the *only* thing we love to do.

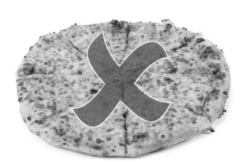

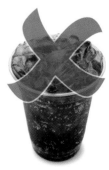

This messed-up way of using food as a pacifier, as a mood-elevator, as an escape mechanism and as a way to relieve tension mimics the way people use drugs and alcohol. Here is a self-reported list of the top reasons teens use alcohol and drugs[1]:

**1** To have a good time with friends

**2** To experiment

**3** To feel good

**4** Because it tastes good

**5** To relax or relieve tension

**6** Boredom

**7** To escape from problems

How many of these come to mind when you think of your relationship with food? Have you found yourself using food for any of these reasons?

## CONTROVERSY

So can a person actually be addicted to food? Experts differ in their opinions on this. Some state that overeating is a compulsion, which is different from an addiction. These experts believe that, since food does not contain any actual drug, a person cannot become addicted to it. However, the April 2011 release of a breakthrough study indicates that the tides are beginning to turn. The study revealed numerous parallels in the brain functioning associated with substance abuse and obesity.[2] This has led the researchers to theorize that addictive processes may be involved in the cause of obesity. Or to put it bluntly, food addiction is (most likely) real. The study involved identifying certain participants as pathological eaters by getting them to fill out a food-addiction questionnaire. All participants were then shown photographs of food. When the

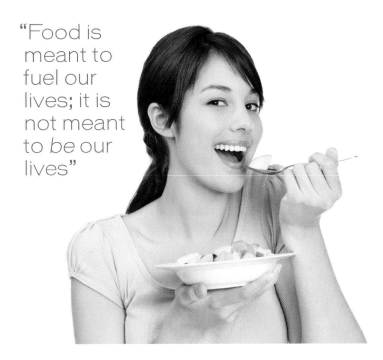

"Food is meant to fuel our lives; it is not meant to *be* our lives"

pathological eaters saw the food photos, brain scans revealed that their brain activity was similar to that of a drug addict who was being shown drugs.

The study noted that food and drug use both result in dopamine release in certain regions of the brain (dopamine is a neurotransmitter associated with pleasure and also with addiction), and went on to state, "The degree of [dopamine] release correlates with subjective reward from both food and drug use." So now that we know this, how can we use it to help people?

There is a saying in some alcoholic circles: Q. What's the difference between a problem drinker and an alcoholic? A. "Problem drinker" is the term used by those who love the alcoholic. While most experts do, in fact, see a difference between a problem drinker and a true alcoholic, this saying illustrates that it's partly a matter of perception. Most counselors seem to use the medical definition of addiction to assess the most effective way to treat an individual. Do you wonder if you are a food addict? Answer the yes or no questions below.

# The Medical Definition of Addiction

**1 TOLERANCE:** Has your consumption of junk food increased over time?

**2 WITHDRAWAL:** Have you ever experienced physical or emotional withdrawal when you've tried to stop eating junk food? Have you had any of the following symptoms when you do not get junk food: irritability, anxiety, shakes, sweats, nausea or vomiting?

**3 DIFFICULTY CONTROLLING YOUR CONSUMPTION:** Do you sometimes eat more or for a longer time than you would like? Do you eat uncontrollably once you begin? Do you tell yourself that you'll just have one cookie, for example, or one piece of pizza, and then keep eating and eating?

**4 NEGATIVE CONSEQUENCES:** Have you continued to eat junk food even though there have been negative consequences to your mood, self-esteem, health, job or family?

**5 PUTTING OFF OR NEGLECTING ACTIVITIES:** Have you ever put off or reduced social, recreational, household or job-related activities because of your eating?

**6 SPENDING SIGNIFICANT TIME OR EMOTIONAL ENERGY:** Have you spent a significant amount of time obtaining, using, concealing, planning or recovering from your eating? Have you spent a lot of time thinking about eating junk food or how/when to obtain it? Have you ever eaten in secret? Have you been dishonest with others (or yourself) about how much you've actually eaten?

**7 DESIRE TO CUT DOWN:** Have you sometimes thought about cutting down or controlling your junk food consumption? Have you ever made unsuccessful attempts to cut down or control your use of junk food?

If you answered yes to at least three of these questions, then you meet the medical definition of addiction according to the World Health Organization and the American Psychiatric Association. This could be a sign you are addicted to the substance in question – in your case, junk food. Keep in mind, though, that alcoholics can quit drinking, and you can stop eating junk!

I don't know and will never know whether I was a full-fledged food addict, but I was definitely headed in that direction. I could have answered "yes" to most of the questions in the quiz above. Regardless of whether I could technically be called an addict, I used food in the way that a drug addict uses drugs, and that's how I ended up weighing 360 pounds at the age of 17. And like an alcoholic or drug addict, I kept "using" long after I realized my behavior was putting my health in danger.

Thankfully, at 17, something finally clicked for me and I made the change that I fully believe saved my life. Now it's your turn.

If you are a true "food addict" you can change your life, just as millions of alcoholics have quit drinking. But you don't have to be at that extreme to make the change. If you are overweight right now, then you must use food in some of the ways I did, or you wouldn't be overweight. (Or you might overuse alcohol, which also contributes to excess weight.) Maybe you eat fine through the week but on weekends let yourself go "because it's the weekend." Maybe you don't pay attention to getting enough nutrition, and just eat for pleasure. Maybe you starve yourself all day and then overeat at night to make up for it. Countless different unhealthy behaviors lead to becoming overweight or obese. I don't know which of these behaviors applies to you, but I do know that if you choose to continue eating the way you have been, then you will continue to gain more and more fat. You will also continue to feel worse and worse, both physically and mentally. Your health will be poorer, your energy level will be lower and you'll be weaker, even as you grow larger. If you choose to make the change then you will be stronger and healthier, you'll have more energy and you'll feel better about yourself.

I once was coaching a 70-year-old Italian priest who not only struggled with his eating habits, but had also once been addicted to alcohol. Many years earlier, he had made the decision to stop drinking. When I asked why, he had a simple answer, "I'm not going to be an alcoholic." In other words, he shifted his perception of himself.

The labels we give ourselves have a huge impact on our behaviors. The most powerful principle in modern psychology is that people will do anything they can to stay in line with the perception they have of themselves. In other words, if you call yourself "fat," a "junk-food junkie" or a "food addict," your behavior is going to reflect that belief! If you tell yourself you have no power over food or the cravings that control you, then you are relinquishing your control. Words are powerful, and by using phrases and terms like this, you are choosing to be powerless.

You must be very careful about the labels you give yourself. You are constantly feeding your subconscious, which doesn't question anything you tell it. If you feed it unhealthy beliefs, it will act on those beliefs and make you behave in a way that supports them. If you catch yourself thinking things that take the control away from you and give control to your negative impulses and behavior, you have to change the words you use. If you hear your inner voice saying, "I shouldn't have this donut but I can't help myself. I have no control over it," then you are not listening to reality. You do have control over whether or not you eat the

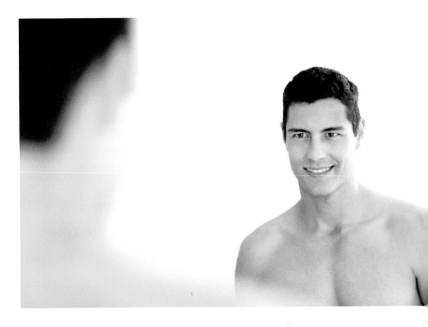

"Instead of calling yourself fat, tell yourself you are fit, healthy, and energetic, but simply carrying around an extra 20, 30, 50, 100 or more pounds of fat."

donut, and you can help yourself. By telling yourself these lies, you are reinforcing the negative identity that is not the real you, and you will continue to act in a way that supports that identity. As Napoleon Hill and W. Clement Stone wrote in *Success Through a Positive Mental Attitude*, "Keep your mind on the things you should and do want, and off the things you shouldn't and don't want." So, instead of calling yourself fat, tell yourself you are fit, healthy and energetic, but simply carrying around an extra 20, 30, 50, 100 or more pounds of fat.

When you begin to believe you are a fit and healthy person, you will start to act as a healthier person. This makes it easy to choose nutritious foods and exercise, because that is the behavior of a fit person and that's what you are! If you call yourself fat and lazy, or ratio-

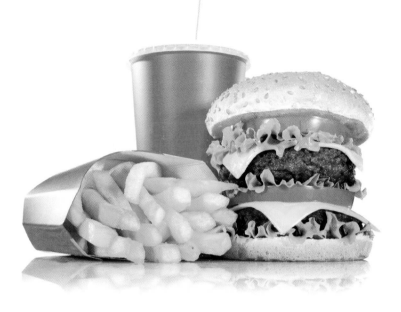

"Food addicts are not addicted to real food that offers nutrition; they are addicted to junk food."

nalize your behavior, shrugging it off because those voices in your head are saying you'll always be fat, then you're going to be stuck in a place you hate. You must change the way you look at yourself if you want others to start to look at you differently and, ultimately, if you want to change your behavior.

The priest I mentioned earlier said something to me after he had lost 70 pounds on my program. I asked him what the most challenging part of his weight-loss journey was. Here are his words: "Charlie, you know when I was having that struggle with alcohol it was easy to quit. I just stopped. Alcohol isn't something the body absolutely needs to survive. The alcoholic can quit drinking. The smoker can quit smoking. The heroin addict can stop using heroin. But the food addict cannot quit eating. We must have food to live." In fact it is this thought that leads a lot of food addicts to give up, or not even try to overcome their addiction.

While it is true that the food addict cannot quit eating in order to get beyond their food addiction, food addicts do not spend the day planning how to get their next meal of wilted spinach with grilled chicken breast. Food addicts are not addicted to real food that offers nutrition; they are addicted to junk food. So while the addict cannot quit eating, he or she can and must quit eating junk. And when you think about it, alcoholics cannot quit drinking, either – they still have to drink nonalcoholic beverages such as water, milk and juice, so it's not that dissimilar.

We can't stop eating, although there are many proponents of all-liquid diets and fasts. I don't personally support that approach unless a person has absolutely no other options. I believe we must stop allowing our negative habits to have control over us and we must take control of our own health. Not eating for a short time isn't going to help us develop new healthier habits. In fact, I believe it does the opposite. Drinking only liquids for months seems to me a difficult, painful and uncomfortable experience. If you're doing something that painful to get to a pleasurable state, what's going to happen once you achieve the pleasure? In other words, once you reach your goal weight, your clothes fit and you hear everyone telling you how great you look and how much they admire you, how would you continue to follow a plan that your brain associates with bringing you pain?

Remember, it's our brain's job to keep us from getting hurt, even when the things it wants us to do don't make sense in the long term. Let me ask you a question. Have you ever been rejected by someone of the opposite sex? I sure have. When that happened to me, my brain quickly adopted the idea that trying to reach out to the opposite sex meant pain. Logically, I know a relationship is the path to the most happy, exciting and fireworks-filled parts of our lives. But my brain didn't see it that way. It associated relationships with pain and rejection. The next time I would think about asking someone out, my brain would remind me of all my past negative experiences in an effort to keep me from the pain I experienced before.

# "The past doesn't equal the future!"

– Tony Robbins

When your brain starts telling you these things, remember what Tony Robbins, a man whose work has had a tremendous influence on me, says, "The past doesn't equal the future!" In other words, just because you got a certain result the first time you tried something doesn't mean you will get the same result the next time you try. You may associate pain with being on a diet or exercise plan because you've been let down before by not seeing the results you desired, or you've disappointed yourself because you didn't stick with it. But in this process you may have learned a thing or two about what works for you and what

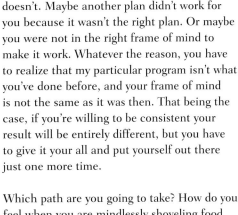

doesn't. Maybe another plan didn't work for you because it wasn't the right plan. Or maybe you were not in the right frame of mind to make it work. Whatever the reason, you have to realize that my particular program isn't what you've done before, and your frame of mind is not the same as it was then. That being the case, if you're willing to be consistent your result will be entirely different, but you have to give it your all and put yourself out there just one more time.

Which path are you going to take? How do you feel when you are mindlessly shoveling food into your mouth? Does it honestly feel good, or do you feel completely out of control, as if something else is in charge of your actions? And afterwards, do you feel satisfied or do you feel depressed? Is the momentary pleasure you get from eating an entire pizza worth the pain it causes you when you lie in bed feeling miserable – maybe even feeling you'd like to die?

So now let's think about the future for a minute. Answer the following questions honestly!

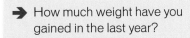

➜ How much weight have you gained in the last year?

➜ How much weight have you gained in the last two years?

Now I want you to close your eyes and fast-forward two years into the future. You wake up in your warm comfy bed. It's not yet fully light outside, but your alarm is beeping annoyingly. You press the "off" button, sit up, put your feet on the floor and sleepily make your way to the bathroom. The house is cool. You realize that winter is coming and this makes you think of last year at the same time. You get to the bathroom and turn on the bright light. As your pupils adjust, you step on the scale. You look down at the number, remembering what you weighed last year at this time. You are shocked at the number staring back at you.

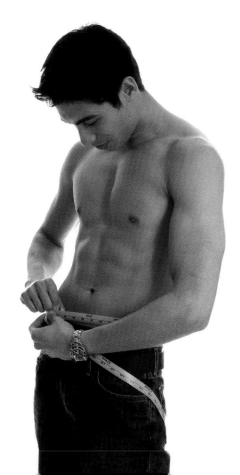

You step off the scale and look into the mirror. Now think about the following questions:

→ How do you think you look with an additional 20 or 30 pounds stuffed on you? Younger? Older?

→ Is your energy level better or worse?

→ Do you feel you present yourself more or less confidently, now that you are unable to fit into your favorite clothes?

→ Is your relationship as gratifying as it once was?

→ Do you think that you will still enjoy going shopping and socializing?

→ How about your health? Do you think your health will be better or worse?

→ How would you feel giving yourself two or more cold, sharp injections of insulin a day, just so your body can operate normally?

Wow, some painful questions to answer, aren't they? The truth is that if you continue to gain weight you will have to deal with these painful issues every single day.

But the great thing is that you don't ever have to get to that point. You can take control of your eating, your exercise habits, your weight and your health. You never have to experience any of this pain. If you have already experienced this pain, you can make sure you never do again. You can live a life you designed, certain the future is yours for the taking!

Remember that addictions and habits can be either positive or negative. Some people use habits or addictions to stop themselves from thinking about what's really bothering them. Some might lose themselves in hour after hour of TV. Others might use drugs or alcohol. Many, like the former me, use food. Other people, like the current me, have replaced the negative behaviors with positive ones. Instead of eating loads of junk food and watching endless TV, I now use activities such as cardio, weight lifting, reading, walking and talking with friends to get the same rush I used to get from sugar and fat. Different habits produce the same feelings, but with positive results instead of negative.

To succeed at this, you must identify the intention of your behavior. Find the "why" behind your negative behavior. Once you can be honest with yourself and answer that question truthfully, you can begin to look for a new behavior to put in its place. Preserve the intention but replace the behavior, and instead of evenings filled with junk food and misery, you'll have evenings filled with energy, excitement and pleasure. You'll be living your dreams.

Do it now!

---

1. Patrick M. O'Malley, Ph.D., Lloyd D. Johnston, Ph.D. and Jerald G. Bachman, Ph.D. "Alcohol Use Among Adolescents." *Alcohol Health & Research World*, Vol 22(2). Table 4, p. 92.

2. Ashley N. Gearhardt, MS, MPhil, et al. "Neural Correlates of Food Addiction." *Arch General Psychiatry*. Published online April 4, 2011.

## *"I wanted to feel comfortable in my own skin."*

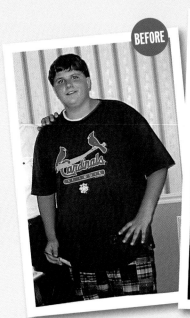

BEFORE

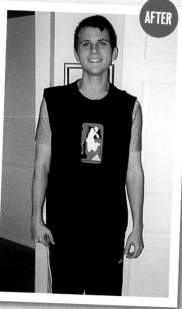

AFTER

**NAME:** Allan Finnegan
**AGE:** 22
**HEIGHT:** 6'
**WEIGHT BEFORE:** 265 lbs
**WEIGHT AFTER:** 165 lbs
**WEIGHT LOSS:** 100 lbs

**ALTHOUGH ALLAN FINNEGAN WAS AN ACTIVE YOUNGSTER, BY THE TIME HE GOT TO HIGH SCHOOL HE HAD STOPPED EXERCISING AND PARTICIPATING IN SPORTS.** Around this time, his eating habits also changed for the worse. He never ate breakfast, had little if any lunch and gorged on huge meals late at night. It was a recipe for disaster, and before he knew it his weight had climbed to 265 pounds.

Allan was extremely unhappy with his appearance and the lack of personal relationships in his life, but it wasn't until his first semester of law school that he realized he needed to make a change. The switch finally went on in his head when he went to a party and noticed that he spent the whole night feeling awkward and uncomfortable. "That was the first time I actually felt embarrassed by who I was and what I looked like," he said. "I wanted to feel comfortable in my own skin, whether

that was something as simple as walking to class every day or if it was going out with my buddies on the weekend."

Allan decided to sign up for a nutrition plan and training sessions with Charles D'Angelo. After an initial setback, Allan eventually lost 100 pounds. Charles then put him on a program to gain healthy weight and muscle mass, and Allan hasn't looked back since! He loves his success and says he is healthier now than he has ever been. He is more athletic and better at sports, and he has even run a couple of half-marathons. All areas of his life – physical, mental and social – have improved dramatically for the better but, most importantly, Allan finally feels comfortable with who he is.

Allan says that without Charles' advice, he would not have had a clue about how to start his journey toward

health and fitness. "I think that is what people need above all else: the knowledge of how to succeed. Charles provided me with the knowledge of how to lose weight healthfully."

These days, to maintain his weight loss and muscle gains, Allan keeps a close eye on his body. He says that keeping track of tangible things like body fat, along with simply looking in the mirror and seeing the difference, are what keep him motivated and going strong.

When he feels like doing something he knows is unhealthy, Allan reminds himself of how far he has come and of all the hours he has spent in the gym working toward his new body. He stays motivated because his life is simply better today than it was before. "Knowing how good life can be – and that the best is yet to come – makes me realize that I never want to go back to where I used to be," he says.

Allan is thankful for the impact Charles made on his whole life, not just his weight. "I've told this to Charles many times; he improved not only my health, but my entire outlook on life more than he or anyone else will ever know, and for that I can't say 'thank you' enough."

# DON'T EAT YOUR HEART OUT!

## Healthy Ways to Deal With Your Feelings

*For years you may have rewarded, comforted and medicated yourself with the very thing that has brought you so much incessant long-term pain – junk food. I overcame this vicious habit by recognizing that it wasn't the food I desired, but the feeling I thought it gave me. The next time you're about to reach for an unhealthy snack, put your focus on the feeling you're looking to get from eating and then remind yourself that food can't fix it. Then you can replace your negative behaviors with positive ones. Below you will find some common reasons my clients give for eating the wrong foods, followed by suggestions that will help you get the feelings you're seeking in positive, healthy and often fun ways!*

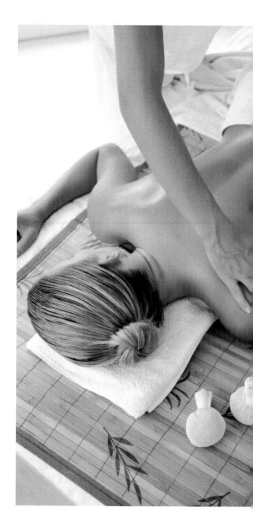

### ♥ "I eat to experience love."

When you are looking to feel love from food, recognize that you can give yourself that love without the calories! Take up the hobby of gathering mementos of times you've felt most appreciated and happy. Put together scrapbooks to review when you're looking to cure your blues. If you have a partner, doing something intimate together can bring about the loving feelings you desire as well. This doesn't have to be sexual – simply going for a walk together can bring about these intense feelings of love.

### ♥ "Eating helps relieve my stress."

The next time you're feeling stressed treat yourself to a massage. Relax and enjoy the feeling of nurturing yourself. Let all your tension slip away. Researchers at Cedars-Sinai Medical Center in Los Angeles discovered that just one deep-tissue massage significantly reduced levels of the stress hormone cortisol and increased the level of lymphocytes, white blood cells that are part of the immune system.[1]

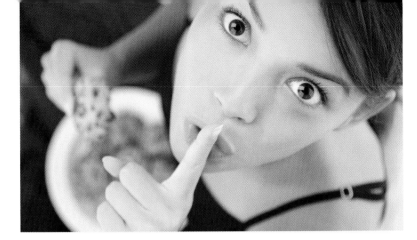

 **"I use food as a distraction."**

Using food as a distraction is a surefire way to blow a week's worth of hard work! Ask yourself why you need distraction. What's bothering you? If it's on your mind then you should handle it now! Don't procrastinate. Remedying the situation will immediately relieve the need to distract yourself with food. If you are eating to distract yourself from something you have absolutely no control over, why worry? You have no control over it! Seek out books or courses on meditation and start practicing – even if it's just 10 minutes a day to start with. Meditation will help you focus on what really matters.

 **"Food helps me feel safe and certain."**

If you are longing to feel secure, open an investment account and commit to saving a certain percentage of every dollar you earn. If possible, put away 10 percent of your income. Financial experts say this is the minimum amount you should save. If this seems too intimidating, even three or five percent is a good start. Arrange for the money to automatically come out of your paycheck or account. Watching your savings accumulate and grow is a great feeling! Whenever you are longing to get a sense of certainty and security, log onto your bank account and take a

look at the tangible result your positive habits have brought about.

 **"It's not a celebration without food!"**

Unhealthy food is used to celebrate so many occasions, from birthdays to retirement parties to holidays to family reunions. Recognize that you're not at the party for the cake – you're there to enjoy the company of your friends and family. Consciously making yourself aware of the distinction is the first step in transforming your mindset and enjoying social situations without feeling the need for unhealthy food. Besides, true celebration emerges from charting your path and fulfilling your destiny, not in a brief moment's enjoyment of chocolate cake and ice cream.

 **"I eat because I'm afraid of reaching my goals."**

Wow! Weird to think we would actually sabotage our own efforts, but sometimes we do. The thought of reaching a goal can bring about anxiety for a number of reasons: fear of the work necessary to maintain your success, fear of losing the "self" you've associated with your fat, fear of failure. It doesn't make any sense, but some people feel that if they don't really try, then they won't have failed.

The way to combat these anxieties is to follow the advice I give in this book: Believe that you have already reached your goals! As the pioneering American psychologist William James said, "Belief creates the actual fact." If you believe you are already a thin person, then you don't need to fear becoming a thin person – you're already there! You will experience a tremendous breakthrough when you finally realize that all you desire is within and you can have it at any moment you choose to give it to yourself.

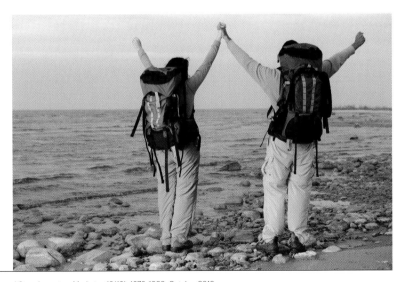

1. Mark Hyman Rapaport et al. *The Journal of Alternative and Complementary Medicine.* 16(10): 1079-1088. October 2010.

# section II

## Your remarkable transformation comes from managing your mind!

# CHAPTER FOUR

## Ignite a Fire that Lasts: Become Motivated!

"Our bodies are our gardens ... our wills are gardeners."
– William Shakespeare

We all have goals and aspirations of being somehow better than we presently are. We dream of waking up with energy, getting dressed and feeling great about the reflection in the mirror, of feeling appreciated and welcome at a satisfying job. We want to go through the day feeling fulfilled. We want to make contributions to other people's lives, and then come home to a warm and welcoming family. Sounds idealistic, doesn't it? Some might call it unrealistic, but I know without question that kind of life is possible.

As a kid I had an ideal vision of the life I would lead. I would have a great body – wide shoulders, a rippling six-pack, plump pecs – and a beautiful girlfriend on my arm. I'd become popular. And one day I would get the job of my dreams, helping others. I had complete conviction that I was going to lead that life. At first, though, things didn't seem to be going as planned. The future seemed bleak and overwhelming. I felt beaten down by the few years of life I had behind me. I'd surrendered my self-control and had almost let go of my dreams.

While we may feel as if the problems that arise in our lives are exclusive to us, life can seem to get in the way for everyone. No one has a smooth and easy life, much as we might think others do. As the great Scottish poet Robbie Burns began and John Steinbeck restated, "The best-laid schemes of mice and men often go awry." Illness, financial and emotional problems, family issues and time constraints tend to drain us of the exciting dreams and ideals we once had, leaving us feeling empty and hopeless if we lose our perspective.

Although everyone experiences a few unexpected bumps in the road of life, we can control whether or not we let them ruin the journey. Unfortunately, I learned this lesson by going through a difficult situation with my mother. During my childhood, she had always been such a source of love and support, but as I got older, the psychological pain of her past began to haunt her and she turned to a heavy mix of prescription drugs and alcohol to self medicate. By the time I was a teen, she was a full-blown alcoholic and prescription drug addict. This affected my daily life in ways I would never have been able to imagine, and I never told a soul about it. I spent so much futile effort trying to change my life by attempting to control my mother's addictions to pills and alcohol, but my life didn't actually change until I realized that the only person I could control was myself. Once I understood that reality, my life changed drastically for the better, and has been improving ever since.

You need to focus on changing *you* – not blaming everyone and everything else for your problems. As Carl Jung said, "Your vision will become clear only when you can look into your own heart. Who looks outside, dreams; who looks inside, awakes." Are you ready to wake up? In this chapter, I will help you look inside by asking you questions that will get you to think about your motivations and goals. I know they are inside of you somewhere – you just need to find them and hold on to them. To make lasting changes, you have to stay on purpose with improving yourself, on a continuous basis. Most people regain the weight they lose because they stop setting goals and they don't continue to condition their identity as a fit and healthy person.

You likely don't think of your finances as having an endpoint. Finances are something you will always have to manage. But for some reason, people look at weight loss as something they have to intensely focus on until it has been handled and then they can relax. What kind of success plan is that? What if you managed your finances intently for six months and then simply stopped?

I will never forget the day I decided I was going to take complete control of my destiny, lose weight and, more importantly, do everything I possibly could to inspire others. In those days, I wore a size 50 pant. I came home from school exhausted, although I hadn't done much. Weighing 360 pounds is draining; just moving is hard. On that day I plopped down on my bed and turned on the TV. While most guys at 17 would be hanging out with girls and other friends after school, I lay alone in bed trying to distract myself with cartoons. When I was heavy, the only thing I used besides food to try and combat my depression was cartoons. But as I lay on my back watching TV that day, I noticed that every time I breathed in, my stomach would inflate to the point that it blocked my view. It was devastating.

I felt warm, wet tears stream down my face. I was miserable. I was tired of being the boy who never went to dances or had any friends. I was fed up with not being able to shop at a mall because they didn't carry clothes in my size. I was sick of being scared to death of approaching a girl, knowing I would automatically be rejected. I was tired of being the last person to be picked to participate in games or other events. I was frustrated with myself for letting food control me. I was done with my life. At this very young age I was confronted with my own mortality and felt true despair. I almost didn't see a positive way out. I whispered to God, "If you help me lose this weight and get the body I deserve, I will do *everything* in my power to help others who are suffering like I am. I promise, God, I will dedicate my life to helping as many people as I can. Just please help me!"

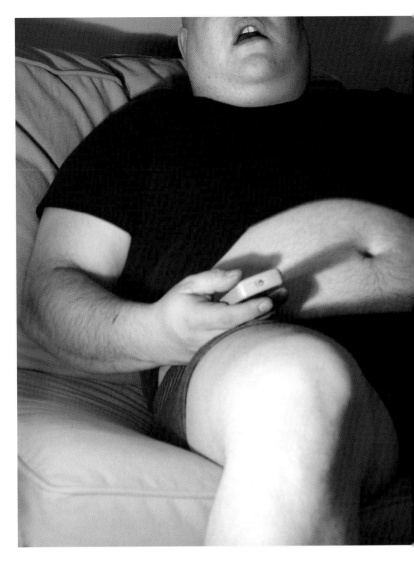

"As I lay on my back watching TV that day, I noticed that every time I breathed in, my stomach would inflate to the point that it blocked my view. It was devastating."

I rolled over on my side, still crying, and drifted off to sleep. When I awoke, I felt a strange calm wash over me. I suddenly knew that things were going to work out because I was ready to assume responsibility and take control. My dreams would be a reality as long as I was willing to do the work to make them happen. This Tony Robbins quote happens to sum up my realization quite well, "I've continued to recognize the power individuals have to change virtually anything and everything in their lives in an instant. I've learned that the resources we need to turn our dreams into reality are within us, merely waiting for the day when we decide to wake up and claim our birthright." And that's exactly what I did. Two years later, after eating healthy foods and exercising every day, I had burned through 160 pounds of fat and was finally living my destiny.

> "I remember saying to myself, 'Wow, I went from being totally ostracized because of my weight to having people fly in from across the country to work with me ... how cool is that?!'"

Now almost a decade after that first day, it really has hit me that I am living life by my own design. I'll tell you about the moment I knew my dream had come true. I was reading emails one morning and a client of mine, who'd lost 46 pounds in just three months, had sent me a message about a friend of his who desperately needed to lose weight. He begged me to help Elaine (not her real name), explaining that she'd tried everything before with no lasting success and was stuck in a place she hated. She couldn't maintain a healthy relationship since she didn't even love herself. My client offered to fly me out on a private jet to see her in Colorado, but even with that offer I needed to speak with her myself before I would com-

mit to helping her. I had learned through my mother's battle with drug and alcohol addiction and my own struggle with obesity that no one can create lasting change in their life until they are ready to totally commit. No amount of begging, crying or cajoling from even the closest of friends or family makes a difference.

I spoke to Elaine about her challenges. I blatantly told her that I wasn't convinced she was ready. She was very wishy-washy about her goals. That all changed when I asked her about her future. I said to her, "Elaine, I know you've put yourself out there and have tried before to no avail, but let me ask you a question. Where will you be in a year if you weigh 360 pounds instead of 300?" She had mentioned to me earlier in the conversation that her work demanded she travel by commercial plane. At her size it was already challenging. She grew silent but finally said, "Oh my God, I wouldn't be able to grow my business anymore, which means I would start to struggle financially!"

Everyone's motivation is different. For Elaine, being diabetic, having high blood pressure and being alone were not enough to cause her to commit to the necessary changes in her life. She loved her business and wanted to be able to express herself through it. When I helped her to discover that she could lose her business unless she changed her lifestyle, she was ready to make that change. I didn't have to fly to Colorado; she flew in to see me and did so every two weeks thereafter. Each flight, her plane voyage got easier and more comfortable as she continued to lose weight. What are your reasons to change?

I remember saying to myself, "Wow, I went from being totally ostracized because of my weight to having people fly in from across the country to work with me ... how cool is that?!" I knew I was creating the life I had always wanted *and* I was keeping my word with God. At that moment I knew I was empowered with the strategies to help people not just locally, but nationally. I had gone from lying in bed alone on Friday nights, feeling I was worthless and that I didn't have the ability to influence anything in my own life, let alone others', to living my dream of helping other people even two states away. And this was all because I made the decision to no longer accept that my destiny was determined by my environment, my family history or my own history. It's never too early or too late to start. Today is your day to begin.

## "It's never too early or too late to start. Today is your day to begin."

You may be wondering how a 17-year-old kid could have made such a powerful change in his own life, and eventually in the lives of others. The answer is profoundly simple. I decided to make myself the priority. I refused to continue to let aspects of life get in the way of my goals. I decided I could do anything I wanted and, most importantly, I took action. I was going to create and commit to a schedule of eating and an exercise routine that worked for me. It all changed the moment I made that decision. Decisions are powerful, yet most people are afraid to make any significant ones.

Since then, I've spent every waking moment doing everything I can to ignite a fire in the people I'm blessed to cross paths with. I start by reminding them about what is possible. I help them reawaken the vision of life they once had, and can still tap into.

We all have an unbelievable amount of personal power to achieve our dreams, yet few of us tap into it. Why? Think about Walt Disney. He almost went bankrupt several times, and at one time he couldn't even afford a pair of shoes. He was betrayed by those he trusted. Yet still he kept his dream alive and never set-tled for anything less than what he envisioned. He built the largest entertainment empire that has ever existed, and has brought so much joy to the world because of his sheer hard-head-edness and determination. He said, "All our dreams can come true, if we have the courage to pursue them." But even when we hear such inspiring and exciting stories and learn what's possible if we reach for our dreams, we can still feel complacent.

Humans certainly are complex! We all know how to lose weight: eat less and exercise more. It's simple math, right? I'll also add that we should eat properly and exercise more regularly. So while we spend millions trying to find the perfect diet, I think the most important question isn't "What diet do I need to follow to lose weight?" but rather, "How do I get myself so ecstatic about what's possible for me that I will stick to whatever plan I embark on?" As Tony Robbins said, "It is not knowing what to do, it's doing what you know." How do you motivate yourself to make that change in your life? And even more importantly, how do you *stay* motivated and keep yourself off the diet roller coaster where, chances are, you will reach your goal only to end up right back where you started – or even heavier – like more than 90 percent of people do?

You may have grown comfortable, even in your misery. Maybe you've accepted that being fat is who you are. If you've built that into your identity, then we have some work to do. To succeed you must get disturbed and uncomfortable with yourself – not the inner you, who you should love, but your out-ward representation.

You may not want to change the way you live your life, but you have to accept that life is all about change. Change is inevitable. You are not the same as you were last year. For better or for worse, you are different. Every member of your family is different than they were 10 years ago, aren't they? You know change

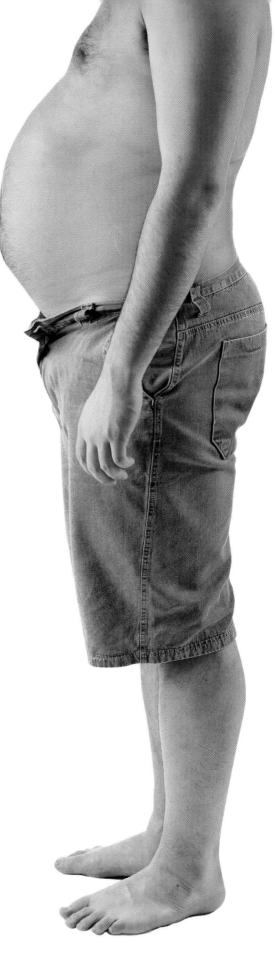

> ## "How will I feel about the reflection staring back in the mirror a year from now if I do not make the necessary changes?"

is inevitable, but if you are not controlling the changes you can control, you are practically guaranteeing that the changes you experience in the future will be negative rather than positive.

You need to ask yourself the following questions:

➜ If I do not change my habits, if I continue making the unhealthy decisions I know I'm making and I continue to gain weight as I have been, then will I have changed for the better or for the worse one year from now?

➜ How will I feel about the reflection staring back in the mirror a year from now if I do not make the necessary changes?

➜ How will my health be in a year if I've gained another 10, 20, 30 or 60 pounds?

➜ If I do not make the necessary changes to my lifestyle, will I be living the life I dreamed about when I was younger?

➜ Am I contributing to the lives of others the way I am able to?

You have your daily routine. You're comfortable. Maybe you're the one who brings donuts to share with your coworkers, and they count on you to bring them. Your dad brings home fried chicken with extra-large fries, two-liter bottles of soda and chocolate pie every Friday night. You and your friends order in pizza and wings every Sunday as you watch football. These are habits that must be changed for you to achieve your goals. As they say, losing weight is simple, but it's not easy.

The first step you must take in order to succeed is to make the decision that you are not a "fat" person. You must clarify this in your mind. Instead of looking at yourself as being a "fat" person, tell yourself that you are a fit person who is presently carrying around a lot of extra fat.

# MOTIVATION

To a scientist, motivation determines all behavior of every species, including humans. If motivation determines everything we do, then it follows that motivation determines whether you remain overweight or whether you will achieve your goal and become the size you want to be. Although I feel it is extremely helpful to figure out what motivated you to become overweight, it is even more important to ensure your motivation for losing weight is strong, and that your motivation to keep the weight off remains strong once you've achieved your goal.

Many people have negative feelings toward dieting because they have found it painful in the past. Deprivation, anxiety, fear and even depression can be associated with making huge changes in the foods you're eating. Vegetables were so foreign to me that I remember vomiting the first time I took a bite of canned peas. Talk about a strong negative association! Granted they're not canned, but now I eat several kinds of vegetables on a daily basis. How did I cross this road? I've conditioned myself to focus on the benefits that action would

create in my life. Instead of indulging in short-term thinking, I've forced myself to look ahead to the future impact of the actions I'm taking today. A rock-hard six-pack, more energy, lasting health … these things all come to my mind when I conjure up the thought of veggies. This is because I have rewired my brain to make a positive association – quite a contrast from the days when I weighed 360 pounds.

# NO PAIN, NO LONG-TERM GAIN

The reason we can have a hard time sticking to a new eating and exercise plan is that we experience pain. We have to either suffer the pain of changing or we have to suffer the pain of staying the way we are now (or getting bigger). We have a choice in which type of pain we must endure, but we must endure one of the two.

The first is the pain that comes from the discipline of changing. It can be painful to alter your current way of doing things. Change can be difficult, but it becomes fun once you replace your old pleasure with a healthier one. The second type of pain isn't so enjoyable. That's the pain of regret. The pain of regret comes when we don't do what our gut (or the little Jiminy Cricket on our shoulder) tells us we should. When we violate our own rules and values by making a decision to seek short-term pleasure, we experience a much longer-lasting pain. Ouch! What I'd like to give you are the strategies that will not only help you create change, but also make those changes last.

"We have to either suffer the pain of changing or we have to suffer the pain of staying the way we are now."

# USING THE THREE R's TO MAKE WEIGHT LOSS HAPPEN - AND LAST!

## THE FIRST "R": REASON

You might want to lose 10 pounds to look your best for a reunion, or you might need to lose 300 pounds to avoid an early death. You may simply wish you looked better in a bikini, or you may want to lose weight so badly that you cry yourself to sleep at night. No matter how badly you want to lose weight, this doesn't mean you feel motivated to do what you've got to do each day in order to succeed. You're looking for results, but you have to ask yourself, "What is the point? What will motivate me to continue even after I have achieved the results I'm after?" If you don't feel motivated, or motivated enough, then how can you *make* yourself feel that way?

> "Stop accepting subpar standards – they'll only bring about subpar results and ultimately a subpar life."

The most important element of motivation is that you have to discover what gets *you* going. Maybe you're on the verge of getting diabetes but that doesn't seem real to you and therefore does not inspire you to change. Maybe the thing that will really get you to change is the fact that you want to get a date. Don't worry about having the "correct" motivation. It does you no good to repeat words that sound impressive but mean nothing to you. Many times, clients come to me and say they don't know what they want. That's a start, because from there we can find out what they *don't* want. Ask yourself those tough questions I listed earlier, and look hard at the reality. If you continue eating the way you do, how will you feel when you look in the mirror next year? What

are the things you'll hear from those you love? If you're in a relationship now but continue to get heavier and loathe yourself even more, will your soul mate still feel the same about you? If you keep getting heavier will you settle for a person not worthy of you just so you can have someone in your life? The answers might be scary to think about, but these are important questions to ask.

## THE SECOND "R": RESULTS

You are a unique and special person. You may dislike things you've done in your life – the people you've hurt, the decisions you've made, the opportunities you've missed – we all do. But by picking up this book you've chosen to take a step in a positive direction. You must decide that since you are a good and unique person, you deserve the best. This means setting your sights on bigger and better things. You deserve to eat foods that nourish your body instead of settling for whatever is easy, convenient and cheap. You deserve to be able to travel in comfort. You deserve not to be talked down to because of your size or the way the fat on your body makes you look. You deserve to be in a relationship that fulfills you, not one in which you are ridiculed or made fun of. You deserve to find the time to exercise and do the things that are helping to bring about the life you desire. Stop accepting subpar standards – they'll only bring about subpar results and ultimately a subpar life.

Take a look at the following list of adjectives and choose 10 that describe you. If you can find more than 10 – all the better! Write those words down on a piece of paper with the words "I am" at the top of the page. Look at that list every day as a reminder of why you deserve to treat yourself properly.

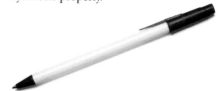

| | | | | |
|---|---|---|---|---|
| adaptable | efficient | honorable | painstaking | splendid |
| agreeable | encouraging | imaginative | peaceful | spontaneous |
| alert | enduring | impartial | placid | steadfast |
| amazing | energetic | incredible | pleasant | stimulating |
| ambitious | entertaining | indestructible | plucky | succinct |
| amusing | enthusiastic | industrious | practical | talented |
| awesome | excellent | instinctive | productive | thoughtful |
| brave | excited | intelligent | protective | thorough |
| bright | exuberant | jolly | proud | thrifty |
| brilliant | fabulous | joyous | punctual | tough |
| calm | fair | keen | quick-thinking | trusting |
| capable | faithful | kind | quiet | trustworthy |
| caring | fantastic | kind-hearted | receptive | unbiased |
| charming | fearless | knowledgeable | reflective | unique |
| cheerful | fine | level-headed | resolute | unusual |
| cooperative | frank | likeable | responsible | upbeat |
| courageous | friendly | lively | rhetorical | valiant |
| creative | funny | loving | righteous | vigorous |
| credible | generous | loyal | selective | vivacious |
| cultured | gentle | mature | self-assured | warm |
| dazzling | glorious | modest | sensible | willing |
| decisive | good | natural | sensitive | wise |
| delightful | grateful | nice | shrewd | witty |
| determined | great | noble | silly | wonderful |
| diligent | happy | obedient | sincere | worthy |
| discreet | harmonious | open-minded | skillful | |
| dynamic | helpful | original | smart | |
| eager | hilarious | outstanding | smiling | |

## USE IMAGERY AND AUTO-SUGGESTION

Close your eyes. Think about how you would like to be. Think of a real, achievable goal. Is it to fit into that old pair of jeans buried in the back of your closet? You know, the ones that used to fit you? Is it to see your blood pressure return to normal? Is it to hear the person you've been dreaming about say "Yes!" when you finally ask him or her out? Is it to feel the warm loving hand of the person you want to spend your life with nestled in yours? Maybe your goal is to be able to spend more quality time with your children. Can you fit on the roller coaster with your son? Whatever your goal is, make it concrete: I will fit into my old jeans and they will not be too tight. My blood pressure will be 120/80. I will have the girl/boy of my dreams. I will not settle. I will ride the roller coaster with my son.

Choose something very important to you, and live that success in your mind. Act as if it's already in your possession. This is an all-important key. In order to put the right energy out in the universe to attract the circumstances you're after, you must begin to act as if your desire is already yours to hold. You have to emotionalize your desire to bring it about. Simply repeating the words "I will be skinny, I will be skinny, I will be skinny," will do nothing! You must have a concrete goal and you have to get charged up about it. Scream it out! You have to make your goal compelling if you're going to stick to it!

Take the image of your desire and make a visual reminder of it. This can be a note you write, a picture from a magazine, an old photo of yourself, a piece of clothing or a dream board. Whatever works for you. Every night

> "Choose something very important to you, and live that success in your mind. Act as if it's already in your possession."

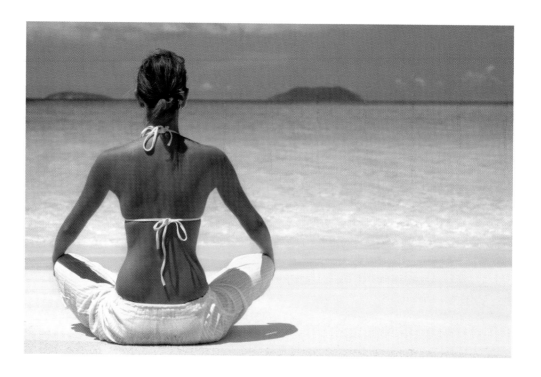

and every morning, remind yourself of your goal by taking a moment to regard this item. I find first thing in the morning and right before bed is ideal. Spend a good 10 to 15 minutes concentrating on this vision. Don't question whether or not you will achieve it. Accept that it is real and that it is waiting for you. This will keep your goal at the top of your mind, helping to reinforce your determination each and every day.

When I have a goal, I follow Napoleon Hill's formula for impressing the subconscious. First, I write down that specific goal and put a copy up everywhere I know I'll see it: the bathroom mirror, the fridge, the TV. Every night before I go to bed and every morning when I wake up, I go to that note. I read it, and then I close my eyes and concentrate. I envision what achieving that goal will feel like. I picture myself already there. I get myself to actually "feel" what it is like knowing my goal is already in my possession. That reinforces my strength to do what I have to do each day to help that vision become reality.

Write your goal out. State what it is you're after, set a definite date for its achievement, write down what you intend to do in exchange for achieving this goal, and end with: "My goal is now awaiting transfer to me in proportion to the amount of focus, dedication, commitment and hard work I'm giving to it!" You must repeat your statement each morning upon waking and every night before bed – *with emotion*. Don't just speed through it without feeling! As Napoleon Hill stated, "If you repeat a million times the famous Émile Coué formula, 'Day by day, in every way, I am getting better and better,' without mixing emotion and faith with your words, you will experience no desirable results. Your subconscious mind recognizes and acts *only* upon thoughts which have been well-mixed with emotion or feeling." Energy is power, and you have to be willing to be excited in order to reach your dreams.

# KEEP YOUR EYES ON THE PRIZE

The practice of goal setting is an important key for keeping motivated and therefore achieving your goal. If you have an arbitrary non-compelling goal like "I want to lose weight" then this is not nearly as powerful as saying "My goal is to weigh 180 pounds and have a 32-inch waist by December 1st!" Think of your long-term goal first, then break that down into short- and medium-term goals, and include these goals in your visual reminders.

Let's use Maria (not her real name) to illustrate this example. Maria weighed 212 pounds at 5'5". As a young teenager she had been, in her words, skinny. She developed a rounded, more "womanly" figure into her late teens and early 20s, which she liked. She married, and says her ideal body was on her wedding day. She weighed 135 pounds. Through the years she had three kids, and with each successive pregnancy she gained more weight, finally ending up at the 212 pounds she weighed when this journey began, at age 34. She wanted to weigh 135 pounds again but each time she'd tried to lose weight she failed and had begun to feel like it was pointless to try. But with the help of a coach she developed a plan, and one year later Maria was back to the 135 pounds she had been on her wedding day.

Here's how Maria used goal setting to reach her desired weight:

**1** She already knew the weight she wanted to be, but when she had dieted before she had always given herself too short a time to reach that goal. She would go on fad diets to try to get there too quickly and when she didn't reach her unrealistic goals she'd give up and her weight would climb right back up. Once she realized that she'd wasted many years getting fatter while trying to lose weight too rapidly, she was more receptive to giving herself the more realistic timeframe of one year.

**Key:** Your goal must be attainable. Losing 80 pounds in three months is an unreasonable goal. If you see that you are not going to achieve that unreasonable goal, you will get a sense of failure from losing 10 pounds in a month, for example, even though that is a huge success! Losing 80 pounds in a year is a reasonable goal that allows time for body-adjusting plateaus, which will inevitably occur.

2 Maria then broke this larger goal into smaller goals. She had daily goals, weekly goals and monthly goals alongside her long-term goal. They say all great journeys start with a single step, and while that's true, it sure helps to have some markers along the way. Maria wrote down all these goals in a notebook, and kept some out as visual cues. She made a collage of images of bodies she not only liked, but also resembled her own. (It can be counterproductive to put up an image of a 5'11" fashion model if your natural shape is 5'2" and curvy.) Then she wrote down her daily and weekly goals and put them up in places that worked for her. Her daily goal went on her bathroom mirror and her weekly goal went up on the fridge.

**Key:** Have attainable goals for every time-frame. A long-term goal can be intimidating and not very immediate. If you focus instead on what you are working toward each day and week, then you are constantly achieving and constantly moving closer to your eventual goal without getting overwhelmed.

3 Maria allowed herself to feel a real sense of accomplishment for every single goal met. Over the years she had got in the common habit of putting herself down and minimizing her successes. This time around she pulled her daily goal down from the mirror each evening, read it and thought about whether she had achieved it. When she concluded she had, she gave herself a big pat on the back. She then put that note in a scrapbook, so she could go back over time to see all she had accomplished. Whenever she

felt down or like she was going nowhere, she got that book out and it invariably made her feel powerful, successful and in control of her destiny.

**Key:** Celebrate your successes, no matter how small. Don't minimize their importance. Every step in the right direction will bring you closer to your goal.

4 Maria did not let occasional slip-ups convince her to go back to her old habits. Those who are consistently thin eat treats sometimes, and may even overeat sometimes. The rest of the time they eat properly. These thin people do not eat a couple of cookies and convince themselves that they're failures so they might as well finish the bag. They enjoy their treat and then go back to their healthy eating plan. Even if they go totally off the rails one evening, and they may feel rotten the next day and even depressed, they do not use that as an excuse to go on a week-long binge. They go back to their healthy eating plan.

**Key:** No one is perfect. Very few people follow any diet plan without the occasional treat or slip-up. If you have that daily goal pasted on your mirror and you do not achieve it, then make doubly sure you achieve it the next day. I list the things I'm not too excited about doing but that I know I have to do on a legal pad each night before going to bed. I then force myself to get those things done first the next day so I know I get to enjoy the rest of the day. The same goes for working out. If I'm not excited about doing a particular exercise, I force myself to get it out of the way first.

5 Maria learned all about the lifestyles of the women who had the type of body she was after. One of the main things she learned was that most of them practiced moderation rather than denial. That was important to her, because she did not want to feel deprived. Once she learned that most thin people stay that way with consistency as opposed to abstinence, she felt she could

really live with this way of life. She stopped looking at a "diet" as a temporary fix and began to see it as a lifelong eating plan – one that included treats in moderation. She also learned that she did not have to exercise every day without fail – something she had found hard to do with her work and family responsibilities. She found that exercising for an hour, four times a week consistently was enough for her and she managed to fit those four hours into her busy schedule.

"If you can discover the reason you overeat, you can find the *intention* of that behavior."

# TYPES OF MOTIVATION

According to psychologists there are two basic types of motivation, intrinsic and extrinsic. To help you figure out the best way to get motivated, let's have a look at them.

*Intrinsic motivation* means you are motivated to perform an action because you get something out of it. To use intrinsic motivation to reach your goal, you need to get to the point where the actions that will bring you to your goal are pleasurable. People who yo-yo diet do so because the method they use to bring about their weight loss is too painful to keep up. Fad diets involve deprivation, low energy, poor mood and even feelings of desperation. It can be scary and painful. This method takes away the perceived pleasure of eating junk food and offers no pleasure in return, so a person would not have any intrinsic motivation to continue.

If you can discover the reason you overeat, you can find the *intention* of that behavior. In other words, what do you get out of it? Once you discover that, you can get to work at preserving the pleasure by simply replacing the negative behavior with a positive behavior. For example, my parents are both smokers. I tell them all the time how much danger they're in because of it, and that there is no question they will get cancer or lung disease if they continue. If they don't quit, then coughing, gagging up phlegm and breathing through oxygen tanks are all inevitably in their future. But guess what? They don't change. Why? Because the pleasure they associate with smoking is stronger than the pain they associate with quitting. The things I talk to them about are things that would make *me* change, but not *them*. My parents' response to me is always, "Well, Uncle Vito smoked until he was 100 without cancer and, besides, when it's your time, it's your time!" For many smokers the motivation is never strong enough until they actually are in the position where cancer is making excruciatingly painful sponges out of their lungs, or until they literally cannot smoke or they will blow up their oxygen tank. But by then it's too late.

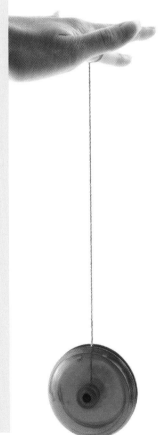

If you struggle with weight, maybe knowing you will likely get diabetes or heart disease isn't enough. Maybe the thought of losing your eyesight isn't real enough. You won't be motivated to change until you find out you have to stick a long, cold, silver needle into your arm to inject insulin. Or maybe the thought of spending $100 or more a week on insulin and other diabetic supplies, just so you won't die, will motivate you. Maybe you don't look at yourself in the mirror anymore because you can't bear the way you appear. Or maybe you find you don't want to go out with your friends anymore because you feel uncomfortable with the way you look. You have to find where your own personal pain is, and irritate yourself with that pain. When you associate pain with your current behavior and at the same time associate pleasure with the necessary changes, it happens! You make the shift instantly.

The trick is finding a positive behavior that will replace the pleasure you receive from your negative behavior. For example, if you distract yourself from the pain you're feeling by eating junk food and watching TV, like I did, then seek out a method to get the same distraction (the pleasure) while propelling yourself toward your goal. Why not go to a gym and watch your favorite TV show while walking on the treadmill instead of watching it while lying on the couch eating Funyuns? You still achieve the pleasurable distraction, but you have replaced the negative behavior with a positive one. If going to the gym is too intimidating for you, or if it's counterproductive because it makes you oversensitive about how much extra fat you have, then put a treadmill or exercise bike in your TV room and exercise there while watching your favorite show. However, I strongly encourage you to get out of the negative environment that has reinforced the bad eating behavior for so long. Sometimes you have to go outside of your comfort zone and get to a place you're not used to. You just may discover you like it! How about simply walking to the museum or art gallery and then walking around inside while you look at our world of wonder? That will help you achieve your goal of distraction while associating pleasure with the positive behavior of walking. Find what you like and create a way to combine a positive behavior with something that gives you pleasure.

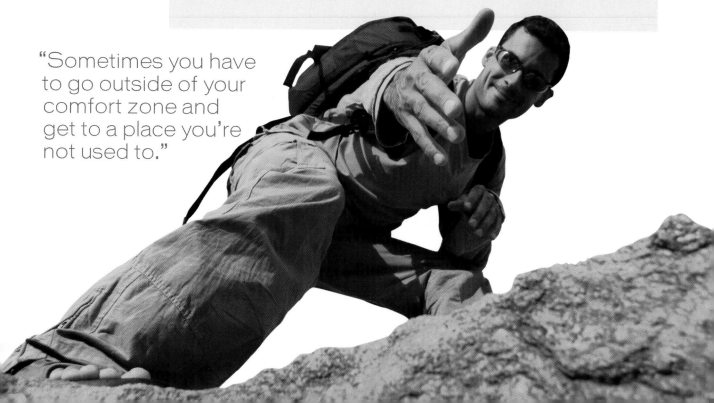

"Sometimes you have to go outside of your comfort zone and get to a place you're not used to."

Many people binge because they get an endorphin rush when they do so. A great way to get an endorphin rush is to exercise. Sure the first few times may hurt, but as you keep doing it and get better at it, you will find you get a feeling of euphoria from exercise far greater than the euphoria you ever experienced from bingeing – and without the regret.

Sports are great for intrinsic motivation. Most people who play soccer, basketball, badminton, football, racquetball or any other sport do so because they enjoy playing these sports, not because they get fans, fame or a sweet endorsement deal. If you can find any sport or game that you like to play, then this is a great replacement for overeating. And you have endless choices. You don't have to play something that needs real exertion to replace the pleasure you feel from overeating. How about table tennis in the basement? With the advent of motion-controlled video games, there's no excuse not to move! Obviously a more active sport or game will be more helpful for weight loss, but as long as your game replaces overeating and you enjoy it, this is a positive step. And you may find as you lose weight you want to try other sports that are more challenging.

There are as many reasons people become overweight as there are overweight people. You will have to figure out your own intrinsic motivation for overeating and under-exercising, and overcome that with an intrinsic motivation for positive behavior.

*Extrinsic motivation* means you are motivated to do something because of a positive or negative message you encounter from outside yourself. Most of us are primarily either "moving-toward" people or "moving-away" people. A "moving-toward" person might go to work each day because she wants to make money. A "moving-away" person might go to work so he won't seem useless (to avoid the pain of disapproval). Perhaps you don't steal from stores because you don't want to get in trouble with the police (moving away). Or you perform on stage because you like the applause and attention you get (moving toward).

In general, intrinsic motivation is stronger than extrinsic motivation, and in fact thinking too much about external motivation rather than internal can be what causes our failure to reach our goals. Our family tells us to lose weight, or we hear other people's negative comments, for example. While these are both motivators, they are extrinsic and therefore don't mean as much to us. Our family members and unkind strangers can't understand why their words do not inspire us to change, but – as with my parents and smoking – we won't lose weight until we find our internal motivation.

Sometimes, however, we are not completely aware of what motivates us. When you binge on an entire container of ice cream, you might say you are doing it because you like the taste. While that might be your motivation for eating a bite or two, what drives you to eat a gallon? In this case, you likely have an unconscious motivation to do so. Seeking help from a counselor is great because he or she can often help you realize the motivations you might be missing. Maybe there is something within you that wants to stay overweight because you have some idea that fat insulates you from the world. Maybe in some way you desire the invisibility you think obesity offers you. Whatever the unconscious reason you eat excessively, the key is to find something stronger that motivates you to *not* eat the ice cream, and use that to propel you.

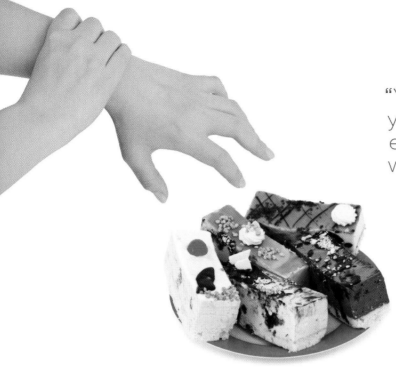

> "You need motivation, and you need motivation strong enough that it will help you with your self-control."

## SELF-CONTROL AND SELF-MOTIVATION

Some people seem to have an internal drive that makes them seek achievement. You likely remember some of these people from your school days – in addition to being the best athletes, they were also the best students and were always the first to raise their hand with the answer. When you thought of them, you likely thought about how lucky they were to have abilities in all areas. But while natural ability may allow a person to do well, it does not enable that person to excel. Excellence is never the result of ability but rather the result of motivation. Excellence requires dedication, which in turn requires both motivation and self-control. Without motivation *and* self-control, the most talented person can end up mediocre, whereas a person with sincere drive, focus and self-control can end up on top – even without so-called natural ability.

You might be saying to yourself right now, "I have motivation, otherwise I wouldn't be reading this book! Of course I want to lose weight!" But wanting to lose weight is very different from having the motivation to do what you

have to do to achieve your weight-loss goal. Millions of people want to be successful, yet so few are willing to commit to the consistent level of action required to achieve the success they desire and deserve. Today you want to lose weight. You might not eat any junk food today. You might join a gym and set up an appointment with a personal trainer. But what about tomorrow, next week, a month from now, three months, six months, or even a year down the road?

The desire to lose weight might get you through a day, but to get through the time it takes to actually lose the weight and keep it off, you need something a little more. You need motivation, and you need motivation strong enough that it will help you with your self-control.

## AND THEN THERE'S MAINTENANCE

What's going to happen after you lose the weight? I assure you there is no doubt in my mind that you can and will lose. The concern I have is this: After you've succeeded in losing weight, will you be as committed to maintaining your weight loss as you were to losing it? Clients who work with me after their weight loss is complete do maintain what they've achieved. Maintenance strategies are powerful, but they must be applied and conditioned consistently. Did you know the best athletes in the world all have coaches? They don't stop using a coach once they've reached the top. They have daily, weekly, monthly and yearly plans, just like they did when they were working toward the goals they eventually achieved. You may not have a personal coach, but use this book as your coach to achieve and maintain the weight loss you desire and deserve.

Once you've achieved your goal, your reason to maintain your health and weight must be so compelling that you continue to make great choices in both food and exercise. No matter which diet you follow, you will have to restrict yourself in the short term because you are correcting the excesses of the past. But as soon as you are back to where you want to be, or maybe at a place you've never been before, lighter than ever, you have to remain goal oriented and find something to focus on other than seeing the number on the scale go down, because that has now stopped. Going back to your bad habits is not an option unless you want to relive that agony. As Aristotle said, "We are what we repeatedly do. Excellence, then, is not an act, but a habit." How are you going to live today to ensure the future is in line with what you want? How are you going to be sure you remain accountable?

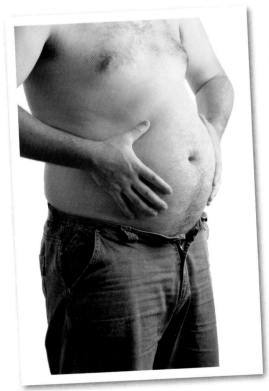

# PICTURE ME AT 17

What was my motivation to lose weight? I wanted to show myself that I wasn't bound by my circumstances or by the labels others had given me. In a way, I was saying to the world, I can be whoever I want to be, do whatever I want to do, achieve anything I decide I'm going to achieve. I wanted to prove that my family's history of addictions and obesity along with the requisite health problems would not be the predictor of my own future.

I grew up in a blue-collar urban environment, where shootings and robberies were common, where not going to college was the path most followed, where eating was usually the highlight of a person's day and healthy choices weren't even considered. Food was food, and you were supposed to be happy that your family could afford to order pizza or go to McDonald's. That was my life.

I remember when I was 17 and 360 pounds, driving past my high school on homecoming night in my little Honda Civic. I was looking at the colored lights flashing through the windows, hearing all the booming party music and watching the shadows of my classmates dancing with their dates behind the clouded gym windows. More and more smiling couples walked in, hand in hand, the doors closing tightly behind them. I sat in my car, all alone, my breath turning to vapor in the cool fall air, saying to myself, "Wow, what an analogy. All the fun and excitement going on inside, and here I am on the outside, separated by huge walls and a door I could easily walk through if I chose to." The one thing holding me back was my belief about myself.

"Going back to your bad habits is not an option unless you want to relive that agony."

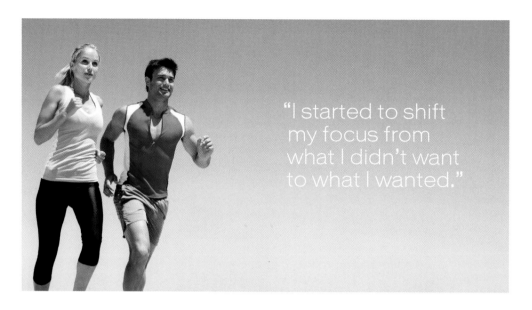

"I started to shift my focus from what I didn't want to what I wanted."

I was tired of being tired. I was sick of not being part of the fun. Of missing out on the greatest feeling in the world – holding the hand of a girl I really loved and who really loved me. Even though I was an awesome piano player, often performing with the jazz band at an all-girls school, I was totally ignored, repeatedly, because of my size. I'd hurry back to the bus in humiliation while all the other guys exchanged numbers with the throngs of female admirers. I would sit on the bus, anxiously wanting to escape the feeling of not being good enough. It was time to change.

I started to shift my focus from what I didn't want to what I wanted. I zeroed in on pictures of guys who had the type of body I wanted. Looking at magazines, watching TV, at the movies – everywhere I looked I found examples of the type of body I was after. In the mall, I would note how fit the models in the Abercrombie & Fitch posters looked. I tried to learn everything I could about those who lived the lifestyle I wanted. I reminded myself that with consistency in a healthy diet and exercise regimen, I could get my body to look that great too.

Your job right this second is to decide exactly what you want, where you're headed, precisely what it's going to take, how you will remain accountable and which foods you need to buy to get there! Once you've decided what you want and are entirely focused on it, something magical will happen – all sorts of opportunities will become apparent. Out of the blue someone will call asking if you'd like to join a gym with them because they want to lose weight; people will be volunteering to help you almost magically; commercials and advertisements will all seem to have a secret message in them just for you. Decide what you want today so the universe can begin to help you find it!

## NO, I DIDN'T FORGET THE THIRD "R"!

You'll have to wait a bit to get to step three. The third "R" stands for "Road" and involves mapping out what you will be eating. This will be covered in Chapters 8 and 9, but hang in there for a bit – we have a little more ground to cover first!

## "I sometimes feel like I have superpowers."

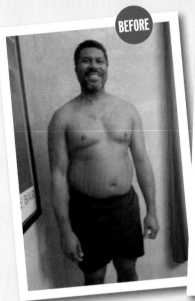

BEFORE

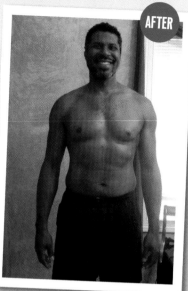

AFTER

**NAME:** Gene Dobbs Bradford
**AGE:** 44
**HEIGHT:** 6'4"
**WEIGHT BEFORE:** 268 lbs
**WEIGHT AFTER:** 219 lbs
**WEIGHT LOSS:** 49 lbs

*"To stay motivated all Gene has to do is look at his before picture. He remembers how much time and effort he dedicated to his weight loss and how easy it is to let it all go."*

**WEIGHT GAIN CAN HAPPEN TO THE BEST OF US – EVEN SERIOUS ATHLETES.** Where do things go wrong? The trouble usually begins when we stop paying attention to what we eat.

Such was the case with Gene Dobbs Bradford. Gene followed a strict exercise routine that included training for kung fu tournaments as well as several triathlons. But when he decided to return to school to work toward his MBA, he had to scale back his two-hour-plus daily fitness routine. Unfortunately, he neglected to scale back his eating habits as well, and he quickly topped the scales at 268 pounds – much more than his 6'4" frame could handle.

As a result of his weight gain, Gene began feeling sluggish and low on energy. Worst of all, he suffered from sleep apnea, which kept both him and his wife tossing and turning. He was forced to use a cumbersome CPAP

machine at night just so he could keep breathing.

Gene knew it was time for a change, so for his 44th birthday present he gave himself one year of good health. Part of this deal included losing the weight he had put on while studying. Although he had lost weight in the past using Weight Watchers, he was never able to get down to his goal weight of 220 pounds. Gene knew that he needed to do something different this time around. As fate would have it, that's exactly when he stumbled upon Charles D'Angelo's plan for success.

After working with Charles, Gene was able to whittle himself down to a svelte 219 pounds. And as the weight disappeared, so did Gene's sleep apnea. He is now sleeping soundly, as is his wife. Best of all, Gene's energy has returned! "I have much more energy than I ever had and I feel like my thinking is getting clearer every day,"

he says. "I am training for a marathon, and I have shaved a full minute off of my previous pace. I sometimes feel like I have superpowers."

To stay motivated all Gene has to do is look at his before picture. He remembers how much time and effort he dedicated to his weight loss and how easy it is to let it all go. Gene never wants to get back there again! He follows Charles' advice to "stay focused" at all times because he knows that it takes solid commitment to achieve the body of your dreams.

# MASTERING YOUR MIND
## Putting a STOP to Ineffective Personality Traits

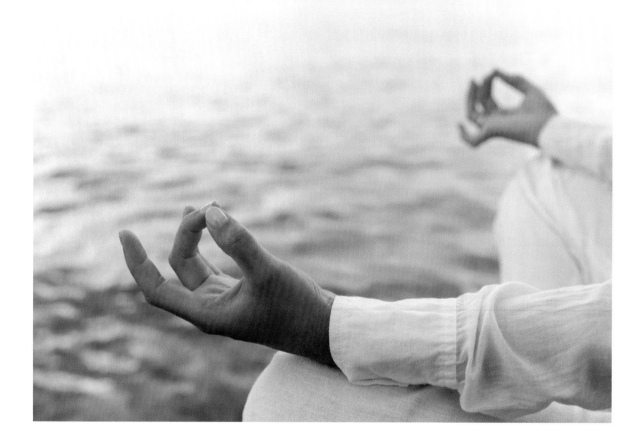

*If you are significantly overweight or even morbidly obese, you may have a lot of anger, hate, despair and other negative feelings stored up inside you, stemming both from what you've done to yourself and what you perceive others to have done to you. If you're like most overweight people (including the old me), these feelings probably cause you to seek solace in food. This is a vicious cycle, and to break out of it you must come to realize that one of the primary causes of your pain is the fact that you often say "yes" to yourself and others when you should be saying "no."*

What am I talking about? I want you to stand up, take responsibility and learn to say no. I want you to say no when you are tempted to deviate from your plan. Say no when you find yourself listening to someone who is trying to pull you off course or belittle your efforts. Say no to thinking you're not good enough. Say no to believing

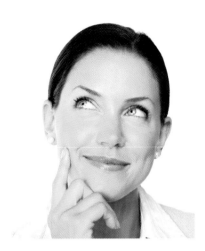

the best is behind you. Instead, I want you to say a big YES! to knowing that a better life lies ahead, that you were created perfectly and that you are destined for great things that only you can achieve. If you don't change your personality habits, your life may change for a while but you'll eventually revert to your old ways (and your old weight!) because you won't find the happiness you're looking for – a happiness that can only be found once you accept and love who you are. Now is the time to take these simple STOP measures to correct the imbalance and restore yourself to a centered place where you can be your best!

### 1 STOP the guilt habit

All day long, whether you're walking through a store, sitting in your cubicle or driving to and from work, you are in constant dialogue with yourself. Most of the time you aren't even aware of these voices in your head, but they are playing a large role in determining your emotions. Thoughts of guilt, learned early on, or hyper-responsibility for others' happiness can force you into the trap of putting your own needs low on your priority list, which ends up making you feel like a victim of life. I

want you to make a conscious effort to pay more attention to these inner voices. The next time they start causing you to feel guilty or anxious, remind yourself of your goals. People who are focused on becoming the best they can be don't have time to indulge in negative self-talk.

### 2 STOP the blame habit

Unless someone was holding a gun to your head, you made the choices that created the life you're currently living. You said yes to countless unhealthy food choices. You said yes to skipping exercise for the umpteenth time. No one made you do either of those things, so stop blaming others and start taking positive action. It's time to harness the power within you and use it to start building a better future. Don't let whatever harmed you earlier in your life continue to harm you now by driving you to overeat and not exercise. Your past will drive you into an early grave – but only if you let it. As the 20th-century Buddhist monk Ajahn Chah said, "If you let go a little, you will have a little peace. If you let go a lot, you will have a lot of peace. If you let go completely, you will have complete peace."

### 3 STOP the habit of avoiding responsibility

Responsibility is power! When you accept responsibility, you achieve an unparalleled power that only you have access to. Once you accept that you are responsible for your actions and their outcomes, your actions take on new meaning. Once you accept that your future is not dictated by what happens to you, and you realize that, instead, you decide your future by how you respond to what happens to you,

then you will see your future is limitless! You will achieve success because you have the power to do so!

### 4 STOP the habit of trying to fit in

How many of us have amazing gifts and abilities but are beaten down by others for being different at an early age? Oh, the things we do to fit in! We try to appear more ordinary, we hide our true greatness from others and we forget that we were created to be perfect in ourselves. By saying that we shouldn't change ourselves to fit in, I'm not implying that being overweight is okay – quite the opposite. In fact, I believe your excess fat is helping you hide from who you really are.

Until you understand that you and you alone are responsible for achieving your potential – not through any short-cut, but instead through hard work, discipline and being yourself – you'll never be truly happy. Only when you learn how to say no to disempowering habits and yes to the things that are going to help you become even more disciplined and focused will you have mastered yourself and set the course for a remarkably fulfilling destiny.

"Once you accept that you are responsible for your actions and their outcomes, your actions take on new meaning."

# CHAPTER FIVE
## Walk Around Like a Rock Star!

> "The human mind may be likened to an electric battery. It may be positive or it may be negative. Self-confidence is the quality with which the mind is recharged and made positive."
>
> – Napoleon Hill, *The Law of Success*

Before you get ready to start my program, you need to learn how to develop outstanding self-confidence. Self-doubt is the one thing that will, without fail, kill your dreams before they are even fully thought out.

Think it's impossible for you to develop huge amounts of self-confidence and achieve your goals? Think again! Times change, and there's no reason you can't change too. Although a huge, deep-rooted oak tree starts out as an acorn, it doesn't look or "act" anything like an acorn as it grows. Tony Robbins often says: "The past doesn't equal the future." Wayne Dyer puts it another way, saying, "The wake of your life is like the wake of a boat. It's nothing more than the trail that's left behind. The wake doesn't drive the boat. The wake is not driving your life." Consider all that is now possible that once wasn't. Items that were once science fiction are now real. Cars are faster than ever and are becoming more and more energy efficient. Imagine what a coal miner of the 1800s would have thought if someone had taken him on a tour of a modern-day nuclear power plant, or explained to him that we can now use energy from the sun and from the ground to provide electricity and heat. Technology is improving and changing at an exponential rate. We can program our appliances to work while we are away; there are high-definition movies and TV; the new version of 3D and incredibly realistic computer graphics that would have excited even Walt Disney. We can even water our real gardens via the Internet. Speaking of the Internet, just the other day I talked with a client via webcam. This client wasn't just in a different state; he was in Israel – all the way across the globe! What do you think people of the 19th century would have thought if you had told them you could both see and talk to someone over 7,000 miles away on a contraption as thick as a small notebook? You would likely have been carted off in a straitjacket and locked up for being insane, and yet here we are in this reality.

Despite all the strides we've made in technology, few people have mastered the one thing that in my opinion makes all the difference to their happiness – their own thinking. Taking control of your emotions so they do not influence your behavior in a negative way is a must. What if Rosa Parks had never stood up and refused to accept the way she was treated because she didn't think herself worthy, or because she was too afraid? When we doubt ourselves, we halt our drive to succeed, in turn creating instant defeat.

I'm sure at some point in your life you have stopped yourself from doing something you wanted to because of fear. At one point fear controlled me. I stopped talking to people and didn't even attempt to socialize because my history was riddled with such painful experiences. I had let fear take charge of my life. It wasn't until I decided I deserved better that everything changed.

To take charge of your weight like I did, and to keep it off long term, you must take control of this and all other destructive emotions. Researchers say that worry (another form of fear) is worse for your body and nervous system than a terrible event actually happening. Because worry creates the chemi-

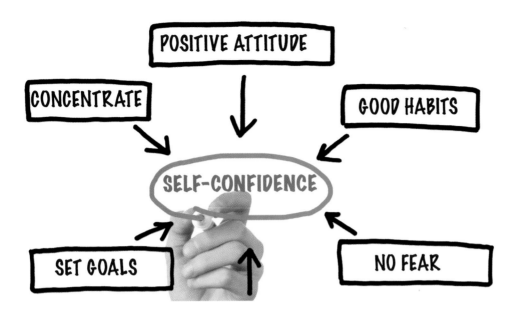

cal thunderstorm fear elicits, each time you worry about something, even though it hasn't happened, you are creating the result in your body over and over again. It's like experiencing a loved one's death, over and over again, even though that person never died! Sometimes we become fearful of what others are going to say if we try another diet or exercise regimen. Maybe we're afraid because we've been criticized for not following through before.

Creating your vision is one thing – putting a plan into action consistently is entirely different and requires you to control your fears. Here I offer to you your contract for unstoppable self-confidence:

## I AGREE:

**1** To realize that the way I think has an impact on my behaviors and in turn on my quality of life. Therefore I admit that I am where I am because of the thoughts I've held consistently and my focus on them. Through this admission, I realize that by shifting my thoughts and focusing on my ability to take charge of my life, I am in complete control of achieving my goals. I will concentrate on maintaining that positive outlook each day, upon waking, at lunch and before bed.

**2** I will write out a vivid, compelling, precise and clear outline of my goals, and I will read them daily – out loud and with confidence! When I go to the bathroom first thing in the morning, I will look in my own eyes and say, "I love you!" because I realize that if I don't love myself, I can't expect others to love me.

**3** I will learn, understand and follow the diet plan Charles outlines in this book or I will find another healthy plan I feel works well for me, a plan that sets out the times I will eat and the food choices I will make at each of those times. I will also follow an exercise routine I enjoy.

**4** I understand that if it's going to be, it's up to me! I will put everything I have into this. No matter how many times I've tried before, this time is different. I will not eat or drink anything that does not agree with the successful quality of life I'm pursuing. I choose to not consume foods or drinks that do not nourish me.

**5** I will keep a positive attitude and make eliminating fear a priority. I will stay on task no matter what the scale reads, or what others say or do. Through my actions, it will be evident that I truly am the person I want to be!

# HABITS

My successful clients and I have all managed to remain confident by developing habits that support our goals. Habits are patterns, and when we form a habit we do so because we've practiced the same "skill" over and over again. At that point, the completion of the action becomes unconscious – we don't have to think about it anymore; we just do it.

> "By gaining control of our emotions, we can see things in a clearer, calmer way and react more rationally to whatever challenges life throws our way."

As a piano player, I can sit and play my favorite songs while talking and laughing with friends. My mind is so locked into the pattern of playing those songs that I don't have to think about playing them. I just play unconsciously. When you begin my program, you have to be willing to establish new habits and patterns. And, yes, this will be challenging at first – no one expects to sit down at the piano the first time and play Rachmaninoff's Concerto No. 3 right off the bat – but with practice it eventually can be done. You may have heard of the "21 Day Habit Theory" developed by Dr. Maxwell Maltz. Dr. Maltz discovered that if you engage in an activity or behavior a few minutes a day for 21 consecutive days, it becomes a habit. And let me assure you, whether it takes 21 days or 200 days, forming new, healthy habits to the point where they just become a part of your personality (and you don't even know you're doing them) is one of the most exciting and invigorating things you can do.

When you start my program or any other, I recommend making the decision to eat the same set of nourishing foods, day in and day out, for at least the first two weeks. Through repetition, you will be training your mind, your taste buds and your body to desire these foods.

(You do have to choose a program that consists of nourishing meals.) Once you have both established these habits and reaped a positive reward (e.g., you've lost weight in those first two weeks and your clothes are loose, people are complimenting you, you're full of energy, you're sleeping better) you will become addicted to the behavior.

Think about how an alcoholic becomes one. Sure there is a genetic component, but would a person with an "alcoholic" gene or family background choose to drink if her first experience was a horrible time that ended with getting her stomach pumped in the emergency room? And if she did try again and the alcohol made her behave in ways that went against her morals and she woke up filled with pain and regret, would she keep drinking? Likely not, because drinking alcohol would have negative and painful associations for her. If, on the other hand, a person spent quality time with his friends, had a great night and met the love of his life the first time he drank alcohol, it's easy to see how this guy could associate good feelings with drinking, even though cognitively

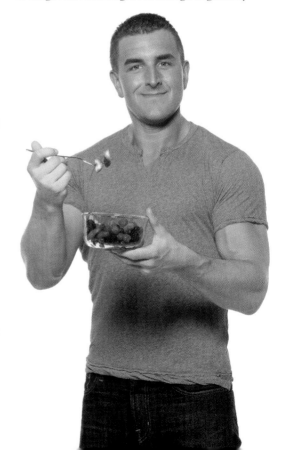

we understand that it was the good times with his friends and not the booze that made the evening fun and enjoyable.

The overweight person can replace "alcohol" with "junk food." If you had negative experiences when you first began eating junk food, you would likely not eat it now. What if your first experience involved watching your parents fight or getting violently ill? If, as is more likely, your first experience eating junk food was a nice time with your family that involved getting a fun new toy, then in your subconscious junk food will continue to be associated with these positive experiences.

To change our habits and thereby gain self-confidence, we have to gain insight into our behaviors and, more importantly, our psychology. Our habits are not always acquired out of desire or out of judgment. Our habits often come about unconsciously because of association, and we react emotionally. By gaining control of our emotions, we can see things in a clearer, calmer way and react more rationally to whatever challenges life throws our way. By the way, I always recommend enlisting a counselor or psychologist who can help you see things in a way you may not have seen them before, if you are in a position to do so. A counselor can also provide you with a positive outlook when you do get caught up in a slump.

Self-confidence comes from a true understanding of yourself. You realize that while you're not perfect, no one is! You recognize what you know and don't know, and then you find out how you are going to gain the

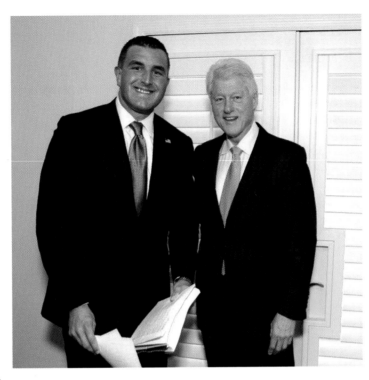

◄ SHARING MY STORY (AND A COPY OF THIS MANUSCRIPT) WITH A MAN I TRULY RESPECT, PRESIDENT CLINTON.

"President Clinton walks into a room and he owns it. He makes every individual feel important. He smiles, offers compliments and listens intently while making eye contact."

knowledge to get what you're after. Think of a confident person you admire. Close your eyes and visualize how that person walks, sounds, dresses, stands and moves. I bet you picture that person striding into a room with purpose, head held high, back straight, shoulders broad, his or her eyes meeting the eyes of those already in the room. When I think of a confident person, the first person that comes to mind is former US President Bill Clinton. One of my goals after losing weight was to meet him and share my story. I finally had the unique privilege of doing just that. President Clinton walks into a room and he owns it. He makes every individual feel important. He smiles, offers compliments and listens intently while making eye contact. You might think,

"Well of course Clinton's got confidence, he was the president. If I was that successful, I'd have confidence too!" But this thinking is backward. Clinton wasn't always the president. He was able to become the president in part because he had confidence. The truth is, you are what you think you are. Or as Buddha put it, "All that we are is the result of what we have thought. The mind is everything. What we think, we become."

One of the most important things you can do is get serious and start expecting more from

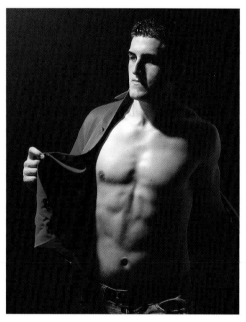

"While others are out eating fattening foods and drinking, I'm at the gym, knowing that I am going the extra mile and will reap the reward for my sacrifice."

yourself than anyone else expects of you. While others are out eating fattening foods and drinking, I'm at the gym, knowing that I am going the extra mile and will reap the reward for my sacrifice.

If you look at yourself as just average or, worse, below average, you will go about your life in such a way that supports this belief. Why would you work hard if you don't think your efforts will pay off? When you have a belief, your brain goes to work to support that belief, whether positive or negative. As Napoleon Hill put it, "There are millions of people who believe themselves 'doomed' to poverty and failure, because of some strange force over which they believe they have no control. They are the creators of their own 'misfortunes' because of their negative belief, which is picked up by subconscious mind and translated into its physical equivalent."

If you believe the economy is terrible, you'll find support for that belief. Everywhere you look you will see the unemployed, you'll see red arrows pointing down, you'll see businesses closing down and people losing their houses. But even in the worst economic times people are thriving and businesses are booming. Even a terrible unemployment rate of 15 percent means 85 percent of people are working. This is not making light of those who are struggling, but it demonstrates how easy it is for your mind to get cluttered when you don't control and direct it. If you choose to focus on how you always mess up or how you never follow through, your brain will go to work to find past experiences that support that belief. And because your brain wants to substantiate its beliefs, it will try to make you behave in ways that prove its case. In other words, you will sabotage yourself without even knowing you are doing so because you're not taking control of your subconscious. Stop allowing your subconscious to choose what you focus on! Take control! Choose to focus on good things about yourself and your confidence can be as high as President Clinton's.

The first step to becoming a success, in weight loss or in any other area, is to realize just how unique and special you are, and expect more from yourself than anyone else could dream. Know that you are so much more than you are allowing yourself to be.

With that outlook, you'll start to talk to yourself in a much more positive way and behave in a way that supports your goals instead of sabotaging them!

Self-confidence brings success, not the other way around. And the path to success in any area is the same as in any other area – the same rules apply. If you wanted to be a successful guitarist, for example, you would go through these steps:

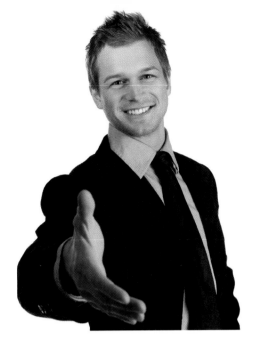

**1** **Consider your goal.** To play guitar well. This goal is more powerful if you choose a specific advanced piece of music as your benchmark.

**2** **Break this goal into smaller units.** This week you will learn the strings, their names, the sound they make, how to tune the guitar, and possibly the scales. Next week you might learn some easy chords. The week after you might learn a song that contains two or three simple chords.

**3** **Make practicing part of your life.** If you "forget" to practice or make excuses to avoid practicing, then you will not achieve the goal of playing the piece of music you'd like to play. This is your brain trying to convince you to behave in a way that supports failure. According to Malcolm Gladwell and accepted the world over, the magic number to become an expert at anything is 10,000 hours. No matter what a person's natural ability is in a given area, if that person spends 10,000 hours working toward it, he or she becomes an expert. The world's greatest violinists, for example, are often spoken of as if they were born with this greatness, but studies show that they have each played for more than 10,000 hours. Violinists who have played for 5,000 hours are considered good, regardless of their natural ability. In his book, *The Tipping Point*, Malcolm Gladwell hypothesizes that famous musicians were able to magnify their gifts through countless hours of practicing and

performing the same songs, hour after hour, long before they ever became famous. So knowing that, ask yourself: "How many hours have I put into practicing healthy living and weight loss?"

## "Self-confidence brings success, not the other way around."

**4** **Stay focused.** If one day you decide to learn guitar, the next day you decide to learn piano and the next you start learning saxophone, you'll end up playing none of these instruments. You may be able to learn all of them over time, but first you will have to focus on one to learn it well.

**5** **Have confidence in your ability.** If you go to each lesson/practice session saying, "I'll never be able to do this," then you never will. If you approach each session with the confidence that you will succeed, then you will, no matter the setbacks. As Henry Ford said, "If you think you can do a thing or think you can't do a thing, you're right."

If you take a good look at these steps, you will see that they apply to any area of your life that you want to improve. Want to earn a better income or have a nest egg to fall back on? Make a goal, figure out the steps you need to get there, carry out these steps every day without getting distracted from your goal and approach it from the start with the confidence that it's already waiting for you!

The simple notion that your goal occurred to you should be proof enough that you deserve it and it's searching for you. Act as if you're already in possession of what you want. This will naturally cause you to do the things that are in alignment with your goal. Want to lose weight? You guessed it. You need to start to act as if you are already in shape. What does that mean, you ask? Eat healthy foods and get off your butt and move! As Tony Robbins has said, "The person who uses the word 'but' all of the time usually has a big one!" You have to believe in order to achieve.

# THE IMPORTANCE OF SELF-CONFIDENCE

Self-confidence is a big problem for those who are overweight, and the more overweight you are the less likely you are to feel confident. It's a vicious spiral, spinning downward faster than you can say McNugget. You gain weight and feel bad about yourself, so you hide away, overeating and avoiding people, and thus gain more weight, so you hide yourself away more, becoming increasingly miserable with each additional pound!

To lose weight, you have to get yourself out of this downward spiral. To do this successfully, you need to develop enough self-confidence to break out of this pattern. So, how do you start? Here's the first step in gaining self-confidence:

Fake it until you make it!

That's right. Think back to all of those confident people you've encountered throughout your life. Want to know a secret? Most of them were probably faking it! For example, most people are terrified of giving speeches or en-gaging in other types of public speaking. They appear confident in that ability because they fake it. But here's the funny thing: The more they fake it, the more confident they become – and not just in the area of public speaking, but in life in general. So, what you need to do is let the world know that you believe in yourself, not by telling them what you're capable of, but by showing them! Here's how:

1 **Perfect posture.** People who are hunched over look like they're trying to protect themselves from the harsh blows of the world; they don't look like they're facing the world head-on. If possible, get someone to take a video of you walking the way you normally do. Note the position of your head and shoulders in particular. Keep your head in line with your spine, keep your shoulders back and yet relaxed and hold your stomach in. Don't look down, but rather ahead of you. Changing your physiology will change your emotions. When you feel depressed, where are you typically looking? Down, of course. Start looking up, not only philosophically, but also physically!

2 **Stride!** Those with self-confidence walk with energy and purpose. Those without confidence walk meekly, slowly, quietly and painfully. They walk like they don't want to be noticed, which is probably true (but it's not what confident people do!). Walk as if you want to be seen, even if you don't.

3 **Dress appropriately.** You may not be able to wear the clothes you really want to at this point, but please don't walk around in sweats and other baggy, shapeless articles of clothing. People often think they look smaller if they wear baggy clothes, but this is not true – they look larger. More importantly, baggy sweats give the impression that you just don't care about how you look – and that screams lack of self-confidence. Conversely, don't wear a size 14 if in reality you wear a size 18. Wearing clothing that doesn't fit you might make you feel better when you look at the tag,

but the resulting bulges make you look fatter, and just … well, worse. Find a few good pieces of clothing in sizes that fit you. If you are too big to find clothing that fits, get a couple of items tailor made. If you feel embarrassed to do this, then use that feeling to spur you on to greater success. Tell yourself: "This is the last time I will ever buy clothing in this size. Next time I buy clothes they will be two sizes smaller because I will have lost that much weight."

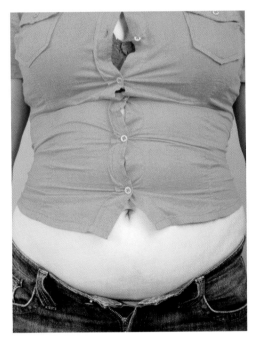

**4** **Exercise.** Yes, exercise contributes to weight loss, but exercise also contributes to feelings of self-confidence, as long as you don't go in expecting too much too soon. First, exercise produces endorphins, otherwise known as the feel-good hormones. Second, as long as you start exercising at an appropriate level for you and gradually increase the intensity, then every time you exercise you will accomplish more and more, which will make you feel very good indeed! Third, every time you exercise you know you are doing something that brings you closer to your goal, and that makes you feel great about yourself.

**5** **Get out of yourself.** Ironically, truly self-confident people are not obsessed with themselves. They don't need to spend all that time thinking about themselves, because they aren't all that worried about what other people think of them. Instead, they spend their time accomplishing things and helping others. As Napoleon Hill said, "It is literally true that

## "Don't wear a size 14 if in reality you wear a size 18. Wearing clothing that doesn't fit you might make you feel better when you look at the tag, but the resulting bulges make you look fatter, and just … well, worse."

you can succeed best and quickest by helping others to succeed." Look at the people around you. Help them feel good about themselves. Stop complaining. Complaining about things, along with belittling others, gossiping and other negative behavior all stem from a lack of self-confidence. Egomaniacs are often hounded by the thing they fear most: criticism. We attract what we focus on. If you keep thinking you will never keep your weight down, pretty soon you'll be doing the very things that will make that fear a reality. Guard your mind and stay focused on helping others. It works!

**6** **Stop hiding.** This can be a tough habit to break. If you don't feel good about yourself, chances are you hide in many ways: you wear baggy clothes, you walk with bad posture, you look at the ground. You may not go to events you would like to because you don't want to be seen or because you will feel uncomfortable around others who are not overweight. You might not want to go the beach with friends, for example, because you think they'll look good and you won't, and you assume that you'll be too uncomfortable to enjoy yourself. But confident people get out there. They go where they want to go and do the things they want to do, and you have to do this too because it's what makes life worth living. Hiding is another form of wallowing in your misery, and just as sitting there thinking about how miserable you feel makes you feel more

> "When I decided to transform my life, the biggest change I made was in my confidence. I decided to have some."

miserable, hiding away because you're overweight makes you gain more weight. You eat more, binge more, do less physical activity and think depressing thoughts, which can cause you to eat to make yourself feel better. Once you start taking part in enjoyable activities instead of hiding away, you'll feel good! Your confidence will grow and your weight will decrease. Just like you have to fake confidence until you feel it, you have to make yourself get out there, smile and have fun even if you're telling yourself you'd rather stay home and watch TV.

If you doubt the difference a little confidence makes, think about Kenan Thompson, Zach Galifianakis, Elizabeth Taylor, Roseanne Barr, John Goodman, Queen Latifah, Aretha Franklin and even Anna Nicole Smith. Large? Yes. Confident? You'd better believe it! Now picture the same people in baggy sweats, slumped over, looking at the ground, shuffling as they walk and mumbling when they speak. All of a sudden they don't look, sound or act like stars anymore, do they? Now, maybe some of these people have made a choice to stay overweight and some have gone up and down on the scale, but their charisma comes from their confidence, their focus on their own unique good qualities and from their belief in themselves and what they want to accomplish. Did you know that Marilyn Monroe (whose own weight went up and down considerably) would choose whether or not people paid attention to her? If she wanted to be recognized she would stand tall and stride confidently, and throngs of people would surround her asking for her autograph. If she wanted to be left alone she would look to the ground, hunch her body inwards and shuffle along, and no one would even recognize her! If people ignored Marilyn Monroe because she didn't look confident, imagine what happens with the rest of us?

When I decided to transform my life, the biggest change I made was in my confidence. I decided to have some. I decided I would be popular, and not because of how great I looked, but because I believed I looked great. I would walk around with a smile, knowing with complete conviction that I was in control of my destiny. No other person's thoughts could negatively affect me unless I allowed them to by accepting their limiting beliefs. I decided that my decisions would determine how far I go in life and how much I would contribute. Only after I stopped blaming other people for my unhappiness and lack of confidence could I take credit for all the wonderful things I've been blessed to achieve and contribute. When you take the responsibility for your future, your actions and your happiness, then your confidence can truly shine.

▼ TIMES SQUARE, NYC

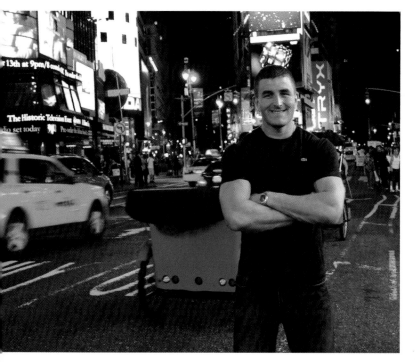

## "I neglected the most important person — myself."

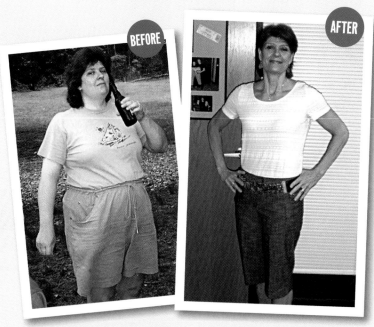

BEFORE

AFTER

**NAME: Sandy Crancer**
**AGE: 51**
**HEIGHT: 5'6"**
**WEIGHT BEFORE: 240 lbs**
**WEIGHT AFTER: 147 lbs**
**WEIGHT LOSS: 93 lbs**

**AFTER TWO PREGNANCIES, DUR-ING THE SECOND OF WHICH HER WEIGHT ESCALATED TO ITS PEAK OF 240 POUNDS, SANDY CRANCER SUFFERED FROM A SEVERE CASE OF MOMMY TUMMY.** And she is the first to admit that the combination of an unhealthy diet, lack of exercise and poor self-care is what got her there. As she explains, "I was always taking care of my family and I neglected the most important person – myself." Although Sandy was lucky enough to have not suffered from any serious weight-related health issues, she was always tired and was experiencing constant back pain. She also couldn't indulge in her passion for fashion because shopping for stylish clothes that fit became a depressing exercise in self-loathing.

It was the relentless lethargy that final-ly prompted Sandy to seek change. She had tried fad diets in the past, but nothing ever stuck. She would find

herself losing 20 to 25 pounds and then gaining back all of the weight she had lost – and then some. One of her biggest obstacles was her skewed perception of the relationship between diet and exercise. "I would change my eating habits but didn't exercise," Sandy says. "Then I would exercise and eat whatever I wanted."

It was Charles D'Angelo who was able to finally help Sandy change her perspective by getting her to realize that exercising and practic-ing good nutrition – simultaneously – are necessary to create a slim and healthy physique. Charles also made it very clear that he expected Sandy to stick to the plan. Accountability for her actions was key to her success. And what a success! Sandy was able to drop an incredible 93 pounds and now wears a slim size 6. Her back pain has disappeared and her energy levels have gone through the roof. With her newfound spark for

life, Sandy is motivated to exercise every day. She has even discovered that she prefers the taste of nutritious foods to their processed, junky coun-terparts. Sandy fully believes that "there is nothing that tastes as good as thin feels," and this keeps her focused on maintaining her healthy lifestyle. Sandy can also enjoy shop-ping again and has filled her closet with the latest fashions. She says, "I don't have to hang my clothes to dry in fear they will shrink."

*"Sandy fully believes that there is nothing that tastes as good as thin feels."*

Sandy stays on track with Charles' continued support. She says his no-nonsense attitude is exactly what she needs. In fact, she believes she would not have been able to achieve her remarkable weight-loss results without Charles' help. "Over my adult life nothing has worked," Sandy says, "Charles' program is the best I have ever done and it really works!"

# MENTAL DIETING
## Unlocking the Power of Positivity

*You've committed to the* **Think and Grow Thin** *program, you've gone shopping for all the right foods and you've bought a treadmill or joined the gym, but you still have to go out and face the world each day, and you're taking "you" with you wherever you go. As I've demonstrated throughout this book, success is more mindset than mechanics. In order for the physical diet and exercise program to work, you need to go on a mental diet. Take the following steps to get your head where it needs to be:*

### 1 Surround yourself with positive peers.

One reason many people fall back into old habits is that their peer group remains the same. Some people can be as toxic as drinking a bottle of bleach! Avoid those who are negative, critical or cynical – not just of you, but also of others. If you surround yourself with negative people, your worldview will likely conform to theirs. Don't let your dreams be restricted by others' lack of faith. Choose a peer group filled with people who inspire you, promote healthy habits and enjoy living well. Sometimes out of fear of loneliness, we allow anyone who shows the slightest bit of affection or attention into our lives. This is not healthy. Choose your close friends wisely. They have a tremendous impact on your mindset, which ultimately affects your ability to tap into your potential.

### 2 Replace any negative thought immediately.

When any thought of doubt, inability or full-out pessimism pops into your mind, force yourself to balance it out with at least two positive revisions of that thought. For example, if you find yourself thinking, "Why do I have to walk 35 minutes on the treadmill again tonight?" change it to this thought: "How can I make walking on the treadmill the

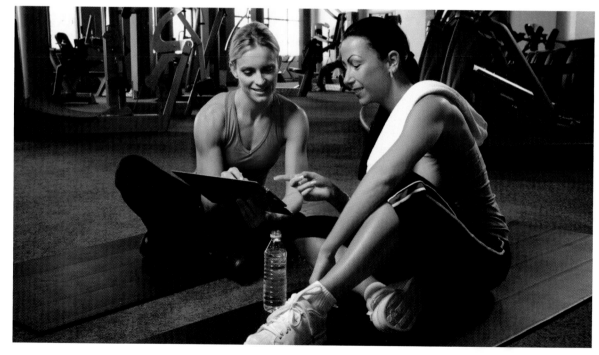

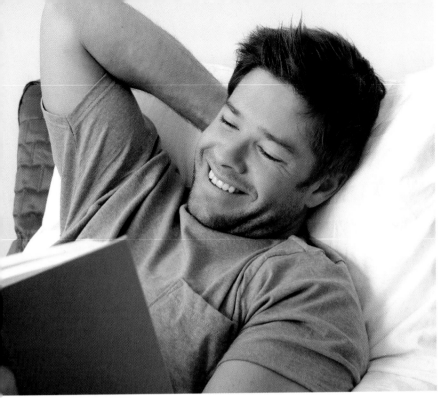

## 5 Make reading positive literature a habit.

As you must feed and exercise your body, you must do the same with your mind. Pick up books by Anthony Robbins, Wayne Dyer, Napoleon Hill, Jack Canfield and other motivational writers, or pick up the autobiography or biography of someone you admire and spend an intimate afternoon "with" them. The cool thing about books is you can have a conversation with someone you've never met, just as we are doing now, and it will change you in positive, life-enriching ways. You can learn valuable lessons about how your heroes and role models overcame obstacles to build happy, fulfilled and successful lives for themselves. Books can be worth their weight in gold several times over!

most enjoyable part of my day?" You will have to force this change to begin with, but it will get easier and easier until eventually you do it by nature. As Tony Robbins and many other motivational masters have said, repetition is the mother of skill.

## 3 Tune out the negativity in the world.

The media feeds off of bad news, and the more sensational it is the better. Tragedy, war, murder, corruption – they all attract more viewers and ultimately increase advertising dollars for TV stations, websites and newspapers. Instead of tuning into a day's worth of bad news before you put your head down on the pillow, try reading something positive instead (See #5 on this list!). You may have to force yourself to do it at first, but you will soon look forward to this nightly ritual. Everything around us is energy, even the news we watch. Choose to watch things that reinforce your new positive outlook. I'm not saying you should pretend there's

no bad in the world; I'm simply saying not to invite it into your life constantly. We choose our realities. Make yours one you've dreamed about today!

## 4 Choose to follow the adage: "If you don't have anything nice to say, don't say anything at all."

We must be the change we want to see in the world, as Gandhi said. By choosing not to even engage in negative talk externally, our internal dialogue shifts as well. The more we focus on stating only the positive things, the more we start noticing and experiencing them in our lives.

## 6 Listen to Mozart.

Classical music is divinely inspired. Simply listening to these masterpieces can free your imagination, providing you with a distraction from eating. A 2010 study showed that listening to classical music can decrease tension and increase feelings of relaxation and calmness.[1]

---

1. Christopher Rea et al. "Listening to Classical, Pop, and Metal Music: An Investigation of Mood." *Empora State Research Studies*, 46 (1), 1-3. 2010.

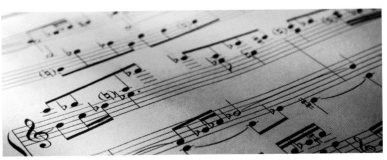

# CHAPTER SIX
## Taking Control of Yourself
### (the one thing you can control!)

"The secret to success is constancy of purpose."

– Benjamin Disraeli

So you've made the decision to change your life. You bought this book. You've chosen a healthy diet. You've joined a gym. You've written your goals out, made your dream board and practiced your self-confidence. That's all amazing and important. But now comes the hard part – carrying it through. Dreams and goals are all well and good, but if you're not willing to take the steps necessary to reach them, you'll be dreaming forever. In other

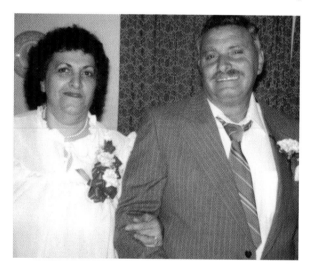

► MY GRANDPARENTS, ROSE AND CHARLIE

words, you need to find the initiative to do what you've got to do in order to get what you want. No matter how enthusiastic you are, you must learn how to direct and control your efforts consistently to achieve those things you've decided on. Controlling your focus and directing it in a balanced way is crucial not only to losing your excess weight, but also to keeping it off.

The will to achieve can be defined as: "The mental faculty by which one deliberately chooses or decides upon a course of action." Deciding isn't enough, though. You must maintain your focus despite the challenges that are certain to arise throughout your journey to getting the body you deserve.

A strong will can make a person succeed when all signals point to failure. I learned this early on in my life. My grandfather wasn't given the privilege of going to school. His father, the sole breadwinner of the family, died of a heart attack when my grandfather was very young. This meant my grandfather and all his brothers had to go to work to support the family, although they were still children. They did a variety of odd jobs and piecemeal work – anything to bring in a little money. Lacking education and learning to associate pleasure with the mere idea of being able to eat, my grandfather's brain quickly associated food with luxury.

My grandfather grew up and married my grandmother, whose father had had a stroke while she was in high school, and so she too had had to go to work without finishing her education. Together they had four sons, including my father. My grandparents successfully made ends meet because they had to. It's true that they didn't have the education to teach my father or his brothers the importance of choosing healthy foods, but they did survive despite the odds against them. This is because they had the will to survive and care for their children. This will was highly emotionalized and, despite their difficulties, they achieved their goals because they kept a constant focus. They never accepted their circumstances and always found a way to provide, no matter what. That need was in their mind at all times.

To succeed, you need to turn your goal into such a burning desire that it is on the same level of your other needs, like shelter and water. In pursuit of your goal, you must never accept less than your best, and you can never convince yourself that not trying hard enough is okay.

Terry Fox is a shining example of this. In 1977 at the age of 18, he was diagnosed with bone cancer. His leg was amputated above the knee. The night before his amputation, he decided he would run about 5,000 miles across Canada to raise money for cancer research. These days we hear about all kinds of people running or biking across countries to raise funds and awareness for a cause, but just two-and-a-half years after his leg amputation Terry Fox was the one who started it all.

People train for months or even years to run one marathon and consider it a big achievement – which it is. But during his "Marathon of Hope," Terry Fox, on one leg and with a heart condition, ran a marathon every single day until cancer struck him down again after he had completed 143 days and 3,339 miles of his journey. One marathon in a lifetime is a lot for an able-bodied person, and yet here was a young man with only one leg and a heart condition who ran close to 143 marathons over as many days. How could he possibly have done it? He did it with will.

## "A strong will can make a person succeed when all signals point to failure."

Terry had shown early on that he had a strong will. In junior high school he was an average-sized, mediocre basketball player who barely made the team, but he was determined to play guard. He didn't lie in bed wishing he could play; he practiced every single day, getting better and better. He became a starting guard a couple of years later and by senior year he was chosen athlete of the year.

Terry's success was not accidental, nor did it come easily to him. He succeeded because every day he did what he had to do to reach his goal. His dream didn't get him where he wanted to be. To get there, he needed the Discipline to practice, the Willpower to practice even if he didn't feel like it, the Consistency to practice regularly rather than in fits and starts

## "Terry Fox was an extraordinary person, but in ability he was utterly ordinary. His exceptional achievements came from his own will and determination, not from any special ability on his part."

or simply whenever he felt like it, and the Focus to keep his eye on his goal – not just for days, weeks or even months, but for years.

He used the same four important traits to get him across those 3,339 miles. First he had the dream – some might say a crazy dream – of running 5,000 miles across the country on one leg. Then he spent 18 months training consistently and with great discipline. Then he dipped his artificial toe in the Atlantic Ocean and set out on the first of his daily marathons. Every day, his foot was covered in blisters and his stump in painful, bleeding cysts. We can only imagine the willpower it took for him to wake up every morning, put on his artificial leg, tie up his shoe and hit the pavement. And then run an entire marathon. Imagine the focus he must have had to tune out the pain and complete the task he had set for himself. In fact, he was so focused on achieving his goal that he said when he was running he felt good, not bad.

Terry Fox's goal was to raise $24 million for cancer research by the time he crossed Canada. Even though he was forced to finish just past the halfway point, the donations kept coming in and Terry raised just over $24 million. The annual Terry Fox runs that take place in his name across the world each year have now raised more than $500 million.

Sure, Terry Fox was an extraordinary person, but in ability he was utterly ordinary. His exceptional achievements came from his own will and determination, not from any special ability on his part. As iconic coach Vince Lombardi once said, "The difference between a successful person and others is not a lack of strength, not a lack of knowledge, but rather a lack of will."

# DISCIPLINE

No question, it takes discipline to go out with friends and stick to your salad and grilled chicken breast when they are all drinking margaritas and eating nachos. It takes discipline to get up and go to the gym on a cold winter morning when you're snuggled under a comforter beside your significant other or favorite pet. But if you want to accomplish your goal of losing weight, then you can't choose when you will and when you won't follow your plan. Your burning desire has to be so great it gets you out of bed in the morning. Knowing that each and every day filled with good decisions

> "If you were to rate your self-discipline on a scale of 1 to 10, where would you put yourself? If you are near the low end, we have work to do! If you are closer to mid-range, congratulations, but to succeed you'll have to move higher up the scale."

is getting you closer and closer to your goal has to be so compelling that, time after time, doing what's right is second nature. Debating with yourself over whether or not to do what's right will leave you struggling with your weight forever, zapping your self-esteem because as soon as you start making progress you will

backslide. If you want to climb a mountain you have to keep moving upward. If you keep having to climb the same 100 feet over and over again you're never going to reach the pinnacle.

Discipline, or self-control, helps you take the actions necessary to accomplish your goals, even though you would rather do something else. For example, instead of staying up to watch a late movie and being too tired to make it to the gym in the morning, you use your self-discipline to turn off the TV and go to sleep at a decent hour. At its core, discipline is maturity. A baby has no self-control. If he wants something, he cries to get it and cries louder if he can't have it. Through the toddler years, a child slowly learns that by waiting he might get more than he would otherwise.

Walter Mischel's marshmallow experiment is a perfect illustration of this. In the late 1960s Mischel, a Stanford psychology professor, conducted a delayed gratification experiment involving four-year-olds. Each child would be put in a room with a marshmallow. A researcher would tell them that if they wanted one marshmallow they could eat it right away, but if they wanted two they would have to wait while he stepped out of the room for a few minutes. The results varied greatly and were often humorous – some children ate the marshmallow immediately while others tried valiantly to wait till the end – but things really started to get interesting as Mischel kept track of these children throughout their lives. He discovered that those who were able to delay gratification and wait for the two marshmallows experienced greater success throughout their entire lives. How much success? On average, the child who could wait 15 minutes had an SAT score that was 210 points higher than the child who could only wait 30 seconds! In fact, more than any other predictor including family income, the longer the child waited for the two marshmallows the more successful he/she was in all areas of life.

As we get older, we get better and better at

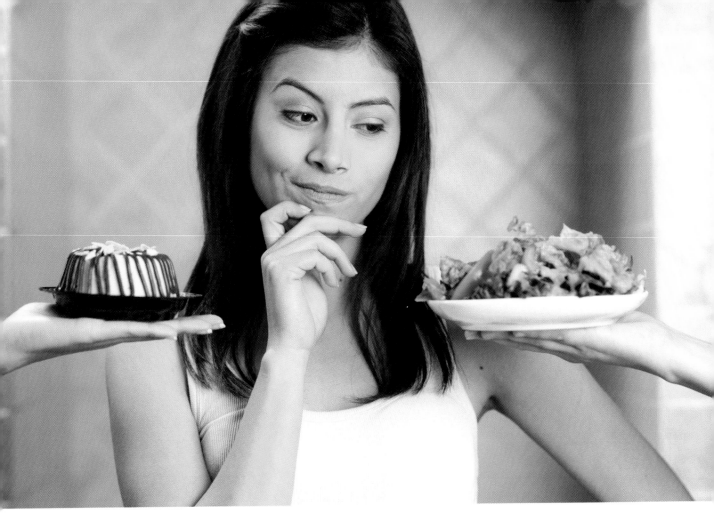

either waiting for what we want, working for what we want or giving up something we want right now in order to get something better later on. Some of us, however, are better at this than others, and these are the ones with the discipline it takes to succeed. If you were to rate your self-discipline on a scale of 1 to 10, where would you put yourself? If you are near the low end, we have work to do! If you are closer to mid-range, congratulations, but to succeed you'll have to move higher up the scale.

Residing at the bottom of this scale normally goes hand in hand with the belief that your circumstances are beyond your control. You believe success comes because of a person's genes or background or because of luck. The further up the self-discipline scale you go the more you are likely to believe in your own ability to determine your success. To succeed, you need discipline. To be disciplined, you must

have faith – not only in the program or person who is helping you to lose weight, but also faith in yourself. As William James, the father of American psychology, said, "The greatest discovery of the 19th century was not in the realm of physical sciences, but the power of the subconscious mind touched by faith. Any individual can tap into an eternal reservoir of power that will enable them to overcome any problem that may arise. All weaknesses can be overcome, bodily healing, financial independence, spiritual awakening, prosperity beyond your wildest dreams. This is the superstructure of happiness."

You do not become healthy by fighting obesity or by fighting the state of being fat, but rather by raising your consciousness and choosing to embrace a healthy lifestyle plan. You will not succeed with a diet plan that fights being fat; you will succeed with a lifestyle plan that pro-

▲ EVENTUALLY, MAKING THE RIGHT CHOICE WILL BECOME SECOND NATURE.

> **"Start to take charge of your life by making conscious decisions each day. Count on yourself more. Stop relying on others to make the change for you. After all, no one can change you but you!"**

motes wellness. In other words, change comes from focusing on a positive solution, not by combating negativity. There is nothing to fight, simply something positive to embrace.

Nothing external has caused you to be overweight. You have made a long series of decisions that have given you the result: the body you now live in. It's time to not only change the way you eat and move, but to change the way you think! You must take responsibility for your result. This book cannot change you. It can influence you in a great way but, ultimately, when you finish reading the final page, it's up to you to make the changes I'm suggesting. Responsible people know that if their life is falling apart, they need to take action. This means they know they can have a positive impact on their own life. It's not what happens to us, it's what we do with what happens that dictates our future.

Some people think mysterious mystical forces have predetermined their fate and they are destined to be overweight and unhappy for one reason or another. These people are forever "the victim." They push people away – even people who would be great assets in their lives – because of their self-pity and misery. They envy others who are successful rather than working toward that success themselves. Because of their negative attitudes they tune into a negative frequency, attracting more and more experiences to support their belief that life is terrible

and they are unlucky. They get so caught up in their moaning that they miss all kinds of opportunities to change and instead get stuck in a place they hate. Some of these people stay in that wretched place their entire lives, never fully understanding they have the key and can escape that prison.

Many overweight people are caught in that pattern. The trick is to break it. You must change your blueprint. Start to take charge of your life by making conscious decisions each day. Count on yourself more. Stop relying on others to make the change for you. After all, no one can change you but you! Going off your program doesn't hurt your trainer. Her butt doesn't get any wider – yours does! Your coach won't develop diabetes if you choose to eat foods loaded with preservatives and soaked in sugar and syrup – you will!

Little things build upon one another to create something great. When I was a kid I enjoyed playing with Lego. When you look at Lego blocks as an adult, you see how tiny each one is. But when put together in the right order and sequence, they can build massive towers, bridges, animals … practically anything in the builder's imagination. The one piece is pretty much useless, but when a person puts the pieces together, a wonderful creation is built. The same is true for you. Every morsel of nutritious food you put in your mouth, every step you take, every day, is a step in the right direction, even if it is not perfect. With each day, you get better and better. After a few months your food and exercise plans will be second nature.

When you find your discipline waning, you have to ask yourself which is more important, having that order of fries right now or losing your excess weight for good? Is it more important to sit on your rear watching TV feeling lazy or is it more important to accomplish your goal of toning up your flabby arms? Where do you really want to be in a year? It might help to picture that little angel and devil on your

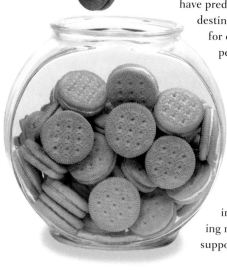

▼ WHAT'S MORE IMPORTANT: ONE LITTLE COOKIE OR LOSING THE WEIGHT FOR GOOD?

shoulders. The devil will tell you whatever he thinks will convince you to do what he wants. He'll be very convincing: "You've followed your eating plan for four days straight. One little cookie won't mess things up." "You've already worked out three times this week. Missing one workout won't matter. You can work out extra hard tomorrow to make up for it." Sounds familiar, doesn't it? After all, you've trained yourself to think that way for a long time! You'll have to tune out that devil and listen to the angel on your shoulder who's telling you to get your butt to the gym if you want to reach

**"You need discipline to go to the gym; you need willpower to not sit in front of the TV. You need discipline to eat the salad and grilled chicken, you need willpower to not eat nachos and drink margaritas."**

the mountaintop instead of slipping back down. Remember the marshmallow test! You're being a more mature person by giving up what you want now (to be lazy and sit in front of the TV) for what you really want but have to both wait and work for (a fabulous body, long-term health, energy).

Some of us were never taught that our decisions mattered. When I was growing up I often changed my mind in restaurants. I would see so many delicious, unhealthy options that I would want them all at once. If I ordered spaghetti and meatballs, for example, and my sister's order of a bacon cheeseburger and onion rings came out first I would think hers looked so good that I'd change my mind and try to switch my order. That kind of behavior is childish, of course. We must make decisions and learn to live with them. Although our parents

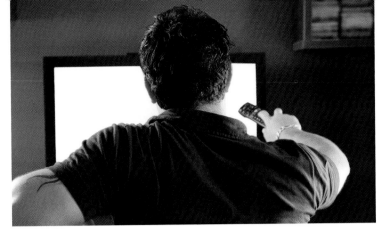

▲ THE ANGEL ON HIS SHOULDER IS SCREAMING, "GET OFF THE COUCH!"

may have meant well, allowing us to change our minds so quickly didn't teach us much about living with the choices we've made.

As Albus Dumbledore said in *Harry Potter and the Chamber of Secrets*, "It is our choices, Harry, that show what we truly are, far more than our abilities." I'm sure you've made some choices you wish you could go back and change, such as the eating and exercise habits that brought you to the point you are now. You are fortunate that this book has come along. As far as your health and body are concerned, it's almost never too late to change things.

God is willing to give you a second, fifth, sixth, or even hundredth shot at changing, but you have to make the decision and use your will to stick to it.

## WILLPOWER

Willpower can be defined as the strength of will to resist barriers to carrying out one's decisions, wishes or plans. This sounds a lot like discipline, and indeed the two are closely related. You could say willpower and discipline are like yin and yang – the balance that equals success. Whereas you need discipline to do what you need to do in order to succeed, you need willpower to not do the things you can't do if you want to succeed. You need discipline to go to the gym; you need willpower to not sit in front of the TV. You need discipline to eat the salad and grilled chicken, you need willpower to not eat nachos and drink margaritas.

But willpower is more than that, too. Will-

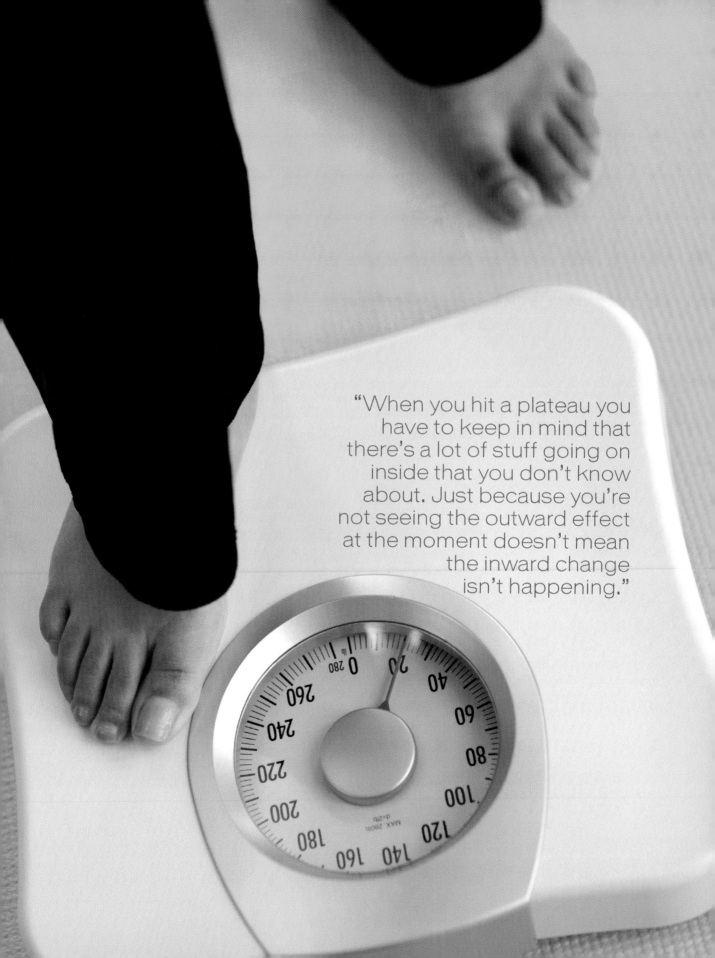

"When you hit a plateau you have to keep in mind that there's a lot of stuff going on inside that you don't know about. Just because you're not seeing the outward effect at the moment doesn't mean the inward change isn't happening."

power is what makes you continue when you feel like giving up, and this is really important when you have difficult times during your weight loss, which you inevitably will, such as the most difficult time of all – the plateau.

Nothing is worse than when you're sticking to your plan, eating exactly as you should, not sneaking any food at all, training with gusto, feeling like a million bucks and then stepping on the scale to find – surprise! – you've gained a pound. What?! How could that happen?

The body is a very complex machine, and we all sometimes experience situations that just don't seem to make sense. When you hit a plateau you have to keep in mind that there's a lot of stuff going on inside that you don't know about. Just because you're not seeing the outward effect at the moment doesn't mean the inward change isn't happening. In fact, normally when people make their way through a tough plateau they'll find that after a few weeks of no weight loss (or even a little weight gain) they'll step on the scale one day and find they've suddenly lost five or six pounds for no apparent reason. While it may not be apparent, the reason for the sudden weight loss is that they stuck it out through the plateau and stayed with the program even though they couldn't see the outward results. And how did they manage to do that? With willpower.

When I was just 17, I decided to change. I had a plan consisting of healthy foods, and I was ready. Unfortunately, my parents had heard that before. To say the least, they were not excited about my new "plan." In fact, I had to save up for my own groceries since most people in my family didn't think I would stick to it. Talk about frustration! I wanted to make the change immediately but had to wait, saving up money from my minimum-wage job until I could buy the healthy food I needed. That would have made a great excuse to prevent me from succeeding if I had not tapped into my willpower.

You cannot expect the world to change be-cause you've changed your eating and exercise habits. When that world and your lifestyle change collide, you will have to prove where your priorities lie. I had to make sacrifices and come up with my own resources to buy a George Foreman Grill, chicken breasts, fresh vegetables and other healthy foods when I was still a high-school student making minimum wage at a part-time job. I had to be very careful with my money. If you are going to be a true success, you too must be willing to do whatever it takes.

# MODIFICATION

Many dieters fail because they have an all-or-nothing attitude. They either stay strictly on their diet at all times and work out in exactly the manner they had planned, or they go completely off the rails. Some dieters even unconsciously (or maybe consciously) look for problems they can use as an excuse. If you really don't want to keep up with an exercise program then an injury is the perfect excuse to stop. But if you have the willpower to continue and the desire to truly succeed, then you can stay with your plan under these types of circumstances by the simple act of modification.

We all have times when the going gets rough and sticking to our original plan is a challenge. We might have to go away on business unexpectedly, or the weather might turn cold and rainy when we had been intending to go for a run, or we get sick or injured, or we come home to find our kids have, for a once-in-a-lifetime event, made dinner, and that dinner is garlic bread with cheese, Caesar salad and Fettuccine Alfredo. These things happen, and while your plans may have to be altered somewhat to deal with them, you cannot let these events dictate your success. You have to find a way to succeed despite them.

You need to take time to think ahead in times you expect travel or to be out of your environment. Through the hundreds of people I've helped to lose tens of thousands of pounds,

> **"If you are planning to go for a run and the weather is cold and rainy, you have any number of choices. Many runners will go out anyway, but if this is not an option for you, then you can go to the gym and run on the treadmill."**

I find the most challenging times for these individuals are when they lose their perceived structure as a result of being out of their environment. You need to organize yourself ahead of time so your success does not become compromised. Call ahead and find out if there is a fitness center in the hotel you plan to stay at or find out if your friend can get you a guest pass at the local gym. Ask if the hotel has rooms with fridges and microwaves – you may even find a whole kitchen. Ask if a blender is available and if not, pick up a travel blender – they're inexpensive and handy! Check online for restaurants at or near the hotel. If you can't find what you need on the menu, give them a call and ask if they'll make your required items for you. Most restaurants have no trouble with special orders.

If you are sent on an unexpected business trip and your hotel does not have a gym, your best bet is to get a day pass at a local gym. But even if you can't do that, you can still work out. You can run in place, skip or go for a jog outside if you're in a safe area. For strength, you can bring along resistance bands if you think ahead. If not, you can use a towel for resistance (yes, that works) and you can do bodyweight exercises. Lunges, squats, pushups, dips on a chair … pick a few exercises such as these and you can have a great circuit-training session. You may even find that by training in a completely different way you work your muscles harder than usual.

If you are planning to go for a run and the weather is cold and rainy, you have any number of choices. Many runners will go out anyway, but if this is not an option for you, then you can go to the gym and run on the treadmill – that's the most obvious substitution. You could stay home and do a skipping workout, or you could climb stairs, use a stationary bike or elliptical trainer or go to an aerobics class. Anything that really gets your heart pumping over an extended period of time is great. What I'm saying is that you have to learn to be flexible. The important thing is that you continue to reinforce the pattern you've grown accustomed to by exercising in some way.

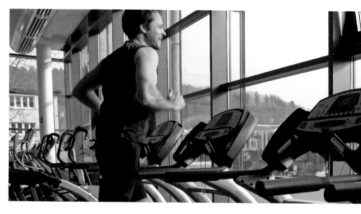

When you are honestly sick, you have to take some time off – no question. Trying to work out when you are sick will stress your immune system, possibly making you sicker. In addition, your training will not be beneficial. You will not be able to put adequate energy into your training and you will not get enough out of it. This refers to sickness such as the flu, not a chronic sickness; most people with chronic illnesses benefit from a modified training program. As for injury, keep in mind that all professional athletes suffer from injury at some point or another. They don't stop training; they train around their injury. If you have a broken ankle, then maybe you'll have to do more upper-body training. For cardio perhaps you can do an upper-body circuit. You can train your non-injured leg with light squats and other leg exercises. Instead of looking at what you can't do, find whatever you can do, and do it.

If you're lucky enough to come home and find that your kids have made dinner, then make the best of it. Have small portions, consider it a treat and get right back on your normal plan the next day. If the heavens have shone on you and your kids start doing this on a regular basis, then you will want to talk to them about which foods you're trying to eat more of and which you're trying to avoid. Ask them to help you out on your journey. If you ask them for help as opposed to telling them to make what you want, then they are much more likely to do what you would like them to.

There were times in my own journey when I couldn't stay on my own food program because of unexpected circumstances. At those times, my creativity served me well. For example, since I was in the habit of eating fast food when I was heavy, I relied on healthier fast-food choices once I made that change. I chose to go to the local sub shop rather than other fast-food establishments because it had healthier options. I could have a grilled chicken sub with no sauce and lots of fresh veggies. I could have a whole wheat bun and ask them to remove part of the inside. If I was out with no food and couldn't find any sub shops, I went back to a place I never thought I would – McDonald's. I would order two grilled chicken sandwiches and toss out the buns. You have to improvise when life presents challenges – it forces you to grow and learn!

Successful people don't let the little things hang them up. They keep their eyes on the ball. They don't get a negative attitude and give up simply because things didn't turn out exactly as they had anticipated. Successful people see the challenges before they occur, when possible, and are ready to find a quick solution when necessary. They are proactive when dealing with challenges, and they move on. They don't look back, keeping their mind stuck on things that went wrong, labeling themselves or their experiences as failures. There is no such thing as failure. Failure comes when you stop trying. Since you've picked up this book, you are not a failure. You haven't stopped trying. People like you, who succeed, will look back on all the challenging times as the times that helped them to grow and get even better, leading them to the moment of change and ultimately to success!

# CONSISTENCY

Think about this hypothetical scenario: You decide you're going to start a diet and exercise program. "This is it!" you think. "This time it's going to work! I'm going to diet and train so hard!" So you start exercising every single day, for two hours each day. Two or three weeks pass and you're feeling tired. You haven't put a day off in your training schedule, so instead you find an excuse to take a day off. That day off feels so good, and now you've broken your

"Successful people see the challenges before they occur, when possible, and are ready to find a quick solution when necessary. They are proactive when dealing with challenges, and they move on."

routine, so you take another day off. Soon your days off become the norm and your training days become the exception. Two months down the road and you're rarely seen at the gym,

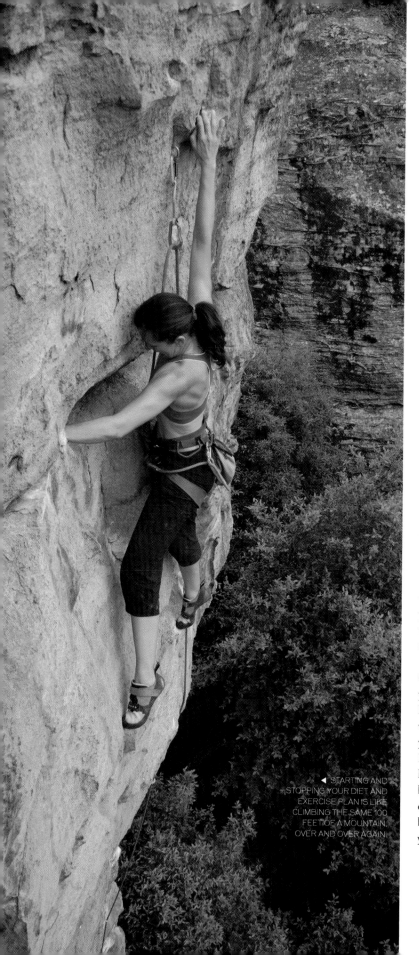

until the next time you decide to transform your life. When I had an office at a gym, throngs of people would flood the gym during the first week of January, but very few of those people would still be around in March. They spent money and invested time and energy, but quickly gave up.

Sound familiar? This may surprise you, but the main reason people quit an exercise program is that they try to do too much too soon. It is far better to set up a program that fits in with your schedule, that gives you time off, both to recuperate and to allow for repair of muscle tissue, and that you can carry out over the long term. In fitness circles they say: "Consistency is king," and with good reason.

An up-and-down exercise program is just like the up-and-down of backsliding down the mountain. Every extended break you take in your exercise program brings you sliding back in the direction you started, so you never get to the point where you are progressing. If you work out once in a while when you feel like it, or work out like mad for a few weeks and then stop, you will never reach the point where your gains endure, and so you are again climbing up and sliding down the same 100 feet of the mountain. If you consistently work out (in a challenging manner) even three or four times a week – consistently – then every week you are building on what you accomplished the week before, and you are progressing up the mountain.

Consistency is also extremely important with your diet. If you consistently eat properly but have a treat now and then, you will lose weight when you need to, and these habits will keep you lean once you succeed at your weight loss. However, if you diet and then binge, or diet, lose the weight and then go "off" the diet and back to your former eating habits, you will either not lose the weight you want to lose, becoming very frustrated and discouraged, or your weight will bounce up and down. Again, you're going up and down the same 100 feet of the mountain. I'm going to guess that you don't want either of those things to happen. Not only do these habits of inconsistency mean you will either not reach your goal or not stay there, inconsistency will also mess up your metabolism, making it harder and harder to get lean.

Perfection in eating is not the goal. Consistent good eating is. Often I am asked how you get yourself to do it even when you are angry, tired, frustrated or excited. I always think of the following note from Napoleon Hill, referring to how he maintains his composure no matter how angry he may be. "[I handle it] in exactly the same way that you would change your manner and the tone of your voice if you were in a heated argument with a member of your family and heard the doorbell ring, warning you that company was about to visit you. You would control yourself because you would desire to do so."

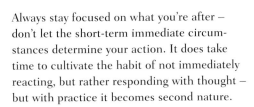

Always stay focused on what you're after – don't let the short-term immediate circumstances determine your action. It does take time to cultivate the habit of not immediately reacting, but rather responding with thought – but with practice it becomes second nature.

# FOCUS

Picture this: You're driving on a busy highway while getting in a fight with your spouse on the cell, eating a meal and putting on your makeup – a disaster waiting to happen. When you drive, you have to focus on your goal of driving where you want to go, or you will crash. Simple, right? But it applies to any goal. If you are not focused on your goal of losing

weight and doing what it takes to get there, then you will end up crashing, and you will never reach your weight-loss destination.

It's easy to slip back into bad habits if you aren't being vigilant. I find the movie theater is a trigger point for many of my clients. I understand this well – when I was overweight there wasn't a more ideal place to be than the movie theater. It was dark, so people couldn't see me well. The seats were large and spacious since the arms lifted up, and it was always kept cool, so I didn't have to worry about perspiring. Couple those attributes with the fact that I could escape to a fictional, happy, movie fantasy world, and I was in heaven. The trouble is, who sees a movie without popcorn

> "Temptation abounds. It's everywhere, from the leftovers on your child's plate to the candy jar on your coworker's desk to the sandwiches and cheese tray on the table at your meetings."

and a soda? Picture this: You start a diet on a Friday morning and go to a movie with your friend that night. Your friend orders an extra-large popcorn to share with you. "A handful won't hurt," you think. The next thing you know you've eaten half the bag, to the tune of about 600 calories if no butter was added, and closer to 1,000 if it was. For half the bag! What went wrong? You lost your focus, that's what. You got distracted by the movie, by your friend and by the fact that you were sitting in a movie theater – and besides, you're *supposed* to eat popcorn there, right?

Temptation abounds. It's everywhere, from the leftovers on your child's plate to the candy jar on your coworker's desk to the sandwiches and cheese tray on the table at your meetings. These are all ways we add hundreds of calories to our daily consumption without even think-

> ## "If you allow yourself to forget your goal, then you will not reach it. When you see the candy or donuts on your coworker's desk, remind yourself of your goal."

ing about it … or counting it, for that matter. Then there are the more obvious temptations: going out for pizza and wings with your friends, or grabbing an iced cappuccino and muffin for your break. Whether the temptation is large or small, obvious or insidious, you will have to stay focused on your goal to beat it.

You will also have to be focused on your goal just to stay on the right path. You may begin the week or day well, but as the hours or days slip by, you unwittingly slip further and further from the plan until you find yourself miserable, feeling like a failure and saying, "Okay, tomorrow I'm starting again."

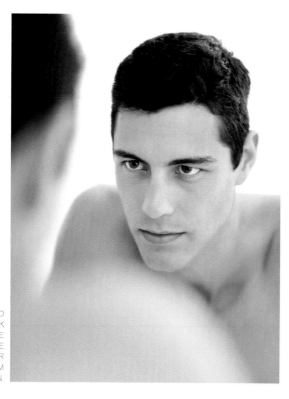

▶ YOU MAY FIND IT HARD TO LOOK YOURSELF IN THE FACE WHEN YOU'VE FALLEN FURTHER AND FURTHER FROM YOUR PLAN.

Just as success builds upon success, failure mounts up upon failure. The key is recognizing patterns and breaking those that are negative. While it's true that tomorrow is another day, you can't go back and live the past differently and you should not beat yourself up if you slip. The fact remains that if every day or week sees you repeating this pattern, then your focus is definitely not clear enough. Give yourself a strong visual reminder every morning, and then remind yourself throughout the day: You have a goal. If you allow yourself to forget your goal, then you will not reach it. When you see the candy or donuts on your coworker's desk, remind yourself of your goal. Before you eat even one bite of any food, ask yourself if that bite moves you toward your goal or brings you away from it. Force yourself to log every single morsel of food you eat in a book and report to a friend. This will be especially helpful if you don't have a person formally coaching you. Make someone else a part of your goal and your fear of disappointing that person will help you to succeed.

Ultimately, you cannot control whether your coworkers bring candy or donuts to work. You do not have total control over whether you get

> ## "Become proactive instead of reactive. Be mature. Recognize that you dictate your future. Stay focused. You will reach your goal."

sick or injured, and you cannot live a life without temptation. You don't even have complete control over how quickly you lose your weight. But you can control how you react to all these challenges on your journey, and the way you react will determine your success. Become proactive instead of reactive. Be mature. Recognize that you dictate your future. Stay focused. You will reach your goal.

## *"Thank you for saving my legs and my life!"*

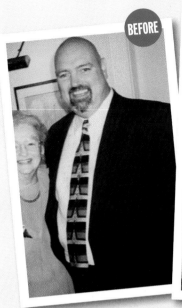

BEFORE

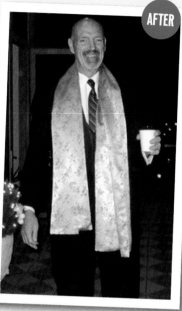

AFTER

NAME: **Patrick Brennan**
AGE: **57**
HEIGHT: **6'5"**
WEIGHT BEFORE: **332 lbs**
WEIGHT AFTER: **220 lbs**
WEIGHT LOSS: **112 lbs**

IT WASN'T UNTIL PATRICK BREN-NAN'S DOCTOR TOLD HIM HE NEEDED TO GET HIS DIABETES UNDER CONTROL OR FACE HAV-ING HIS FEET AMPUTATED THAT PATRICK FOUND THE MOTIVATION HE NEEDED TO LOSE WEIGHT. Patrick's overeating, lack of exercise and overall sedentary lifestyle had all contributed to his development of type 2 diabetes. For 13 years, Patrick struggled to get his condition under control, often ending up in the hospital because of his cellulitis – a bacterial infection of the skin common in those with diabetes. The doctor's dire diagnosis of amputation was due to the fact that Patrick's diabetes was interfering with the medication being used to treat the cellulitis.

With an aching back, sore feet and a major medical condition, Patrick walked into Charles D'Angelo's office looking for a miracle. And that is exactly what he found. Charles helped

Patrick regain his health and retain his limbs by teaching him how to pair excellent nutrition with exercise. Charles taught Patrick that there is no room for excuses. In fact, Patrick had to ditch his excuses at the door and make a total commitment to Charles' plan. It was tough at times, but Patrick persevered and discovered this

## *"Patrick had to ditch his excuses at the door and make a total commitment."*

lifestyle was one definitely worth living. With sound guidance and advice based on his own personal experiences, Charles helped Patrick drop 112 pounds. According to Patrick, hard work and the fact that Charles'

experience resonated with him ended up being "the right combination at the right time."

Patrick has received a new lease on life. He sleeps better, he has more energy, his knees and back don't ache, he can shop at regular clothing stores, he can get in and out of his car with ease and he can even run! This year he competed in a five-mile St. Patrick's Day run with his three sons. Patrick is setting an excellent example for them, as well as for the rest of his family and friends. Best of all, Patrick has managed to eliminate all of the diabetes medications from his life, which saves him more than $2,000 dollars a year on co-pays alone!

All that extra cash piling up in his pocket is a great motivator, but Patrick also stays on track by picking up two 50-pound weights and walking around with them to remind his mind and body of what it was like to carry around all that extra weight. But the most powerful motivator of all is that Patrick no longer has to make regular trips to the doctor, hospital and drug store. He does not want to return to his former way of life. And for all of those gifts, here is what Patrick has to say to Charles: "THANK YOU, THANK YOU, THANK YOU, for saving my legs and my life!"

# THERE'S NO TIME LIKE THE PRESENT

## Focusing on Your Success in the NOW!

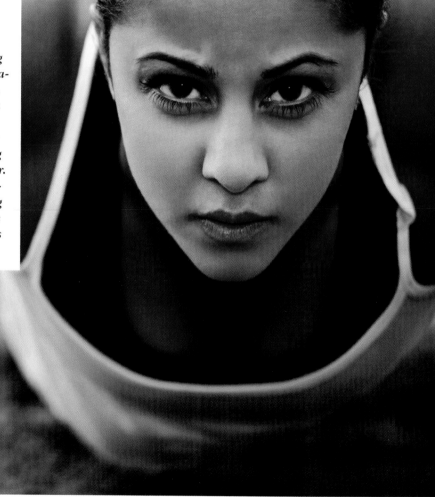

*If you're human, I'm going to guess you've spent at least one night of your life lying in bed, wide awake, with your mind racing from thought to terrifying thought. One moment you're analyzing your failed first marriage, the next you're wondering why a key client hasn't returned your latest email, and the next you're worrying about how you're going to afford new brakes for your car. The Buddhists call this the monkey mind because our chattering thoughts are jumping from topic to topic like a bunch of monkeys swinging from tree to tree.*

"You must train yourself to keep your mind entirely in the present moment."

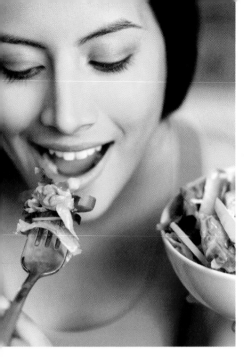

So many people get caught up in the habit of causing themselves undue anguish and stress by making a big deal out of things that really aren't such a big deal. As in the example given, when your mind is stuck worrying about the past or future, you become distracted from your true mission of achieving your dreams. To avoid this type of constant worry and pain, you need to stay in the present moment. Here are three simple ways to make that happen!

### 1 Automate your life.

Many 12-step programs promote the idea of staying in the present and taking things one day at a time. I'll go one further: You need to take it one moment, one hour, one day, one week, one month, one year at a time. A powerful part of my Scary-Easy Weight-Loss Plan is that your food and exercise life is now automated. You make the decision once you circle the options you're going to have, and you stick to just those foods for two weeks – day in and day out, no matter who or what gets in your way. This takes all of the guesswork and worry surrounding eating out of the picture.

### 2 Erase the negative past.

Eckhart Tolle, a modern spiritual teacher, wrote an entire book on this very subject called *The Power of Now*. In this book (which I recommend), he promotes the idea that pain, worry and anguish – any negative emotion, really – are a result of our minds leaving the present moment and traveling to lament over the past or worry about the future. He goes on to say that we have no control over the past, and the future depends on the now!

Think about the following statement: All pain comes from leaving this present moment. While it is so simple, it is profound. How many times have you been so focused on the tasks of the day ahead that you don't remember a thing about driving somewhere? We are blessed with a remarkable ability to forget – if you can manage to forget an entire car ride, you can definitely forget about your perceived past failures and other memories that are causing you to overeat and under-exercise!

### 3 Focus on the positives, no matter how small.

Yes, here I go again with the importance of gratitude! Be grateful you had the ability to buy this book (or be grateful for the library card that allowed you to borrow it or the friend who cared enough to get it for you). Applaud yourself for getting to the gym today, for going to a restaurant and staying on track, for staying with this plan in such a committed way, for making yourself a priority. All are major breakthroughs! Focus on these instead of a silly number on the scale.

You must train yourself to keep your mind entirely in the present moment. This very second, the moment you are reading this, you cannot experience pain, worry, fear, anger or anything that would trigger you to veer away from your program. Simple yet unbelievable – and true! Right now you are a success!

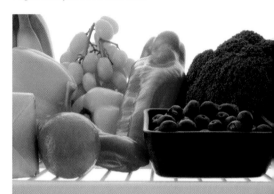

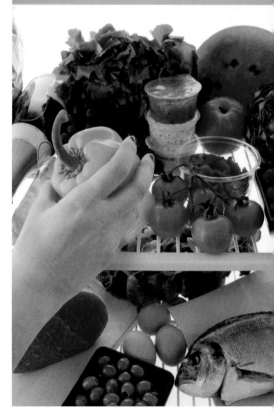

# CHAPTER SEVEN
## Designing Your Destiny

"Be thankful for the defeat which men call failure, because if you can survive it and keep on trying, it gives you a chance to prove your ability to rise to the heights of achievement."

– Napoleon Hill, *The Law of Success*

How many times have you said, or heard someone else say, "I've tried every diet out there, and haven't found anything that works! I've tried to lose before, but my body just won't let me." Come on, now! If we never tried again because we didn't succeed the first time – or even the first number of times – we'd never do anything. It takes time and practice to get good at something. Wasn't there a time when you were terrible at something that you're great at now? Can you knit? Cook? Play Scrabble? You could do none of these things the first time you tried. You had to keep trying and trying, getting a little better each time.

One day when I was just nine years old and overweight, I was sitting in my grandparents' kitchen. My grandmother was baking Christmas cookies with the radio on. Suddenly, a song came on that really caught my ear. My grandmother told me it was Elton John's song "Bennie and the Jets." I was struck by the piano in the song and immediately decided I had to learn how to play. I had always loved music class in school and sometimes would catch our teacher, who was from the Ukraine, playing rock songs on the piano during his lunch hour. I would go in and sit, entranced.

I found that my parents owned some of Elton John's music, including a tape that contained the song I'd heard. One afternoon I took it up to my bedroom, put it in my stereo system, lay on my bed with my Casio keyboard in front of me, and listened, and listened, and listened. I didn't come out of my room for over five hours. At the end of the five hours, I had decoded the opening riff that was so catchy to my ear. I continued to decode more songs and would watch experienced piano players play, often buying videos where I could see Elton John's or Billy Joel's hands. I would practice until I sounded just like them. I was obsessed with it, and I wouldn't stop practicing until I had the sound exactly as it was on the recording. I had no formal training and no one in my family played, but I made it happen. Why? Because I didn't accept the notion that it had to be done in some certain way. I believed that if I was willing to do whatever it took, I could play just like Elton and Billy. Eventually I got so good that when strangers heard me play they often asked if I played in either Billy Joel's or Elton John's bands!

Why do I bring up piano playing in a weight-loss book? Because you must believe that you can achieve whatever goal you have, whether that goal is playing piano or losing weight. It doesn't matter what's happened in the past, or if you have a thyroid issue, or if you don't have the endurance to walk half an hour on a treadmill. If you truly want to succeed and you're willing to work at it, you will overcome any and all obstacles in your way. What would the outcome have been if I had stopped trying after realizing that I couldn't just sit down and play like Elton John my first time at the piano? I would never have found such an incredible outlet for my creativity – an outlet that has not only brought me great joy, but has also brought pleasure to countless others who have heard me play.

Think about a baby. When that baby starts trying to move himself, it takes him days or even weeks of constant attempts before he can move even an inch. Does he stop trying because he's "failing"? How many attempts would you give your child before you give up on him? One, two, ten, a hundred? Of course not – the thought is ridiculous! To help your child achieve, you would do whatever it takes and be as patient as needed. Eventually, that baby learns to crawl, walk, run and speak. Would he accomplish all these things if he stopped trying after his first attempt or two? How about later on, when a young girl is learning to tie her shoes, button her coat and even ride a bike? If you as a parent gave up on her, would she still learn how to do these things? Why are you so willing to give up on yourself but not on others?

You may be thinking right now that I'm crazy for comparing a baby or young child to you and your dieting and exercising. But why is that crazy? Whatever we're attempting, whether it is learning to walk or talk, learning a new skill such as playing an instrument or a sport, or going after any other accomplishment such as losing weight, we are going to experience times when things are not going so well. In fact, there will be times we want to quit. When we're young we expect to have to keep trying and therefore we do so. For some reason, as we get older and supposedly more intelligent, we feel we shouldn't have to try more than once to succeed at something. Isn't that crazy? Perhaps when we turn 21 and are considered "an adult" we figure, okay – now that I'm all grown up I should just know how to do everything right.

Yet those who succeed are the ones who keep trying. According to research, the average number of times it takes a smoker to finally quit is about 10. What if after the 9th attempt a smoker decides he's just not going to try anymore? Edison famously said of his light bulb, "I had to succeed; I was running out of ways to fail." He also said, "I have not failed. I've just found 10,000 ways that won't work." and "Many of life's failures are men who did not realize how close they were to success when they gave up." But you are not one of those failures! You are going to try again, and succeed this time!

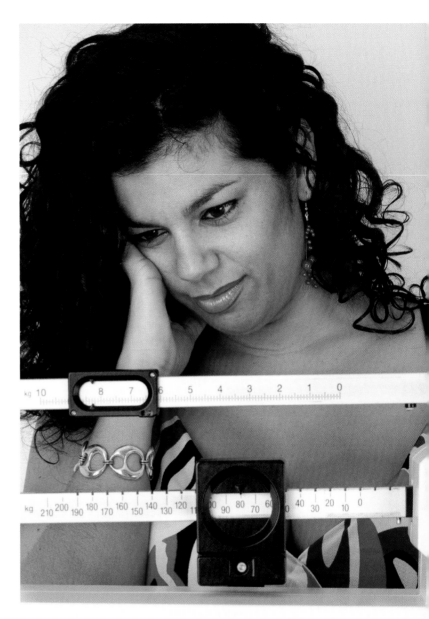

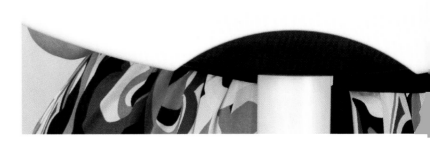

So why do people give up, or decide not to try again? They do this because they fear failure. The irony is that when people give up, they guarantee their failure by not trying again. In fact, the only sure way to fail at doing something such as losing weight is to not try. As Shakespeare so elegantly put it, "Our doubts are traitors, and make us lose the good we oft win by fearing to attempt." But you should try, and try again, because with each successive attempt you get better at succeeding, just like Edison. You learn what does not work for you.

Here's a typical example: Sarah (not her real name) first started dieting when she was 14. She wasn't happy with the womanly figure she had developed the previous year. She couldn't wear her clothes anymore, and for the first time this wasn't because she had grown taller, but because her pants wouldn't fit over her newly rounded hips and her tops pulled tightly across her chest. She was miserable, and her father didn't make things any better when he (no doubt uncomfortable himself about his daughter's blossoming) made a comment that she was getting a little chubby. Devastated, Sarah started looking into diets. Being an impatient teen, she decided on a "lose 10 pounds in seven days" diet she saw in a women's weekly magazine.

She went on the diet and did indeed lose 10 pounds in seven days. Most of the weight lost was water, but she didn't realize that. She also didn't realize that she'd just turned her metabolism down by putting herself into a state of near starvation. Within days she had gained back those 10 pounds,

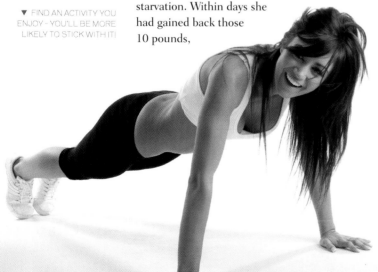

and after a month of skipping meals and then overeating and other unhealthy practices, she ended up a few pounds heavier than she had been before she'd begun to diet.

Over the years Sarah went on and off many diets, and by the time she reached the age of 32, she really was overweight. By this time she had been on the low-carb diet, the low-fat diet, the vegan diet, the high-fat diet and many others. Sometimes she stuck to these diets and lost weight, and sometimes she didn't manage to stick to them for long enough to lose much weight at all. She felt like a failure when it came to losing weight and keeping it off. She read about diets and looked at before and after pictures with envy, but felt it was really not possible to succeed.

But then she sat down with a piece of paper. She tried to remember every diet she'd been on, how easy or difficult it was to follow these diets, why she was able to follow them or not, and what her reaction was after finishing them. She figured out all the things that didn't work for her and what she might take from each one that could work for her. She made a chart like this:

**LOW-FAT DIET** Food didn't taste great. Worked moderately well but I felt hungry all the time. Could maybe cut fat down but not as much as this particular diet says.

**LOW-CARB DIET** Craved sweets, felt tired all the time, made me obsessed with food ... couldn't stop thinking about bread! Seemed to work well except that I couldn't follow it for very long. Maybe I could cut out simple carbs and have a moderate amount of complex carbs this time around.

**VEGETARIAN DIET** Had a hard time not eating any animal products. Found I was not satisfied after meals and so would crave other foods or eat way too much cheese. Could eat some meat-free meals and cut meat servings down but fill up on other proteins like protein shakes, quinoa and beans.

After all was said and done, Sarah ended up finding a program that combined pretty much everything that worked for her, and added the missing link – exercise – into the bargain. What is even more important is that she realized that all these fad diets she'd been following simply did not work. Her "failures" brought her to the understanding that a "diet" had to be a plan she could follow for life rather than something she followed for a short time and then binged her way out of. She also came to the understanding that in always trying to lose weight quickly, she ended up spending year after year getting fatter and fatter. Even if it took her a longer time to lose her excess fat by following a reasonable and moderate eating plan, she could follow it long term and thereby achieve long-term success. So we could look at Sarah's earlier diet attempts as failures, or we could look at them as steps on her path to success. It's not whether you've won or lost in the past, it's whether you are willing to do what you have to do to succeed in the future.

For argument's sake, let's say you have never tried to lose weight before. You feel, like I did, that you were meant to be large. You've always been overweight. Your family is overweight. You could allow yourself to accept that you were destined to be fat, but you shouldn't. You have to wake up and realize you are not doomed to follow in your family's footsteps. In fact, one of the reasons I succeeded was that I was determined to prove I didn't have to end up obese, with diabetes and dying of a heart attack at a young age, just because my family history included all these health problems. You decide your destiny, and your choices move you in whichever direction you have decided on.

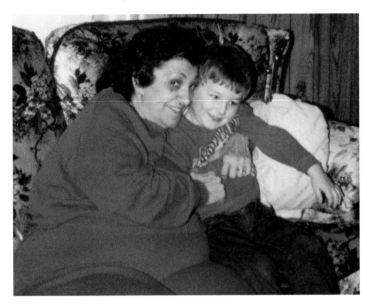

◀ GROWING UP, I SPENT A LOT OF TIME WITH MY GRANDMA ROSE.

What path are you on right now? If you continue to do the things you're doing now, will you be where you want to be one year from

**"You've always been overweight. Your family is overweight. You could allow yourself to accept that you were destined to be fat, but you shouldn't. You have to wake up and realize you are not doomed to follow in your family's footsteps."**

today? You control whether that is your reality or whether you step on that scale a year from now and see the number you want to see. If you adopt the idea that your weight is outside of your control, you'll never change it. You must realize that the things you initiate, such as your weight gain, are completely within your control to change. You were the cause, and you alone can make the change.

You have a gift, and you have power. The question is whether or not you're ready to tap into either of these things. If you don't believe you are able to achieve the goals you've set, then you won't tap into any of the dormant potential you have, you won't go after your goal wholeheartedly and you'll end up in the same place you started – or more likely worse off than before. If you can transmute your challenges into opportunities, your life will blossom. Ask yourself such questions as, "What

> "You can do this. It is math and science. Fewer calories consumed and more calories burned. "

type of program will work for me? Is this something I can stick to?" These questions will lead you to useful answers instead of keeping you in this endless loop of self-doubt and pity.

It doesn't matter what your weight, diet and exercise history are. If you decide to change your life today, you can succeed. Don't worry that you don't know exactly how to do it. Don't worry that you're breaking new ground. Don't worry that you're afraid. Just look in the direction you want to go and start going there. You can do this. It is math and science. Fewer calories consumed and more calories burned. A bit later in the book I outline an exact plan that will tell you more than you want to know about what you need to do – just do it!

In the following chapters, I'll present the third "R." I'll tell you all about what foods to eat (if you want to understand why I suggest what I do) or, if you are overwhelmed by a lot of information, you can just follow the exact plan I've given to thousands of people who have experienced extreme weight-loss success. This plan has worked for all those who have chosen to stick to it. The key is being consistent, as we covered in the last chapter. Are you ready to follow it? Are you ready to make this the moment that changes the rest of your life? I am ready to help you. Make this the second that it all clicks for you, and then follow through, creating the life you deserve!

You have to approach this program with the determination to succeed. There will be challenges. There will be times you don't feel like eating these foods. There will be times you don't want to go to the gym. There will be times your closest loved ones will try to deter you. There will be times when you are doing everything you're supposed to and your weight isn't budging. All these events are likely to occur. Remember it's not what happens in life, but how you choose to deal with what happens that determines whether you succeed. You need to have never-ending resolve! I expect the best from you, and I hope you expect the best from yourself too. Join me and the thousands of others who've made my approach the one that has physically, emotionally and spiritually changed everything about their lives.

## SLIP-UPS AND FALLING OFF THE WAGON

Let's see if this scenario sounds familiar: You start a diet on Monday. You follow it to the letter on Monday, Tuesday and Wednesday, but by Friday you feel like you've been dieting forever. Someone brings in a cake for a coworker's birthday and you say, "Okay, I'll just have one little bite. That can't hurt." But oh, that bite tastes good. And you're a little hungry. Next thing you know, you've eaten the whole piece and scraped the extra icing from the plate and eaten that too. Well, your diet is shot for the day now, right? You give yourself permission to have pizza for dinner that night. After all, you already screwed up anyway. You say to yourself, "I'll

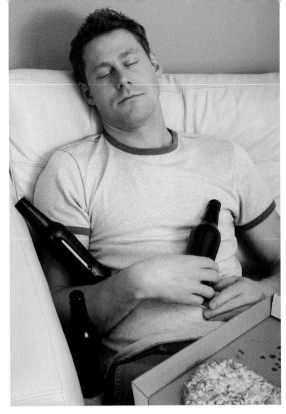

start again tomorrow. I'll even do a little extra exercise to make up for it." At dinner that night you have pizza and you might as well have some beer, too. You're starting your diet again tomorrow, so you should enjoy yourself tonight. This is it – the last time you'll be eating this stuff. From tomorrow on, you'll be so strict. You decide not only to have your pizza and a couple of beers, but you also add a few nacho chips. And just one cookie. A large pizza, a six-pack of beer, a bag of nacho chips and box of cookies later, you collapse into bed on the downside of your fat and sugar high. When you wake up in the morning you feel disgusting. You weigh yourself and find that overnight you've gained not only the two pounds you had lost the week prior, but another two on top. Feeling so discouraged and depressed after a whole week's work was ruined in a few hours, you decide that it's not worth it so you give up altogether.

You may or may not have gone through a scenario like this, but believe me a lot of people have. I can't count the number of clients who've told me a story that matches that example almost to the letter. Now let's revisit the "model" day I presented and find out how many times you could have salvaged your weight loss:

• After the first bite of cake you could have recognized that you were actually hungry, thrown the rest of it out and had a healthy snack or a protein shake.

• After eating the whole piece along with the icing from the plate you could have said, "Well, that was probably not a good idea but I'm going to make sure I get right back on the plan. One piece of cake can't derail me! Tonight's dinner will be exactly what it should be, and next time I'll be more careful."

• After eating the pizza you could have said, "Wow, I really made some bad choices today but that's no reason to completely throw the day away. Time to go to bed."

• The most important time to make a good decision was the next morning. Sure you felt terrible that you messed up, and maybe gained back all you lost throughout the week and then some (much of the overnight weight gain

"After the first bite of cake you could have recognized that you were actually hungry, thrown the rest of it out and had a healthy snack or a protein shake."

would be just water retained from all that sodium, along with the weight of the actual food). But one night of bad decisions is definitely no reason to give up altogether. Remember that giving up is the only sure route to failure. As long as you are traveling in the right direction, you'll eventually get there.

You had been on the right path up until making some mistakes on Friday, and by making

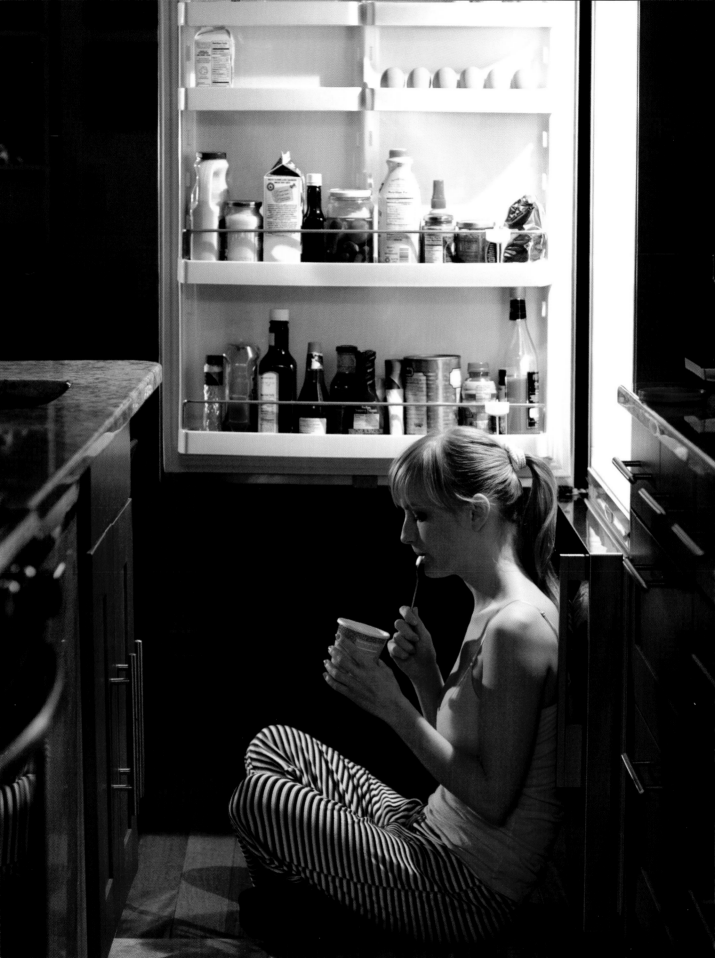

the decision to get right back on your plan the next day you would bring yourself closer than ever to your eventual goal. Getting right back on your plan means you have made the breakthrough that it's not all or nothing. You can slip up occasionally, as long as you are doing the right things for the majority of the time. We are a product of what we've done consistently, not what we've done some of the time. When we're overweight, we often think very negatively since our life experiences are negative. We beat ourselves up instead of looking at the bigger picture and realizing that our bad choices do not define us. Just because we acted in an immature or even stupid way doesn't mean that's who we are. We all make bad choices on occasion. The important thing is to realize your bad choices are not your identity. Often we allow our brains to ignore or delete many of the good things we do. In college, I remember walking out after exams, obsessed about the couple of questions I didn't know the answers to, worrying myself to death over it and forgetting all about the 90 questions that I did know the answers to! Make a conscious effort to acknowledge and remember your successes.

## GOING THE DISTANCE

Let's say you want to drive to the beach for a vacation. At some point on your journey you read the directions incorrectly and end up heading in the wrong direction. Do you then tell your family something like this: "Sorry kids, I turned the wrong way back there, so the vacation is canceled. I'm driving back home. In fact, since I messed up this time I may never take a vacation again." What a ridiculous thought! If you take a wrong turn then you figure out where you went wrong and how to get back on the right road so you can reach your destination. You must have first had a desire to go on vacation, then made a decision where you wanted to go, found a map to get you from your starting location to where you wanted to end up, and finally if you found you

misread the map, you had to get some help getting back on the correct road. That's what this book is all about: Defining where you are, helping you see the world that's truly out there and giving you a very specific map to get there.

## "If you're the type of person who cannot have one serving of certain unhealthy foods without bingeing or otherwise going off your plan, then do not have even a taste of those trigger foods."

If you do make a wrong turn and eat a piece of cake, or even spend an entire day eating junk food, you still want to reach your destination. Giving up at that point is ridiculous. Instead of giving up, find out where you went wrong (starting to eat the piece of cake when I was hungry). Think about how to get back on the right road (start following the program again even if reaching my goal might take a little bit longer), and learn how better to stay on the right road next time (eat some good food before indulging in a bite of birthday cake so I'm not hungry, and always make sure to have some good choices on hand in case of emergency) and enjoy your vacation (enjoy reaching my goal weight and looking amazing)! You can do this!

During your journey, you have to watch out for trigger foods, which can send you careening out of control into oncoming traffic. If you're the type of person who cannot have one serving of certain unhealthy foods without bingeing or otherwise going off your plan, then do not have even a taste of those trigger foods. For many people, these emotionally charged foods are the main cause of weight gain. One little bite makes you feel so good at first, but before you know it you've been rendered powerless to escape the sugary, fatty, starchy clutches, and you end up lying in a guilty heap on the floor. The best way to manage these triggers is by identifying them and avoiding them altogether. I know it sounds severe, but you need to treat this as an addiction and follow the plan I prescribe later in the book to the letter, without deviation. It's normal to feel you shouldn't have to do this, that you should be allowed to have treats or cheat meals, but the reality is that being that strict is the most effective way for you to develop enough momentum to make unbelievable progress. Do not allow yourself even the idea you are allowed to have foods that are off limits. Don't give yourself an inch to fail!

## STEPS TO ENSURING SUCCESS, WHATEVER YOUR PAST HAS BEEN

1   Remember that the past is a great tool to learn from, but it does not dictate the future. Try to look at past mistakes like Edison did, as learning experiences. Figure out

why your former plan didn't work. It might have been the plan itself, or it might have been the way you were thinking at the time. Find that reason and look at it objectively. Don't lay blame on yourself or on others, but accept that you are indeed responsible for the current level of health you experience. Figure out what not to do in the future. Logical and accurate thought is essential to long-term success. Ask yourself, "What can I learn from that experience that will help me make Charles' plan the absolute most effective thing I've ever done?"

2   Remind yourself of your definite goal. Just because you've had a setback, it doesn't mean your goal will disappear. You might get there a little later than expected, but you will get there in time. Learning anything new takes time. I'm asking you to become one of my students. You need to take time to truly "get" what I'm saying. Don't be discouraged if it takes a couple of reads. Getting a touchdown in a football game is rarely if ever the result of a 100-yard pass or run; it's the result of a series of short plays, some of which worked and some of which did not. What matters is not how many plays it took to get to the end zone; what matters is that the ball gets there. If the players lost sight of the goal line at the other end, a touchdown would never result. When plays don't go as anticipated, the team doesn't disband. They watch tape of the game with their coach, looking for errors, asking why they occurred and figuring out how to avoid those errors next time.

3   Open yourself to new experiences. The behavior that has brought you to where you are now will not be what gets you to where you want to be. Consider the oft-repeated definition of insanity: "doing the same thing over and over again and expecting different results." You will not change the way you are by staying the same or by thinking with the same negative thought patterns. Try new foods or a new diet program. Try my Scary-Easy Plan. It

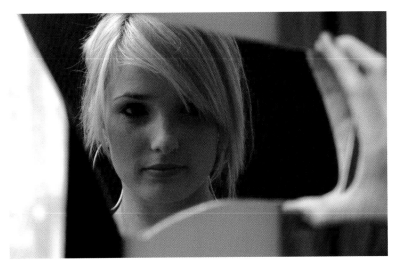

tells you exactly what to eat, when to eat, which exercises to do … everything you need. All you have to do is take consistent action. The fact is, any healthy diet will work if you consistently follow it. If you eat less and burn more you'll lose weight. The key is having the correct mindset. Don't like certain foods very much? Try them again. The more often we try a new food, the more we like it. Marketing studies have found that when a person is exposed to a stimulus repeatedly over time his or her liking for it increases exponentially. We humans have survived and thrived for so many millennia with far fewer choices in food than we have today because we are able to adapt to the foods that are around us.

Try new experiences. Never been for a hike? Go on one. Don't know how to swim? Take lessons. There is a huge world out there full of activities you could never imagine yourself doing. Do them. I understand you may feel out of place initially. I did too. Allow yourself to be a beginner. Find opportunities where everyone is a beginner at first. Challenge yourself by starting to love yourself more.

**4** Be your success. Change your identity internally. You must start to look at yourself in a new way. That new way has to match the lifestyle you want to live. If you think you're poor, you are going to attract more of that poverty because you don't seem successful. As I mentioned in Chapter 5, there's a saying, "Fake it until you make it," similar to faking confidence until you feel it. That's what I did and it worked really well for me. As you know, I wasn't always in shape and successful. My success came when I decided I was not "the fat guy" but rather a fit guy who

happened to have extra fat on top of his muscles. When I was 360 pounds I certainly didn't fit in with the guys with rippling six packs at the gym, but by believing I really was like them on the inside, I was willing to work just as hard as they did, if not harder, and that made me become one of them. In fact, now I'm in even better shape than many of them!

If you can shift your belief system about yourself and your capabilities, you will change your life in an unbelievable way. Imagine that the last time you saw a computer was in 1946, when the 30-ton ENIAC (which had the

> "I wasn't always in shape and successful. My success came when I decided I was not 'the fat guy' but rather a fit guy who happened to have extra fat on top of his muscles."

programming capability of a small calculator) was unveiled. Then one day someone puts a 4.8-ounce smartphone in your hand and shows you a streaming webcast of a music festival taking place on the other side of the planet. Your world would change in an instant after seeing what's possible! That's part of what this book is meant to do: Open your mind and change your world by showing you what I've been able to achieve by simply changing the way I think about food. Allow yourself to become the person you want to be. If you decide you are a lean, healthy person, you will become a lean and healthy person because your habits will fall in line with who you believe you are. Identity is the strongest force in human psychology. We will do all we can to stay true to the definition we have given ourselves. Make sure the definition you have of yourself is that of a person you want to be!

5 Find out where you want to go and keep moving in that direction. Most of us fall off the path now and again. What determines your success is whether you get back on. It only makes sense that to get somewhere you

## "Look ahead toward where you want to go and you'll soon be there."

have to keep moving in that direction. Going off course from time to time is inevitable – no road is that straight – but you must make sure to always get your bearings, turn back to the right direction and move toward your destination. Keep your eye on where you want to be,

not on where you don't want to be. So often we get caught up worrying about needless things that become noise and distraction, when if we were to laser our focus in, we would achieve our goals faster than we ever dreamed. Do you drive down the highway looking out the back window? Of course not! Look ahead toward where you want to go and you'll soon be there.

I care immensely about you and your success. While you may feel unimportant and unloved, as if perhaps everyone has given up on you, please know that I truly love you and so does God. We haven't given up on you. He wants you to enjoy your life and be the happiest you can be – and so do I. The rest is up to you. Follow my plan. Be prepared for the challenges that will arise. And, most importantly, don't give up! There is nothing stronger than you or greater than your ability to achieve. The human spirit is a remarkably resilient thing. Give your heart up to this and to God. We won't let you down. I promise.

▶ I THINK MY CAMARO MATCHES MY PERSONALITY – TRANSFORMER!

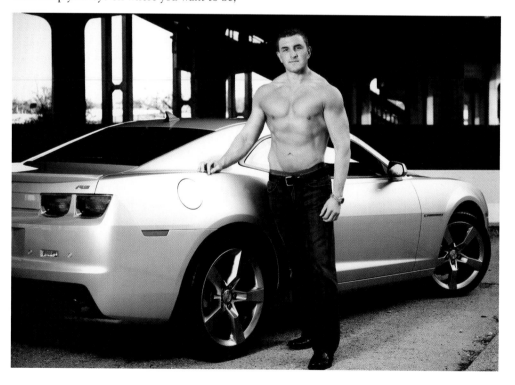

## *"Charles helped me realize that this was up to me."*

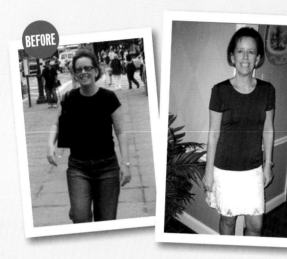

BEFORE

AFTER

**NAME:** Nancy Spewak
**AGE:** 51
**HEIGHT:** 5'2"
**WEIGHT BEFORE:** 148 lbs
**WEIGHT AFTER:** 108 lbs
**WEIGHT LOSS: 40 lbs**

**NANCY SPEWAK WOULD EAT WHETHER SHE WAS HAPPY, SAD, BORED OR ANGRY.** "It didn't matter if it was a tough day or a great day," she says. "I believed that I 'deserved' it."

Nancy's emotional eating brought her to the point where her first thought each day was, "How much do I weigh?" The scale determined her mood and attitude toward food. If her weight was down a bit, she'd eat with abandon, and if it was high she'd eat more lightly. This cycle repeated itself day in and day out.

Nancy was now confronted with a crushing despair each time she opened the closet door. She would make efforts to camouflage the extra weight by wearing basic black and white and then using fancy shoes and jewelry to distract the eye. But then she would catch a glimpse of herself in the mirror and disappointment always followed.

One day Nancy realized she had been trying to lose the same 20 pounds for more than a year. She knew at that moment that she did not want to live the rest of her life ruled by the scale, that it was not about always being on some fad diet, constantly depriving yourself, restricting food groups or buying prepackaged foods. She now saw that those products aren't real; they aren't everyday life. It was after this epiphany that she found Charles. Charles taught Nancy that she could eat real food and be healthy.

"Charles just tells it like it is." She knew he would not pamper her or allow her to make excuses. "He helped me realize that this was up to me. He could tell me what to do, but this would only work if I was willing to commit." His straightforward approach helped Nancy see she alone was responsible for her choices. If she made wise choices and planned ahead, she would lose the weight. And lose it she did. The pounds fell off as Nancy realized her weight issue

had been all about control. Before she met with Charles, she had let her weight control her attitudes and emotions. After following Charles' plan, she was the one in control.

Now, after dropping 40 pounds, Nancy is back at the weight she was in high school. Losing weight and exercising have completely changed her body, and she feels great about her new appearance. She now wakes up excited every morning, looking forward to getting dressed in her new designer clothes. Her energy level is high, and she has dropped back into a normal blood pressure range. Whenever she starts to lose focus with eating or exercise she thinks about how hard she worked to get to where she is now. She no longer gets upset if the scale goes up a pound or two since she knows that eating responsibly will keep her where she wants to be.

Nancy thanks Charles every day for helping to turn her life around. For anyone considering weight loss, Nancy says, "Charles has the key to lifelong weight maintenance and he will give it to you if you have the courage to commit!"

# TAPPING INTO YOUR HIGHER POWER

## 3 Ways to Develop Faith In Yourself

*"A true spiritual teacher does not have anything to teach in the conventional sense of the word, does not have anything to give or add to you, such as new information, beliefs or rules of conduct. The only function of such a teacher is to help you remove that which separates you from the truth of who you are and what you already know ... The words are no more than signposts."*
— Eckhart Tolle, *Stillness Speaks*

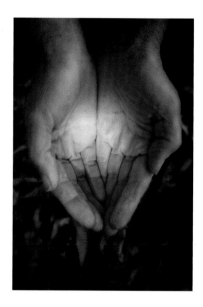

With faith, all things are possible. Doubt is the absolute opposite of faith. Doubt comes about when you need a level of certainty that no one and nothing else can provide. Some people – not knowing that this level of certainty can only come from an inner knowledge of their highest self and their purpose for being here – use food, drugs, partying or sex to try to eliminate doubt. As you know, I was once one of those people. I mistakenly believed that those late night junk food marathons would give me all of the certainty and reassurance I craved. Boy, was I ever wrong!

Where does faith in yourself come from? Some believe it's a force we're born with that is taken from us through years of being told we're not smart enough, good looking enough, tall enough, committed enough and so on. Funny that all of these enoughs never

even originated from within us! Faith comes from developing good references about yourself and your abilities. When we don't feel good about ourselves, we need to get to work on rethinking the meaning we gave to our past experiences. You can start off by asking yourself these questions: What am I good at? What is something I could like about myself? What is something about me that I like in others?

We all go through times of great trial and uncertainty, in our relationships, with friends and coworkers, with regard to making career decisions and in our finances. There are many unpredictable elements to life, but that unpredictability isn't bad – it forces us to grow and adapt. Once you have developed faith in yourself, you will be able to overcome any of the obstacles life puts in your path. We learn and

grow from those things we may find challenging in the moment. This growth is what helps us eventually realize our true potential.

Here are three steps to tapping into your higher power to develop faith in yourself:

### 1 Surrender.

This is not about letting go of responsibility, but rather, focusing on the moment and purpose – doing what's right for your life – instead of the outcome. When we surrender, we are saying we have faith that divinity is present in every moment of our lives. This mindset will allow all of God's graces to flow to us. As soon as you let go of your attachment to outcome and begin to concentrate on purpose, everything you need, like this book, will appear at the moment you need it. The inner feeling that this book and program is right for you is a sign that divinity is at work, giving you a spark and awakening your higher self.

## 2 Get in tune with your Higher Power.

Realizing that you can't do this alone, and that only with the help of a higher power will you achieve your goal, gives you an immense power. God's presence is in the car as you drive to the gym, walking alongside you on the treadmill and watching you as you catch a glimpse of yourself in the mirror. Joining a church or spiritual group where like-minded people congregate for a greater good is a huge step toward achieving your goals. It is also a great way to develop relationships with potential mentors.

## 3 Stay in a state of gratitude.

It's challenging to be grateful when things aren't going your way, but you must come to understand that everything is perfect as it is and you are exactly where you should be. Everything that has happened, whether you've labeled it good or bad, was perfect in and of itself and brought you to where you are today. Be grateful knowing that even more blessings are to come. When you disconnect from negativity, you release a positive flow in your life and miracles begin to show up, making life what you and God have always wanted it to be.

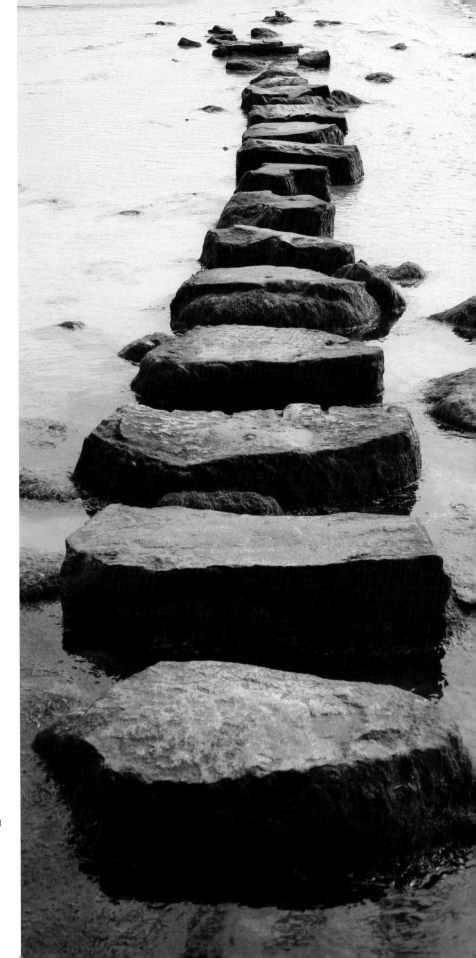

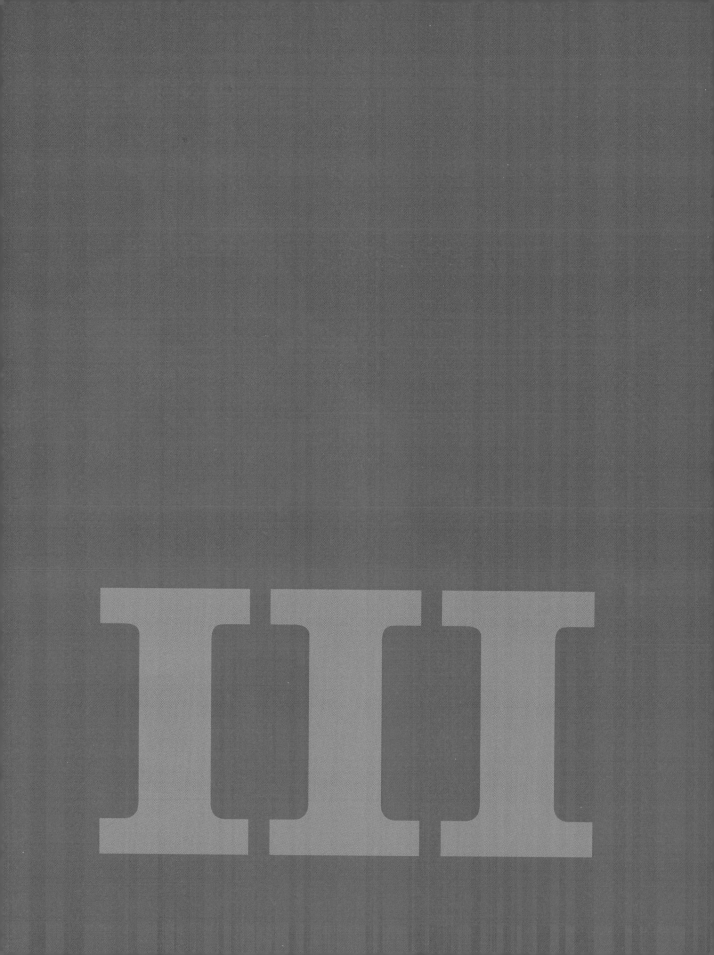

# section III

The Tools
You Need to
Transform
TODAY!

# CHAPTER EIGHT
## The Third "R":
## Road - The Key to Fat Loss

"When you come to that inspiring moment when you choose your Definite Major Purpose, do not become discouraged if relatives or friends who are nearest to you call you a 'dreamer.' Just remember that the dreamers have been the forerunners of all human progress."

– Napoleon Hill, *The Master-Key to Riches*

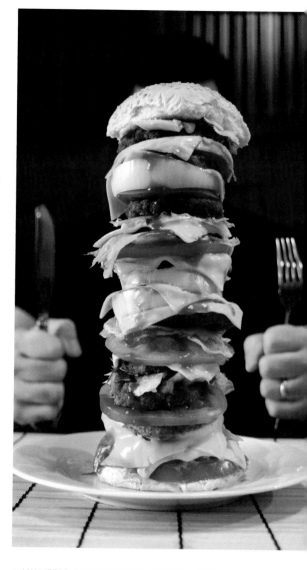

▲ MANY PEOPLE MISTAKENLY BELIEVE THAT BECAUSE THEY WORK OUT, THEY CAN EAT WHATEVER THEY WANT.

A common misconception these days is that exercise is the key to losing fat. While exercise is undoubtedly an important piece of the puzzle, without a proper diet you will not achieve your goals, period. This brings us to the third "R" – Road (See? I didn't forget!). When I first decided to change my life, I weighed 360 pounds. I joined a gym and started going there every night after a long day at school. I worked so hard that I had to put towels on the treadmills on either side of me so they would appear already occupied. This may sound a bit inconsiderate, but it was actually the opposite. I didn't want anyone around me because I knew they would end up getting drenched by the steady stream of sweat flowing off my body. By the end of my workout, my thighs would be chapped from rubbing together so vigorously. I would have to go home and put Vaseline on them, both at night and the next morning. This not only felt disgusting, but it was also embarrassing because the oil would leave huge blotches in the crotch of my pants, making it look like I'd had an accident! (Imagine walking the halls of high school, much larger than everyone else and with a huge oily

stain at your crotch!) Despite all of my efforts, after one month I had lost only three pounds. I couldn't understand! How could I have lost only three pounds after a whole month of working so hard?

I started to seek out as much information as I could on the subject of getting results. However, and maybe you've experienced something similar, I quickly became frustrated and overwhelmed! The wide array of diet plans often contradicted one another, with each one offering more choices than the last and very little structure. Although I'm sure the information was given with the best of intentions, none of it addressed the true underlying problem – my thinking. Most diets can bring about short-term weight loss, but if they don't address the emotional issues tied into the bad behaviors, then permanent change will not occur. It was only when I realized that I had to come up with a way to correct the root cause of the overweight person's issues that I was able to fix the unhealthy habits that had caused my own problem.

The truth was, as I learned, I had been working furiously at the gym only to totally destroy my hard work by heading over to a fast-food place to satisfy my ravenous appetite. I didn't know it at the time, but my muscles were crying out for healthy lean proteins and complex carbs, and instead I shoveled in massive amounts of unhealthy simple carbs and bad fats in an attempt to fill the craving. Once my body got through that swampy mess of food, the cravings came back (because I hadn't actually given my body what it needed), and so again I would fill it with the wrong things. I might have been burning 500 calories in my workout, but then I would go and stuff myself with 1,200 calories of junk! I can't tell you how many times I hear this statement from new clients: "I work out every day but I just can't lose this extra 10 [or 15, 20, 50 or 100] pounds and I don't know why!" Well I know why and now you will know too. It's because they are not making changes in their diets. Even worse – sometimes they feel that because they are exercising they can eat more or whatever they want, like I once believed.

## TOO MUCH INFORMATION?

When I was at my heaviest, I would become overwhelmed by all of the information about nutrition, healthy fats, good carbs, protein,

sugar, etc. I certainly don't want you to give up because you feel overloaded with information. If you're ready to change, accept that diet is important and be willing to try the same program I have my clients do, then you can head straight to "Charles D'Angelo's Scary-Easy Weight-Loss Plan" in the next chapter. If you do head there now, you will want to come back to this section sometime in the future. Understanding why you are doing what you're doing will help you to stay lean and fit once your goal has been reached.

If you're not yet excited about this plan, you should be! It's transformed thousands of lives and is referred to as "scary easy" by the major-

"I didn't know it at the time, but my muscles were crying out for healthy lean proteins and complex carbs, and instead I shoveled in massive amounts of unhealthy simple carbs and bad fats in an attempt to fill the craving."

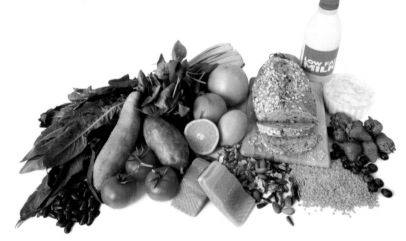

ity of my clients. That's because it's a specific methodology I personally developed to recondition your mind's relationship with food and exercise. All the decisions are made ahead of time. You just have to do it. If you don't want to have to think about what to eat and are looking for a straight-to-the-point regimen to follow, this is it. I will tell you what, when and how much to eat. You must know that there isn't much variety or choice, but the results will be remarkable for you. I've also included a maintenance plan so you can learn how to work variety back into the equation.

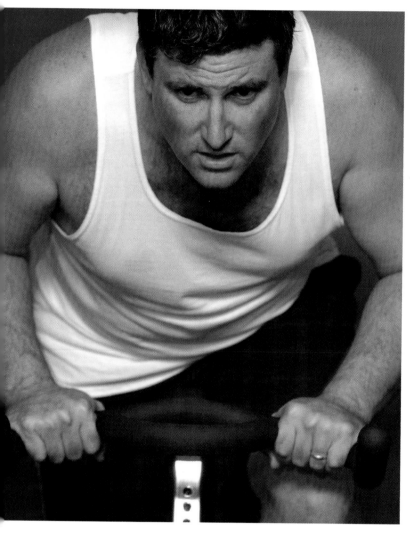

If you are a person who likes lots of information, or you want to understand why I suggest what I do, keep reading the rest of this chapter. Action is the key, but knowledge is very important. To truly be a master at this, you must understand why you do what you do.

## WHY EXERCISE ALONE DOESN'T WORK

So, you've decided to stay and learn. Good! If you want to know why exercise is not the key to weight loss, then read on. Cardio does use some energy, and so does weight training. And yes, building muscles makes your metabolism burn brighter, stronger and longer, meaning you use more energy (calories), even when you're at rest. But now let's take a look at how much energy the average person uses every day:

It takes a surprising amount of energy just to keep you alive. If an average person burns 2,000 calories in a day, about 1,200 to 1,400 of those calories are used to fuel basic life functions: keeping your body temperature regulated, keeping all of your bodily processes working, digesting your food and repairing cells. The amount of calories you use just by staying alive is called your Basal Metabolic Rate, or BMR. If you are a sedentary person, your BMR makes up about 60 to 75 percent of your caloric requirements. If you add, say, four or five fairly strenuous exercise sessions each week, then your BMR will make up about 80 percent of your calorie expenditure each day. A difference, yes – but not enough of a difference to mean you can now pig out on fries. Adding four or five 45-minute to one-hour workouts each week, but keeping your activity level and diet the same the rest of the time means your caloric requirement increases by only about 250 calories a day. If your diet were to stay exactly the same, then this exercise would result in a weight loss of about one pound every two weeks.

And that's assuming that your diet stays the same. Often if people do not consider their diets when they begin an exercise program, they begin eating more – they may subconsciously think the exercise allows them more food or they may justify their extra eating by saying "I worked out, therefore I deserve this creamy milkshake." Remember, I used to do this. I would convince myself that after all this hard, sweaty exercise I needed a meal at Burger King. I know a woman who started a swimming program to lose weight, and after her first month she was shocked to discover that she'd actually gained weight. After talking to her for a bit, I found that she and her friend would putter around the pool for a half-hour and then go for a muffin and coffee. The first mistake she made was thinking that simply being in a pool floating about was somehow using great amounts of energy, and the second mistake was thinking that the 600-calorie, sugar- and fat-laden muffin she was eating was a healthy treat after all that "energy expenditure"!

# CALORIES IN VS. CALORIES OUT

Okay, so let's go back to you. If you've been sedentary and you are now exercising for an hour, four or five days a week, that means you

**"If you are very overweight you will likely have no trouble decreasing by 750 calories because your calorie consumption is already very high. But if you are in fairly good shape and just want to lose 10 or 15 pounds, it may be harder to cut back on calories."**

are using up about an extra 1,750 calories each week. (To learn how to calculate your actual BMR and daily calorie needs, see p. 169.) One pound of fat equals 3,500 calories, so you've used up about a half-pound of fat with that exercise. But you want to see more

weight loss than that! Of course, you no longer want to lose 10 pounds in a week, because you know that's not really possible or healthy either. You want to lose an average of two pounds a week. That's a nice weight-loss rate that a) means you're actually losing fat and not water and b) can be carried out over the long term, meaning you are more likely to stick to it. That means each week you need to consume 7,000 fewer calories than what is required to maintain your weight. (I'll mention here that this formula, known as "the bucket theory" of weight loss, is not completely accurate because your body reacts to different foods in different ways, but it does work fairly well in practice, so we'll go with that.)

To consume 7,000 fewer calories than your maintenance level each week, you'll need to eat about 5,250 fewer calories, since you're using up 1,750 calories for your exercise. This means you need to reduce your calories by about 750 each day on average. This is quite a lot, and depending on how much you've been eating and how much you have to lose, you may want to reconsider your goals at this point. If you are very overweight you will likely have no trouble decreasing by 750 calories because your calorie consumption is already very high. But if you are in fairly good shape and just want to lose 10 or 15 pounds, it may be harder to cut back on calories. In that case, you might want to consider changing your goal to one pound per week. To make this process a little easier and a little faster, you can also increase your activity level in general. Someone once said, in order to lose weight: "Don't lie down if you can sit; don't sit if you can stand; don't stand if you can walk; don't walk if you can run." Even small activities like parking your car at the far end of lot and walking or

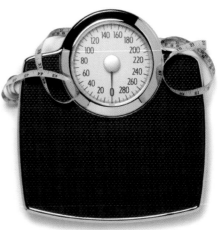

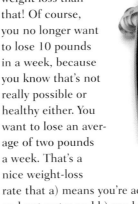

▲ LOSING AN AVERAGE OF ABOUT TWO POUNDS PER WEEK IS IDEAL.

taking a short walk during your lunch hour can make a difference. In fact, inserting more activity into your everyday life can mean an extra 1,500 calories a week or so, which means you will only have to decrease your calories by 500 each day to lose those same two pounds.

## CRAZY WEEKENDS CAN MAKE YOU FAT!

When planning your week of eating, make sure you consider all seven days of the week. This may sound obvious, but lots of people eat fairly well throughout the week and then go crazy on the weekends. They feel like this should keep them slim, and they're shocked when I point out that the weekend (Friday evening, Saturday and Sunday) actually makes up an entire third of the week. You do the math: If you eat your proper calories for two-thirds of your life and go crazy overboard

> "Bill takes in an extra 5,000 calories each week although he indulges only on the weekend. Over the course of a year, if he continued to eat 5,000 calories more than he needs each week, he would be 74 pounds above his optimal weight!"

for a full third, then you're not going to be the size you want to be! Let's have a look at an example:

Bill's an active guy, and he needs about 2,800 calories a day to stay at his optimal weight. Monday to Thursday he stays pretty close to that number. Friday though, is the weekend. His Friday breakfast is just his usual breakfast of an egg sandwich from a fast-food restaurant (300 calories) with orange juice

(150 calories) and coffee with cream and sugar (75 calories), but he often goes out for lunch on Friday. His typical lunch is a large cola (200 calories), Philly steak sandwich (940 calories) and cream of potato soup (400 calories). After work, he goes to his favorite sports bar for dinner with friends. He has a few beers (725 calories), a Caesar salad without chicken (600 calories), a bacon cheeseburger (1,250 calories) and fries (400 calories). While waiting for his meal to arrive, he often nibbles on the nacho chips (400 calories) they put on the table. His caloric total for Friday is 5,440.

Saturdays start off pretty well, but Bill usually skips lunch and then is starving by dinnertime. He starts nibbling before dinner, eats more dinner than he normally would because he's starving, and then sits on the couch with his wife eating potato chips and drinking soda while watching movies. A typical Saturday's caloric total would be about 3,800. Sunday begins with a brunch buffet, moves on to football with beer, wings and pizza, and ends up in the range of 4,200 calories.

So you can see that Bill takes in an extra 5,000 calories each week although he indulges only on the weekend. Over the course of a year, if he continued to eat 5,000 calories more than he needs each week, he would be 74 pounds above his optimal weight!

I'm not saying you can never enjoy a burger, fries, pizza or beer again. That is simply not true. If you consistently eat well then an occasional meal that includes options you wouldn't normally eat on your plan is fine and possibly even desired, depending on your own relationship with food and whether or not your good habits are well established. The trouble comes when these poor food choices outweigh your good choices and you end up not losing weight or, worse, gaining it back.

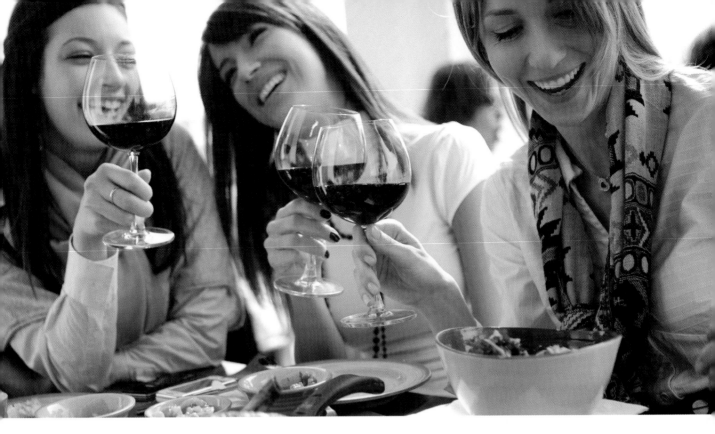

Allowing yourself to have an occasional treat or special meal can also help you avoid the cake scenario described in the previous chapter, whereby because you ate one food you were not planning on, you go hog wild, have a binge and end up going off your diet altogether. If you've been following your program all week and, through lack of planning or for whatever other reason, you have a piece of cake or a plate of fries you had not been planning on, just tell yourself, "Okay, that was my treat this week." And it's all good.

So now that you know about calories and how much you have to rely on your diet for fat loss and weight maintenance, what should you be eating?

## DIET AND NUTRITION IN MORE DEPTH

If you decide you want to learn all you can about your new healthy way of life or if you want to create your own diet plan, this sec-tion offers some great information to help you get started.

Every calorie you consume is made up of one of three macronutrients: carbohydrates, protein or fat. For your body to function properly you need to consume all three. Fad diets often severely limit one (or more) of these important mac-ronutrients, but this is not a good way to lose weight. For one thing, it is hard to stay on an eating plan that does not give your body what it requires, and therefore you are more likely to go off your diet. In addition, a diet such as this is not possible to follow over the long term, which means that if you do manage to stay on track until you reach your goal, you will soon find the weight creeping (or rushing) back on as soon as you revert to your former eating patterns.

## CARBOHYDRATES

Every 25 years or so, a diet comes along that tells people carbs are the reason they gain weight, and the way to lose weight is to severely restrict them. This is an easy theory to market, because restricting carbs immediately results in an impressive loss of a few pounds. These few pounds are almost completely made up of water, but it feels great to get on the scale and see a quick loss. The trouble is our bodies need carbs to function properly. In fact, carbohydrates are the brain's main energy source, and I feel they should make up 40 to 50 percent of your caloric intake.

Diets that are too low in carbs normally end up in failure because they are just too hard to stick to – with good reason. When you deprive yourself of carbs, your muscles, brain and other parts of your body start to crave them so badly that your body tries to get you to eat the very worst carbs possible (simple sugars), because they are broken down and digested very quickly. This leads to cheating and bingeing, and, not surprisingly, rapid weight gain.

However, keep in mind that all carbs are not created equal. In general, we can divide them into the categories of simple and complex. Another word for simple carbs is "sugars," and these should be avoided. But don't be misled by the term "sugar." Although table sugar, high fructose corn syrup and other sweet offerings do fall into this category, as you'd expect, so do items that might surprise you. Refined grains such as white flour are considered sugars. So are fruit juices, even those without added sugars. Many packaged cereals are considered simple sugars, and so are most types of pasta because they are made with white flour.

Huh? Pasta is a sugar? Yup! Natural fruit juice is a sugar? Sure is. Bread is a sugar? If it's made with refined grains it is. The reason these items are classified as sugars is that their molecules have been broken down to such a degree, and their fiber and other nutrients removed to such a degree (all through processing), that we digest these foods very quickly. Eating them causes a spike in our blood sugar, and eating too much ends up causing not only weight gain, but also diabetes.

Contrast those simple carbs with the types of carbs that should make up roughly 40 to 50 percent of your daily calories: complex carbs. Vegetables are all complex carbs. Whole grains are also complex carbs. In fact, the foods you always hear you should eat more of are almost invariably complex carbs. Here's a short list to give you an idea (I'll get into more detail later on):

➡ Unsweetened, whole grain hot cereals such as oatmeal
➡ Unsweetened whole grain cold cereals such as Shredded Wheat
➡ Whole grain breads and wraps
➡ Brown rice
➡ Wild rice
➡ Barley
➡ Sweet potatoes
➡ Corn
➡ Peas
➡ Root vegetables such as carrots, beets and turnips
➡ Leafy green vegetables such as spinach, kale and lettuce
➡ Cucumbers
➡ Green beans
➡ Cruciferous vegetables such as broccoli, cauliflower and cabbage
➡ Bananas
➡ Berries
➡ Apples
➡ Pears
➡ Oranges
➡ Grapefruit

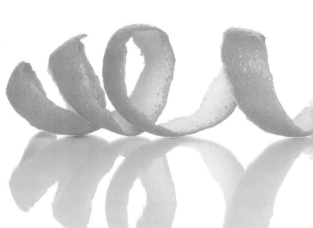

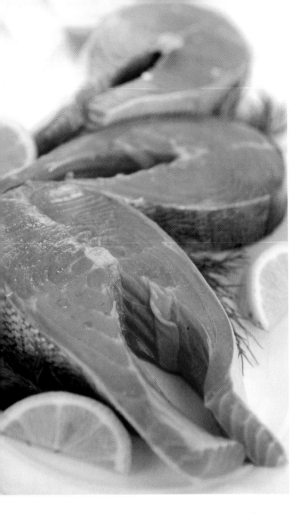

"If you are a muscular person who exercises a lot, your protein needs will be much higher than a non-muscular, sedentary person."

Our protein needs vary quite a bit from person to person, depending on many factors but mainly on an individual's muscle mass and activity levels. If you are a muscular person who exercises a lot, your protein needs will be much higher than a non-muscular, sedentary person. If you are an endurance athlete your protein needs are higher still. But in general, protein should make up about 15 to 25 percent of the calories in your daily diet.

Many of us get too much protein, especially if we are sedentary. Too much protein can result in kidney problems, dehydration and a general stress on your organs, especially if a high-protein diet is followed for a long period of time and, more importantly, if the protein sources are not healthy and the individual does not get enough fiber. That being said, it's important

"Grains also contain protein, as do milk products, nuts, seeds and lentils. Quinoa and soy are both great plant-based protein sources and they are loaded with other healthful ingredients."

to have enough high-quality protein in your diet, especially if you work out regularly. The key words here are "high quality." Most of the protein we eat in this country is from low-quality, processed meats filled with saturated fats and fillers.

You should eat some high-quality, nutrient-rich protein each day, and even at each meal. This protein does not have to come from meat, although meat, seafood and eggs are the sources with the most readily available protein. Grains also contain protein, as do milk products, nuts,

You don't need to ever eat candy, refined bread, refined pasta, donuts, soda or any other simple carb in order to get enough carbs in your diet. You can fulfill all your carbohydrate needs from whole, natural, complex carbs – it seemed to work pretty well for our ancestors!

Keep in mind that starchy carbohydrate sources are more apt to cause weight gain and should be limited for weight loss. These include grains and grain products, potatoes, corn, bananas and winter squash.

## PROTEIN

You hear a lot about protein when discussing weight loss and fitness. That's because protein is what the body uses for building muscle and to repair tissue. It's also because the popular low-carb diets are, almost by definition, high-protein diets.

seeds and lentils. Quinoa and soy are both great plant-based protein sources and they are loaded with other healthful ingredients.

# FATS

In the 1980s and 1990s, the most common refrain in weight loss was: Fat makes you fat. Every product became "low fat" and even products that had never contained much fat were labeled that way. Did you tune in when Oprah hauled out a wheelbarrow full of it? It was argued that because fat has nine calories per gram and protein and carbohydrates contain only four, then common sense dictated that avoiding fat would make you lean. As with low-carb diets, low-fat diets seemed to work – meaning people lost weight. But if you look at whether those people kept the weight off and stayed healthy, it's an entirely different matter.

The fact is we need fats for our bodies to function properly, just as we need carbs. Without fats, our brains will not function properly, our organs will not be protected and our skin and hair get brittle and dry. Our eyes will get weaker, and our immune system function will be reduced. When deprived of fats, our bodies have a hard time creating the substance that insulates our nerves, preventing misfiring. Fats also help us process vitamins and phytonutri-

> "As with low-carb diets, low-fat diets seemed to work – meaning people lost weight. But if you look at whether those people kept the weight off and stayed healthy, it's an entirely different matter."

ents. In fact, some nutritionists recommend taking vitamin supplements along with a fat in order to ensure better absorption. And strangely, a diet too low in fat seems to make us fatter in the long run.

One way to explain this is that, as with carbs, our bodies make us crave fats when we are not eating enough of them, and therefore we start bingeing. Another theory is that when our bodies sense they are not getting enough fats from foods, they begin to hoard body fat. Both of these theories seem to make sense and will

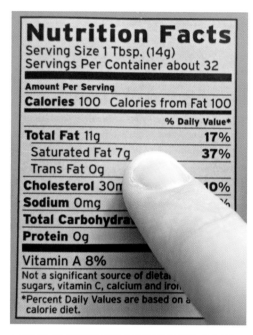

▲ PAY CLOSE ATTENTION TO THE SERVING SIZE – IT IS OFTEN QUITE SMALL.

help you remember that some fats are important for optimal health and for your long-term goal of losing excess fat and keeping it off.

You probably know what's coming now … yes, you need to be eating the right types of fats in order to end up lean and healthy in the long term, and you do need to eat the proper quantities as well. Most of the foods that make us fat are filled with trans and saturated fats. These fats should be avoided, especially trans fats.

Trans fats are oils that have been chemically altered in a lab to create a texture we humans enjoy. Early in the last century, chemists discovered that if they added a hydrogen atom to a molecule of unsaturated fat, they could cre-

**"When you fry starches such as potatoes, tortillas or the batter on fried chicken or fish, a toxic chemical called acrylamide is produced in the food. This toxin can cause everything from reproductive disorders to cancer."**

ate a whole new type of fat – one that acts like a more-expensive saturated fat. Not only did consumers love trans fats, but these fats also greatly extended the shelf life of the products they were added to. You can imagine how exciting this discovery was for food manufacturers. They could take cheap oils and transform them into an almost addictive substance, and then that substance would extend the shelf life of a given product from a few days to a weeks or months! Miraculous! Talk about a cash cow!

Over the next century or so, trans fats became more and more common. They were used in everything from crackers to pudding to baked goods to snack foods, including commercial peanut butter. Throughout much of that time, trans fats were considered healthier than saturated fats because they had been made from unsaturated oils. No one seemed to be listening to researchers such as Dr. Catherine Kousmine who, as far back as the 1940s, suspected trans fats caused or exacerbated disease.

Now that the public is finally aware of the horrors of trans fats, we see "trans fat free" labels on loads of products. The trouble is, this is often not the case. The laws dictate that companies are allowed to call their products "trans fat free" if they contain less than half a gram per serving, but the serving sizes are often very misleading. Your best bet is to read the ingredient label on everything. If you see the words "hydrogenated" or "partially hydrogenated" that means the product contains trans fat, no matter what the label says, and you should avoid it.

Deep-fried foods are especially bad for you. Not only do they usually contain trans fats, depending on the laws of the area in which you eat them, but when you fry starches such as potatoes, tortillas or the batter on fried

▼ THE PROCESS OF DEEP-FRYING CAUSES SOME FOODS TO BECOME CARCINOGENIC.

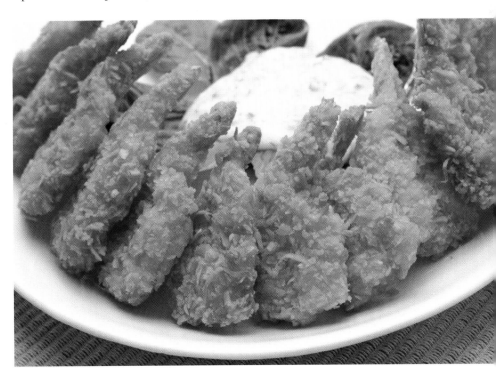

chicken or fish, a toxic chemical called acrylamide is produced in the food. This toxin can cause everything from reproductive disorders to cancer.

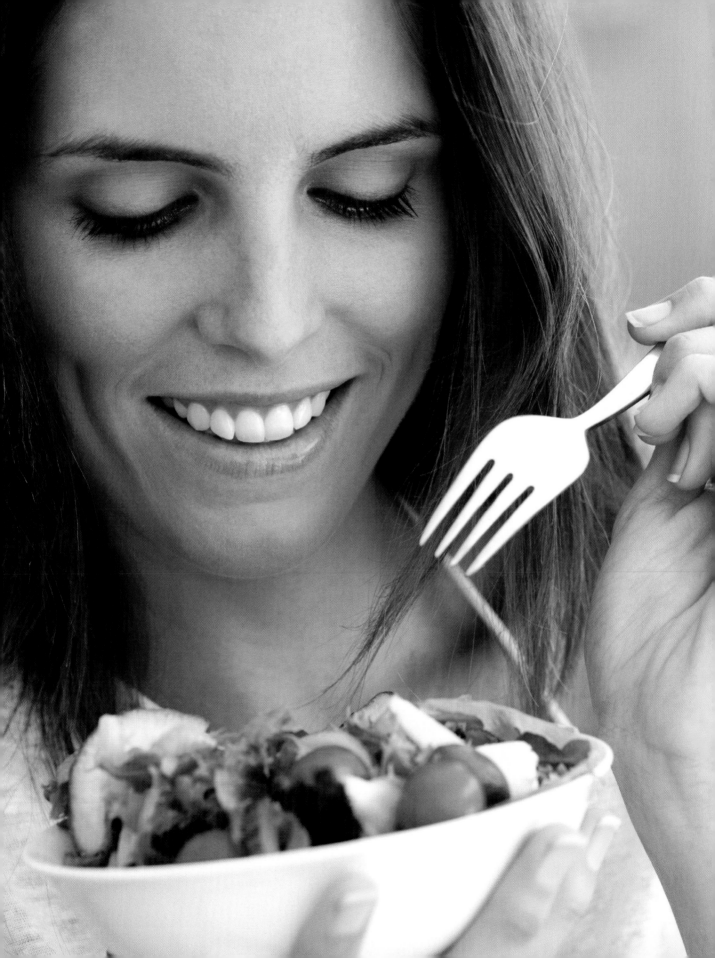

"Omega-3 is the only essential fatty acid that we really have to concentrate on getting into our diet. Good sources of omega-3 fatty acids include flaxseeds, walnuts, salmon, sardines, soybeans, halibut, shrimp, tofu and grass-fed beef."

Saturated fats, too, should be avoided whenever possible. You will not manage to keep all saturated fats out of your diet, but try to keep them to a minimum. Saturated fats are solid at room temperature, and come mainly from meat and dairy, although palm kernel oil, cocoa butter and coconut butter/oil are also sources of saturated fat. Coconut oil and butter, although they are saturated, are good choices because they are medium-chain triglycerides, which are rapidly absorbed and burned as energy. The rest of these saturated fats should be avoided.

Unsaturated fats should make up the majority of fats in your diet. These come from vegetable products and fish. Extra virgin olive oil, avocado oil, canola oil, seeds, nuts and natural nut butters (without added sugars, chemicals or hydrogenation), and cold-water fish such as wild salmon, herring and mackerel should provide most of the fats in your diet. These healthy fat sources are all high in omega-3 fatty acids, which I'm sure you've heard a lot about.

The three essential fats are omega-3, omega-6 and omega-9. Our bodies create omega-9 and we can easily get enough from our diets, so we don't really have to seek it out. We tend to eat far too much of omega-6, mainly because we

eat excessive amounts of grains and fats. In particular, we eat too much omega-6 relative to our consumption of omega-3. Omega-3 is the only essential fatty acid that we really have to concentrate on getting into our diet. Good sources of omega-3 fatty acids include flaxseeds, walnuts, salmon, sardines, soybeans, halibut, shrimp, tofu and grass-fed beef.

Calories from fats should make up about 20 to 35 percent of the calories in your diet. This may sound like a lot, but fats are fairly easy to consume too much of, because their calories are more concentrated in two ways. First, they have more than twice the calories of either protein or carbohydrate per gram. Second, sources of protein and carbohydrates normally contain a great deal of water whereas many fat sources are a more concentrated food consisting mainly or totally of fat.

If a fat is solid at room temperature, that's a good bet you shouldn't eat it, because it's either a saturated or trans fat (with the exception of coconut oil). Make sure to store fats properly – in a cool, dark place and preferably the fridge. You should not eat these fats if they go rancid.

## BEST FOODS FOR HEALTH AND WEIGHT LOSS

If you've made it this far, you now know the three macronutrients – protein, fat and carbohydrates – intimately. The following listing includes serving guidelines and several examples of the good, the bad and the ugly foods in each macronutrient category and subcategory. I'm providing this list to give you some background on good food choices (and not-so-good ones). The specifics of my Scary-Easy Weight-Loss Plan will follow in the next chapter.

NOTE: Serving sizes are given in ranges as a person's daily allowance depends on sex, age and level of physical activity.

# NON-STARCHY CARBOHYDRATES

Minimum of five servings per day, preferably more
(1 serving = ½ to 1 cup)

### BEST CHOICES

You can eat unlimited amounts of these vegetables but should have a minimum of three servings per day.

- Artichokes
- Arugula
- Asparagus
- Beet greens
- Bok choy
- Broccoli
- Brussels sprouts
- Cabbage
- Cauliflower
- Celeriac
- Celery
- Chard
- Chicory
- Cilantro
- Collard greens
- Cress
- Cucumber
- Endive
- Fennel root
- Fiddlehead greens
- Fresh herbs
- Garlic
- Green beans
- Kale
- Kohlrabi
- Leeks
- Lettuce
- Long beans
- Mushrooms
- Okra
- Onions
- Parsley
- Purslane
- Radicchio

- Spinach
- Sprouts
- Zucchini or other summer squash

### GOOD CHOICES

These vegetables and fruits are good choices, but because they have a higher sugar or starch content you should stick to four servings in total per day.

- Apples
- Beets
- Berries (any kind)
- Carrots
- Citrus fruits (clementines, grapefruit, lemons, limes, mandarins, oranges)
- Daikon
- Jerusalem artichokes
- Jicama
- Melons
- Papaya
- Parsnips
- Peas
- Pears
- Radishes
- Sweet bell peppers
- Tomato
- Yellow (wax) beans

### ACCEPTABLE CHOICES

These are highly nutritious but have a higher concentration of calories. Stick to one serving per day.

- Apricots
- Cherries
- Fresh figs
- Grapes
- Guava
- Jackfruit
- Lychees
- Mango
- Pineapple

### ⊗ RESTRICTED

These are okay to use as a sweetener or flavor-enhancer, but should not be eaten in any great quantity, and definitely not as a snack.

- Dried apples
- Dried blueberries
- Dried cranberries
- Dried mango
- Dried papaya
- Dried pineapple
- Raisins

### SEVERELY RESTRICTED

These should be used very sparingly – try to avoid them altogether.

- Honey
- Maple syrup
- Dehydrated cane syrup

### FORBIDDEN

Do not let these pass your lips at all, unless you're having a rare treat!

- Dextrose
- Fructose
- Glucose
- High-fructose corn syrup
- Invert sugar
- Maltose
- Table sugar (sucrose)

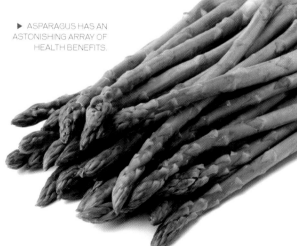

▶ ASPARAGUS HAS AN ASTONISHING ARRAY OF HEALTH BENEFITS.

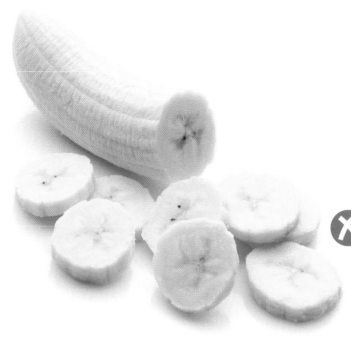

- Quick oats
- Whole grain breads and bread products
- Whole grain pasta
- Whole grain, unsweetened cereal such as Shredded Wheat
- Whole grain couscous

 ## RESTRICTED

These should not be part of your everyday diet and should be avoided.

- Cold cereals (virtually all of them)
- Muffins
- White breads and bread products
- White couscous
- White pasta
- White rice

▼ QUINOA, CONSIDERED A SUPERFOOD, OFFERS HEALTHY CARBOHYDRATES, COMPLETE PROTEIN AND OMEGA-3 FATTY ACIDS.

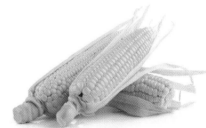

## FORBIDDEN

These items can be eaten only on very, very rare occasions as a treat.

- Cakes
- Donuts
- French fries
- Nacho chips
- Pastry
- Potato chips

# STARCHY CARBOHYDRATES

**Up to four servings per day**
**(1 serving = ½ to 1 cup)**

 ## BEST CHOICES

Try to get most of your starchy carbs from these sources:

- Bananas
- Barley (whole, not pearl)
- Brown and wild rice
- Corn
- Millet
- Oats (steel cut or rolled)
- Potatoes

- Quinoa (Bonus! Quinoa is high in protein and omega-3 fatty acids!)
- Rutabaga
- Sweet potatoes
- Turnips
- Wheat berries
- Winter squash
- Yams (true yam)

## ACCEPTABLE CHOICES

Try not to have too many starchy carbs from this category, as they are inferior to those above.

- Cream of Wheat
- Popcorn

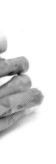

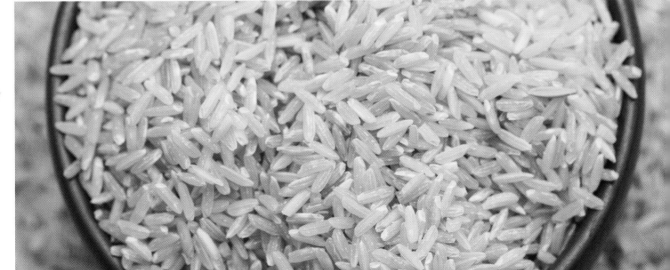

# HIGH-PROTEIN CARBOHYDRATES

These carb sources are unique in that they also offer the considerable benefit of protein. How much you eat will depend on how much meat, fish and other animal products you consume.

 **VEGETARIANS:** 6 servings per day (1 serving = ½ to 1 cup)

**MEAT EATERS:** Up to 4 servings per day (1 serving = ½ to 1 cup)

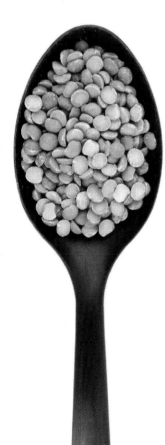

- Adzuki beans
- Black beans
- Black-eyed peas
- Broad beans (fava beans)
- Butter beans
- Calico beans
- Cannellini beans
- Chickpeas (garbanzo beans)
- Edamame
- Great Northern beans
- Italian beans
- Kidney beans
- Lentils
- Lima beans
- Mung beans
- Navy beans
- Pinto beans
- Soy beans
- Split peas
- White beans

# DAIRY

Up to three servings per day (1 serving = ½ to 1 cup)

 ## BEST CHOICES
- Nonfat or 1% buttermilk
- Nonfat or 1% cottage cheese
- Nonfat or 1% kefir
- Nonfat or 1% milk
- Nonfat or 1% plain, sugar-free yogurt
- Whey

## POOR CHOICES

Even when labeled low in fat, these choices contain too much fat to eat more than on rare occasions.

- Higher-fat cottage cheese
- Higher-fat plain yogurt
- Higher-fat milk
- Low-fat cream cheese
- Low-fat hard cheese
- Mascarpone
- Ricotta

## RESTRICTED

These cheeses are very high in fat (usually at least 70% of calories are from fat). Eat only on very rare occasions.

- Cream cheese
- Full-fat hard cheese (e.g., cheddar, mozzarella, Swiss, Monterey Jack)
- Full-fat soft cheese (e.g., Bousault, Brie, Camembert)
- Processed cheese

## FORBIDDEN

These items are high in sugars and/or fats and should be eaten only as a rare treat.

- Cheesecake
- Fruited yogurt (even if low in fat)
- Frozen yogurt
- Ice cream
- Ice milk
- Milk shakes

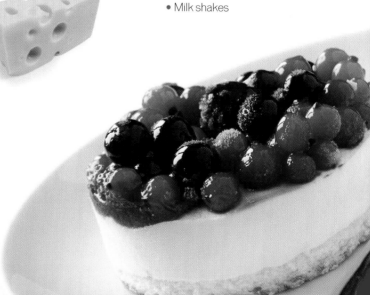

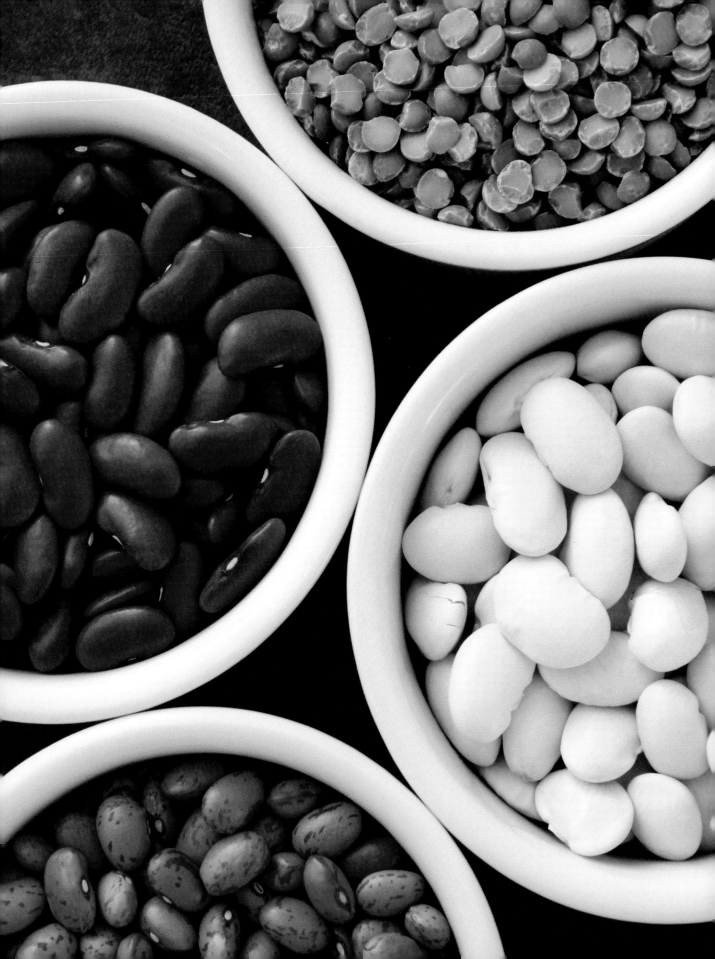

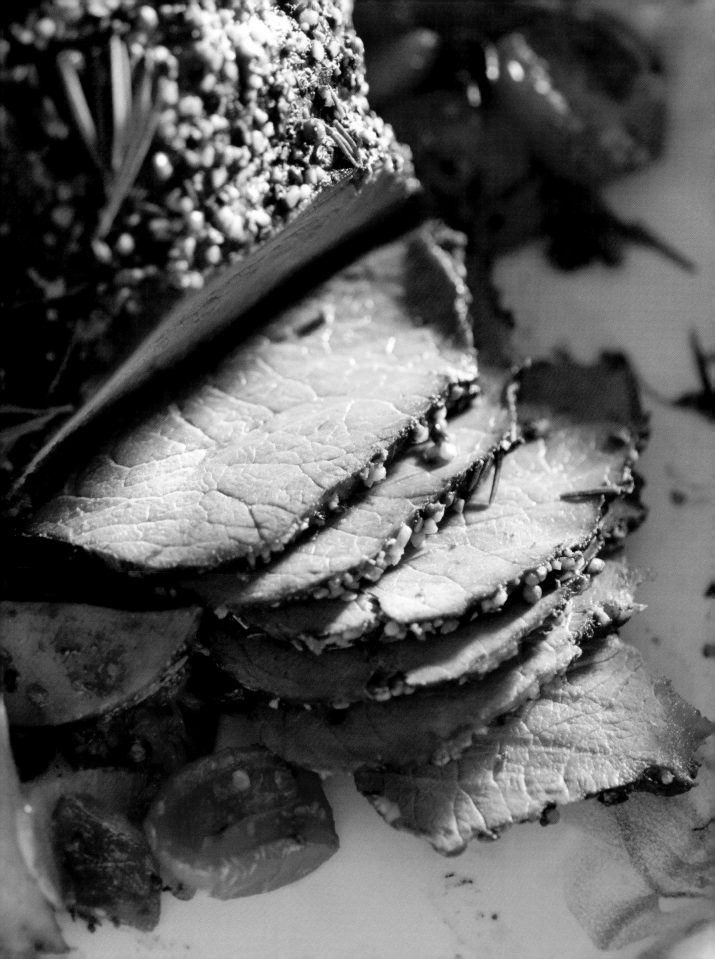

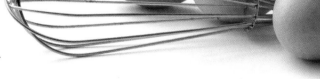

# ANIMAL PROTEIN
Up to 3 servings per day
(1 serving = 4 to 6 oz)

 **BEST CHOICES**
Try to get your protein almost exclusively from these choices. These should be cooked without batters, breading or fats.

- Beef (lean, no visible fat)
- Bison
- Chicken breast (without the fat or skin)
- Cod
- Egg whites
- Extra lean ground chicken (white meat only)
- Extra lean ground turkey (white meat only)
- Halibut
- Herring
- Mackerel
- Pork tenderloin
- Salmon (wild is best)

▲ WILD SALMON IS A GREAT SOURCE OF PROTEIN AND OMEGA-3 FATTY ACIDS.

- Sardines
- Shellfish (skip the butter)
- Tilapia
- Tuna
- Turkey breast (without the fat or skin)
- Whitefish
- Venison

**ACCEPTABLE CHOICES**
Stick to once or twice a week – these choices are higher in saturated fat. These items are to be made without batters, breading or additional fat.

- Chicken (dark meat)
- Corned beef
- Duck
- Extra lean ground beef
- Extra lean ham
- Goose
- Lamb
- Lean ground chicken (white meat only)
- Lean ground turkey (white meat only)
- Prime rib
- Steak
- Turkey (dark meat)
- Whole eggs
- Veal

 **RESTRICTED**
These items are high in fat and/or sugars and should not be eaten as part of your regular diet. They are not good sources of protein.

- Bacon – pork or turkey (well cooked till crisp and drained)
- Chicken wings (baked)
- Lean ground beef or pork
- Lean ham

- Lean luncheon meats
- Pan-fried meats (including chicken breast)
- Pork ribs
- Sausages (lean)

**FORBIDDEN**
These items can be eaten only on very rare occasions as a treat.

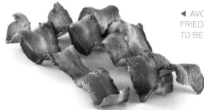

◄ AVOID FATTY AND DEEP-FRIED MEATS IF YOU WANT TO BE LEAN AND HEALTHY.

- Bacon (lightly cooked)
- Breaded and pan-fried meats or fish of any kind
- Deep-fried meats or fish of any kind
- Hot dogs
- Regular ham
- Regular luncheon meats of any kind
- Sausage (regular fat)
- Regular ground beef or pork

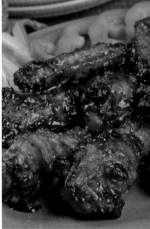

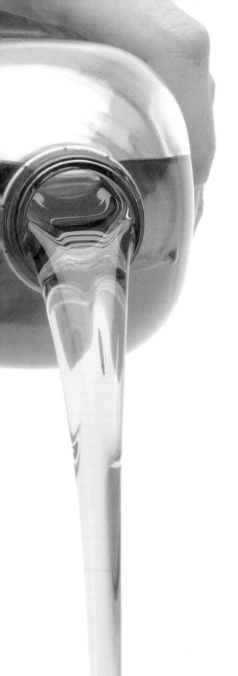

# FATS

Up to three servings
per day
(1 serving = 1-2 Tbsp oil,
⅛-¼ cup nuts or seeds,
4-7 oz fatty fish)

 **BEST CHOICES**

Try to get almost all fats in
your diet from these sources.

- Avocado oil
- Coconut oil/butter (although
  this is a saturated fat, it has
  many healthful qualities)
- Canola oil
- Extra-virgin olive oil
- Cold-pressed oils made from
  nuts and seeds
- Cold-water fatty fish (salmon,
  mackerel, herring, sardines)
- Natural nut butters (without
  hydrogenated oils, added
  sugar or other additives)
- Nuts, especially almonds and
  walnuts (raw, unsalted)
- Seeds, especially flax, hemp
  and chia (raw, unsalted)

## ACCEPTABLE CHOICES

These choices are acceptable
in moderation, but use those
from the list above instead,
if possible. Some of these
choices contain excessive
omega-6.

- Corn oil
- Grapeseed oil

- Safflower oil
- Sunflower oil

 **POOR CHOICES**

These are most commonly
found as ingredients in
other foods.

- Butter
- High-fat dairy products
- High-fat meat products

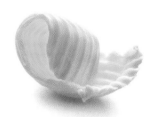

- Palm kernel oil
- Palm oil
- Lard

## FORBIDDEN

Make an effort to never eat
these products.

- Deep-fried foods, including
  nachos, potato chips, fries, etc.
- Hydrogenated vegetable oils
- Partially hydrogenated
  vegetable oils
- Shortening

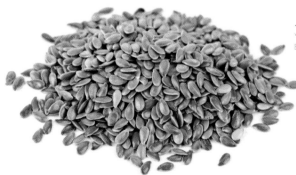

◀ MAKE SURE TO GRIND
YOUR FLAX SEEDS JUST
BEFORE EATING THEM.

## *"My comfort zone has expanded."*

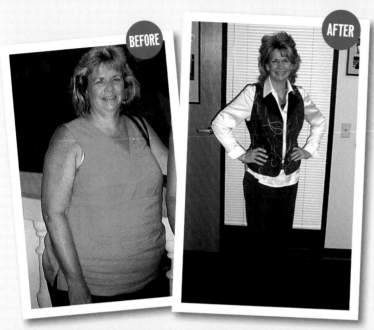

BEFORE

AFTER

**NAME: Bonnie Vemmer**
**AGE: 50**
**HEIGHT: 5'6"**
**WEIGHT BEFORE: 218 lbs**
**WEIGHT AFTER: 138 lbs**
**WEIGHT LOSS: 80 lbs**

**COMING ACROSS A BOTTLE OF ADVIL IN YOUR MEDICINE CABINET HARDLY SEEMS LIKE AN EPIPHANY-EVOKING SCENARIO,** but for the newly thin Bonnie Vemmer, it was exactly that. Upon seeing the little bottle of painkillers, she suddenly realized that she couldn't remember the last time she had needed one – "or four," as she says – because she was no longer experiencing the everyday aches and pains that came from being overweight.

At her heaviest, Bonnie had weighed 218 pounds, and she was well aware that her sedentary lifestyle and diet heavy in fried foods were the culprits. Although she admits she spent most of her life on one diet or another, always trying to lose weight for parties, weddings and vacations, these events came and went and her weight only increased with each passing year.

To make Bonnie's situation even worse, she was trapped in a prison to which she knew she held the key. In fact, Bonnie is the first to acknowledge that she knew she'd feel better about herself if she lost weight. "I have friends who are overweight and claim it does not prevent them from doing things they enjoy," Bonnie says. "That wasn't my case. I just felt very self conscious about my weight and I knew I was allowing it to hold me back." Bonnie was also aware that her weight was something she had complete control over – she just didn't know how to get started.

Fortuitously, that's when Charles D'Angelo entered the picture. At their first meeting, Bonnie soon learned that Charles would only take on clients who would be as committed to his program as he was. There was something about this, and his energy, that made her realize that she was ready to change her life for real this time. Bonnie also liked the fact that that her weight-loss goal was connected to a timeframe. "I was motivated by knowing I would see results within a certain period of time," she says. Charles' program also provided Bonnie with the structure she could never find in other programs. She loves knowing exactly what she's supposed to eat and when.

Now that she's lost 80 pounds, Bonnie can't get over the many ways in which her life has transformed. Would the old Bonnie have been able to climb the 17 flights of stairs to get to her office? No! But the new Bonnie is bursting with energy and vitality. "I'm much healthier at 50 than I was at 40 – and maybe even 30," she says. "I feel happier on the inside. I say 'yes' more often. My comfort zone has expanded."

Bonnie is immensely grateful to Charles for helping her change her perceptions about eating while also teaching her how to have a completely different – and healthy – relationship with food. Because Bonnie's mindset has changed, food does not make her feel the way it used to, and she no longer uses it for comfort or as a stress reliever. "My life had always been good," she says, "but now it is much better. It's so true that it's not about what you lose. It's about all that you gain."

# BALANCING ACT
## Choosing the Best Supplements for Overall Health

*Now that you're embarking on your new, healthy lifestyle, you'll want to think about the best ways to help your body get its daily nutrients. Taking supplements is one way to do this, but are they really necessary?*

*Ideally, no, but it is a good idea to add supplements to your diet when you're not getting adequate amounts of certain nutrients. Think of them like shots of espresso – you may want them for a quick boost, but you may not need them all the time. In other words, you shouldn't rely solely on pills to give your body what it needs. Instead, try to focus on getting most of your nutrients from the healthy foods we all should be eating.*

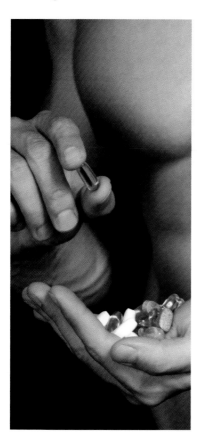

Food is the best source of vitamins, minerals, proteins, healthy fats and carbs, all of which your body needs to function at its best. When you eat a variety of foods, they work together in amazing ways to help nutrients become more active in your body. For example, the vitamin C found in dark leafy greens and citrus fruits helps the body absorb the iron found in lean meats and some veggies. So, as you can see, there is a reason whole foods are the way to go – they have all you need in a convenient little package that tastes delicious, keeps you free of disease and gives you the energy to stay active all day long. Buying food is also much cheaper than buying tons of supplements, which means you'll have some extra cash in your pocket as well!

Sometimes, despite your best efforts to eat a variety of healthy foods, there might be times when you will have to get the nutrients you need from pills. To make things a bit easier for you,

I've listed some of the most important supplements below. Just remember, these are only suggestions. It's best to talk to a dietician or naturopath to find out which supplements you need (if any) and what the proper dosage should be.

## 1 A Good-Quality Multivitamin

The jury is out on the effectiveness of these multi-taskers, but I still think taking them is a good idea – especially during your weight-loss program. You've been mistreating your body for a long time and you're now starting a restrictive diet. Once you have a solid understanding of nutrition and what you need to eat each day, you can decide whether to continue taking them.

## 2 Vitamin D

One of the main roles of vitamin D is to help the body absorb calcium. Also known as the sunshine vitamin (because it is produced in the body when we are exposed to sunlight), this one tops the list of must-have supplements. That's because a lot of us spend most of our time cooped up at the office or at school. In some northern countries, rickets (a bone-softening disease) is making a comeback thanks to the lack of sun and widespread use of sunblock! To get your daily dose, you can sit outside in the sun for 15 minutes or take 1,000 to 2,000 mg of vitamin D.

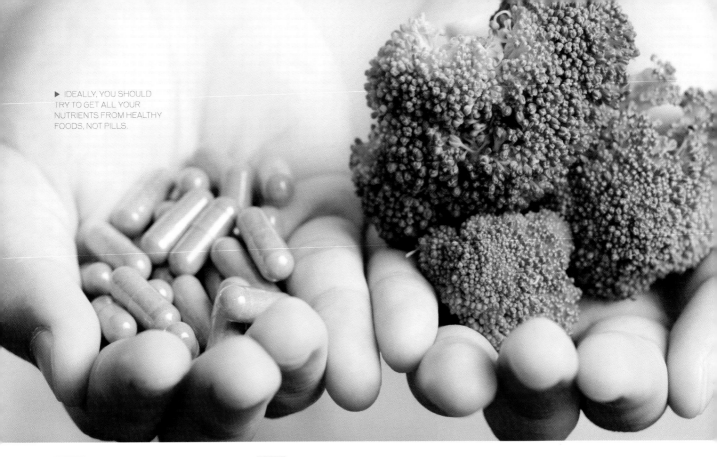

▶ IDEALLY, YOU SHOULD TRY TO GET ALL YOUR NUTRIENTS FROM HEALTHY FOODS, NOT PILLS.

### 3 Fish Oil

Getting enough fish oil may keep your mood in top form in addition to your body and mind. Some health professionals are using doses of fish oil to fight mild depression, inflammation, heart disease and even macular degeneration. All you need each day is 2g of a quality omega-3 fish oil supplement. Make sure the supplement you choose contains a higher concentration of docosahexaenoic acid (DHA) than eicosapentaenoic acid (EPA).

### 4 Probiotics

Probiotics refill your intestines with friendly bacteria, which help break down food and promote nutrient absorption. These tough little guys also help regulate the immune system and keep you healthy by guarding your body against harmful disease-causing bacteria. You can take one capsule three times daily with meals or just follow the bottle directions.

### 5 Hydrochloric Acid

This is the acid sloshing around in your stomach, working hard to break down your food before it enters your intestines. Why am I recommending it? The reality is most people don't create enough stomach acid. We may walk around hopped up on antacids, thinking our heartburn is caused by too much stomach acid, but it's actually caused by the weakening of the muscle that keeps the acid from escaping from your stomach and entering your esophagus. So, regardless of how well you eat, if you don't have enough acid, you can't break down your food optimally. Taking a hydrochloric acid supplement will help fix this problem.

### 6 Calcium

This important mineral does more than build bones and teeth. To learn more about it, see page 164.

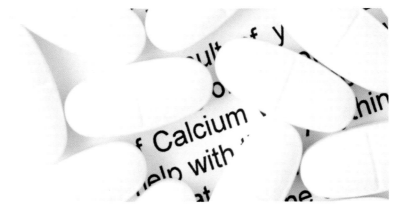

# CHAPTER NINE
## Charles D'Angelo's Scary-Easy Weight-Loss Plan

"Concentrate all your thoughts upon the work at hand. The sun's rays do not burn until brought to a focus."

– Alexander Graham Bell

Here is my plan for you to follow. It doesn't have much variety, but it's straightforward and is certain to work if you stick to it. I even built in what's called a "Refuel Meal," so you can eat a small portion of something you've been craving.

First, you will be eating six times a day – upon waking and every three hours after. I've scheduled the meals to start at 5:30 am each day since many parents, students and employees wake up around then. If you're one of the lucky ones who don't have to wake up this early, then adjust all the mealtimes by moving them forward. For example, if you wake up at 8:00 am, all your meals will be two-and-a-half hours later than shown in the meal-plan chart that follows. Don't worry about eating too late in the day. As long as you are eating these specific six meals a day, you'll do fine no matter what time you eat your last meal. The important thing is to keep your metabolism as active as possible. Eating every three hours and eating as soon as you can upon waking to break your fast (that's where the word breakfast comes from!) will help. Going for long periods of time without food – even four hours – slows down your metabolism. Your eating times need to be consistent, so choose times you can stick with for at least the next two weeks.

You will need to get cardiovascular exercise at least five times a week on my program. If you can do more than five days a week that's great (and I recommend it), but five is all we need. That might mean just walking on a treadmill, depending on your fitness level. If you are a beginner, I recommend starting at a four percent incline at a speed that causes you to perspire. It should be an uphill walk. You don't need to run or jog, but if you are in good enough shape and would enjoy jogging, go ahead. If someone told me I had to run or jog when I first attempted to lose weight, I wouldn't have even tried because I'd have been afraid. Jogging is not necessary for you to lose the weight you deserve to lose.

For now, let's schedule a time in each day that cannot be interrupted. This is the time that you will dedicate to your cardio. Make it as important as taking care of your basic hygiene. It has to be a priority that you don't let others infringe on – at all. If that means first thing in the morning, then get up an hour earlier. (Try to go to bed an hour earlier to make up for the lost sleep). I will never ask you to do more than an hour. Give yourself the whole hour right from the beginning, even though you will start with just 35 minutes of cardio. When you are starting out, don't do more than this. You will gradually increase your time every couple of weeks until you reach your goal weight or until you can go for the full hour, whichever comes first.

Now I have two different plans to offer. If you want to lose more than 50 pounds, go to page 150 for your plan to make it happen. If you want to lose fewer than 50 pounds, go to the next page for your plan. After you've reached your goal, be sure to check out chapter 10, my chapter on the maintenance program so you can make the changes last.

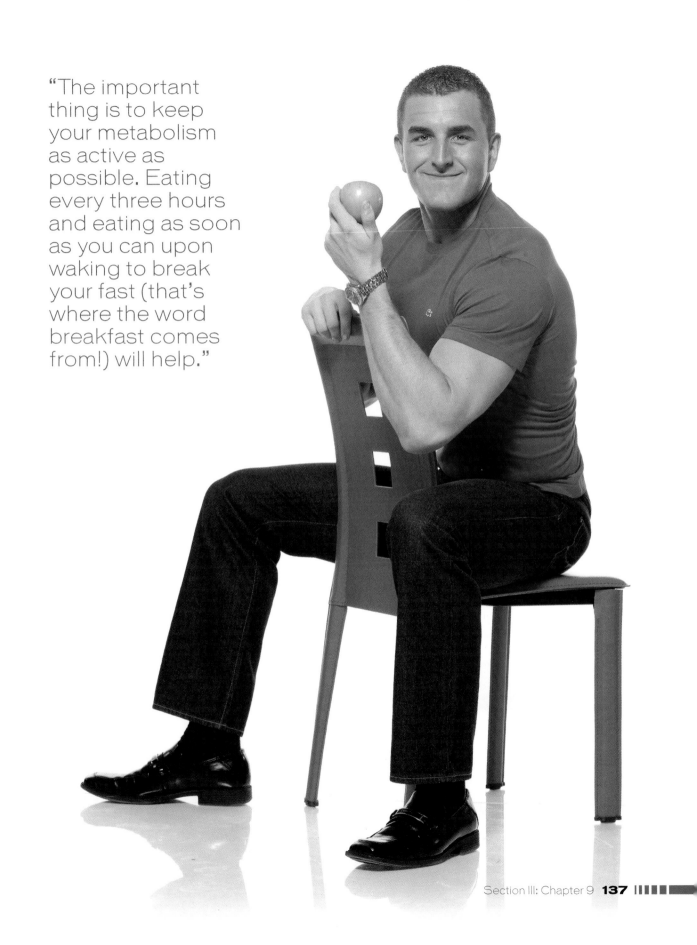

"The important thing is to keep your metabolism as active as possible. Eating every three hours and eating as soon as you can upon waking to break your fast (that's where the word breakfast comes from!) will help."

# Charles D'Angelo's Scary Easy Plan to Lose 50 Pounds or Less

This plan is broken down into six two-week sections. For the duration of each section, you will eat the same foods each day, at the same times each day. If the times don't work for you, you can readjust them as I instructed on page 136. I offer a couple of options for each meal, but this does not mean you can make a different choice each meal! **You must choose which option to follow before beginning the program and then stick to that choice for the duration of each two-week section.** I know this sounds limited, but eating the same foods will help reinforce healthy habits to the point where you will be making decisions automatically. You'll know you are eating the right thing without investing a lot of time and thought (and worry) into deciding what to eat. It also helps break negative thought patterns, and even makes grocery shopping easier!

**NOTE:** *For the entire duration of this plan, drink only zero-calorie beverages such as water, black coffee or tea, herbal teas, unsweetened iced tea, sparkling water, zero-calorie diet sodas, zero-calorie sports drinks or zero-calorie enhanced waters.*

## Berry Good

For your breakfast shake, you can choose up to ¾ cup of any type of berries in place of the 6 strawberries. I recommend strawberries, though, because they are easiest to measure. If you do choose a different fruit, remember that that will be the fruit choice you must eat consistently throughout the plan.

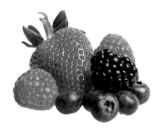

| Weeks 1-2 | |
|---|---|
| **Time** | **Meal Options** |
| **5:30-6:00 am** | ***Protein Shake:*** <br><br>**Option 1:** <br>• 8 oz water <br>• 1 tsp flaxseed oil <br>• 6 frozen strawberries (see sidebar, left) <br>• 2 scoops whey protein (1 scoop for females) (see sidebars, pages 139, 152) <br>*Blend first three ingredients, add whey and blend again.* | **Option 2:** <br>You can use a different type of protein powder or choose a different fruit or choice of fruits up to ¾ cup. Fruit choices: blueberries, raspberries, mango, kiwi, papaya. |
| **8:30-9:00 am** | **Option 1:** <br>• 20 raw natural almonds (non-roasted, no added salt) (see sidebar, page 154) <br><br>**Option 2:** <br>• 1 oz dry roasted soybeans (also known as "soy nuts") or cashews | **Option 3:** <br>• 2 plain rice cakes, each with 1 slice tomato and 1 slice avocado |
| **11:30 am-12:00 pm** | **Option 1:** <br>• Grilled turkey or chicken sandwich made at home with 4-6 oz chicken or turkey meat, mustard, dark green lettuce and whole grain bread <br>***Toppings:*** *lettuce, spinach leaves, onion, tomato, mustard, vinegar and pepper* <br><br>**Option 2:** <br>• 6" turkey breast sub on whole wheat, double meat (4-6 oz meat) | **Option 3:** <br>• 4-oz serving vegetable, beef vegetable or chicken vegetable soup with small whole grain roll or one slice whole grain bread <br><br>**Side options:** <br>• 1 oz bag of baked potato chips (about 15 chips) or 1 banana (choose one side for the entire two-week period.) |

| Weeks 1-2 | |
|---|---|
| Time | Meal Options |
| **2:30- 3:00 pm** | **Option 1:**<br>• 6 oz nonfat, no-sugar-added yogurt<br><br>**Option 2:**<br>• 1 oz dry roasted soybeans or raw cashews | **Option 3:**<br>• 2 plain rice cakes, each with 1 slice tomato and 1 slice avocado |
| **5:30- 6:00 pm** | **Option 1:**<br>• 6-8 oz boneless, skinless chicken or turkey breast, cooked without added fat or salt<br>• 1 Tbsp nonfat sauce, if desired<br>• 2 cups of one or a combination of: asparagus, shredded raw spinach, kale, broccoli, green cabbage<br><br>**Option 2:**<br>• 6-8 oz white fish, cooked without added fat or salt<br>• 1 Tbsp nonfat sauce, if desired<br>• 2 cups of one or a combination of: asparagus, shredded raw spinach, kale, broccoli, green cabbage | **Option 3:**<br>• 6-8 oz tofu cooked without added fat or salt<br>• 1 Tbsp nonfat sauce, if desired<br>• 2 cups of one or a combination of: asparagus, shredded raw spinach, kale, broccoli, green cabbage<br><br>**Option 4:**<br>• 1 cup lentils or beans cooked without added fat or salt<br>• 1 Tbsp nonfat sauce, if desired<br>• 2 cups of one or a combination of: asparagus, shredded raw spinach, kale, broccoli, green cabbage |
| **9:00 pm** | **Option 1:**<br>• 1 all-natural no-sugar-added frozen fruit bar | **Option 2:**<br>Choose any one of the following, and stick with that choice throughout the two-week period:<br>• ½ apple        • 1 clementine<br>• ½ pear         • 1 mango<br>• 1 peach |

Drink only zero-calorie beverages (see note on page 138)

➔ **Saturday Dinner:** Refuel Meal (see page 140)

# Protein 101

➔ You can find protein powder at nutrition stores and many supermarkets.

➔ Most brands include a scoop that usually holds about 24 grams – check the one you purchase.

➔ If you have an allergy to whey protein, or if you travel too often to get to a blender, you may elect to have a two-egg white omelet with diced peppers and onions, and one slice of whole grain bread (or half of a whole grain bagel) at breakfast throughout the program instead of the shake. Just remember, if this is what you choose, this is the option that you have to stick with the whole time!

# Treadmill Tips

If doing 5-6% incline is too much for you, start at 0% or 1% and work your way up toward 5%. The same goes for your speed, if 3.5 mph is too fast, start slower until your aerobic capacity and endurance improves. Once you feel you are more than capable of the recommended speeds and incline, you can increase the incline along with the speed, but don't run! For now, we just want it to be a steady uphill walk that gets you sweating.

If you can't afford a gym or don't have access to equipment, walking outside in your neighborhood for the recommended time and speed is fine – as long as you GET MOVING!

# WEEKS 1-2 EXERCISE
**(5 days per week)**

35 minutes on treadmill, 5% to 6% incline, 3.5 to 4 mph

**Work up a sweat.**

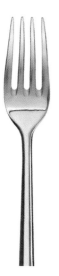

# What is a Refuel Meal?

On every Saturday night throughout my Scary-Easy Weight-Loss Plan, I have included something called a Refuel Meal. This will give you a weekly opportunity to allow yourself to eat more healthy carbohydrates than you've been eating on the plan. The Refuel Meal is not a binge or cheat meal, but a chance to add a bit more variety and flexibility to your life. I offer you this analogy: If you just got your new car washed, waxed and detailed would you then decide to take it off-roading? Of course not! So don't use the Refuel Meal as an excuse to take your new body into the muddy depths of some all-you-can-eat buffet!

By allowing yourself to eat something you've been craving (hopefully healthy carbs) and then realizing that you can get right back on track the next day, you are proving that you are still in control of yourself and your choices. Often when my clients decide to eat a small amount of a forbidden food that was once a source of pleasure for them, they realize that a) the special food isn't nearly as tasty as they had imagined it would be; b) the food makes them feel ill because they are no longer used to eating that way; and c) deviating from the program will not derail them, if they plan for it.

## Refuel Meal Dos and Don'ts

→ **Do** eat a combination of proteins and healthy carbohydrates (both starchy and non-starchy) at every Refuel Meal. Refer to page 126 for a listing of the best choices under each category.

→ **Don't** drink alcohol.

→ **Do** stop eating when you are satisfied (not stuffed).

→ **Don't** eat fried, sugary or high-fat foods.

→ **Do** feel comfortable going off the plan.

→ **Don't** supersize your portions!

| Weeks 3-4 | | |
|---|---|---|
| **Time** | **Meal Options** | |
| 5:30-6:00 am | **Option 1:**<br>***Protein Shake:***<br>• 8 oz water<br>• 1 tsp flaxseed oil<br>• 6 frozen strawberries<br>• 2 scoops whey protein (1 scoop for females)<br>*Blend first three ingredients, add whey and blend again.* | **Option 2:**<br>You can use a different protein powder or choose a different fruit or choice of fruits up to ¾ cup. Fruit choices: blueberries, raspberries, mango, kiwi, papaya. |
| 8:30-9:00 am | **Option 1:**<br>• 20 raw natural almonds (non-roasted, no added salt) | **Option 2:**<br>• 1 oz dry roasted soybeans or cashews<br><br>**Option 3:**<br>• 2 plain rice cakes, each with one slice tomato and one slice avocado |
| 11:30 am-12:00 pm | **Option 1:**<br>• Grilled turkey or chicken sandwich made at home with 4-6 oz chicken or turkey meat, mustard, dark green lettuce and whole grain bread<br>• No more baked potato chips or banana, but you can have raw celery, broccoli or asparagus. So if you chose the "make at home" option, and have been making your own lunch, eliminate the chips too! | **Option 2:**<br>• 6" turkey breast sub on whole wheat, double meat (4-6 oz of turkey on sandwich)<br>***Toppings:*** *lettuce, tomato, onion, spinach leaves, mustard, vinegar and pepper*<br><br>**Option 3:**<br>• 14-oz serving vegetable, beef vegetable or chicken vegetable soup with small whole grain roll or one slice whole grain bread |

## Weeks 3-4

| Time | Meal Options |
|---|---|
| **2:30-3:00 pm** | **Option 1:**<br>• 6 oz nonfat, no-sugar-added yogurt<br><br>**Option 2:**<br>• 1 oz dry roasted soybeans or cashews<br><br>**Option 3:**<br>• 2 plain rice cakes, each with one slice tomato and one slice avocado |
| **5:30-6:00 pm** | **Option 1:**<br>• 6-8 oz boneless, skinless chicken or turkey breast, cooked without added fat or salt<br>• 1 Tbsp nonfat sauce, if desired<br>• 2 cups asparagus<br>(**Exception!** Choose one dish to have throughout the two-week period and then you can have the sirloin steak option only twice per week.)<br><br>**Option 2:**<br>• 8 oz sirloin steak, cooked without added fat or salt<br>• 2 Tbsp nonfat sauce, if desired<br>• 2 cups one or a combination of: asparagus, shredded raw spinach, kale, broccoli, green cabbage, green beans<br><br>**Option 3:**<br>• 8 oz white fish, cooked without added fat or salt<br>• 2 Tbsp nonfat sauce, if desired<br>• 2 cups of one or a combination of: asparagus, shredded raw spinach, kale, broccoli, green cabbage, green beans<br><br>**Option 4:**<br>• 8 oz marinated tofu cooked without added fat or salt<br>• 2 Tbsp nonfat sauce, if desired<br>• 2 cups of one or a combination of: asparagus, shredded raw spinach, kale, broccoli, green cabbage<br><br>**Option 5:**<br>• 1½ cups lentils or beans cooked without added fat or salt<br>• 2 Tbsp nonfat sauce, if desired<br>• 2 cups of one or a combination of: asparagus, shredded raw spinach, kale, broccoli, green cabbage |
| **9:00 pm** | **Option 1:**<br>• 1 or 2 all-natural no-sugar-added frozen fruit bars<br><br>**Option 2:**<br>Choose any one of the following and stick with that choice throughout the two-week period:<br>• ½ apple<br>• ½ pear<br>• 1 peach<br>• 1 clementine<br>• 1 mango |

Drink only zero-calorie beverages

➡ **Saturday Dinner:** Refuel Meal

---

**HERE ARE SOME EXAMPLES OF HEALTHY REFUEL MEALS:**

**Steak Dinner**

- Tenderloin, sirloin or bison steak
- Brown rice
- Salad
- Whole grain dinner roll

**Pasta Night**

- Whole grain pasta with shrimp sauce
- Bruschetta on whole grain bread
- Salad

**Comfort Food Craving**

- Chili mac casserole (made with whole grain pasta, low-fat cheese, tomato-based chili and extra-lean ground beef)
- Salad

**WEEKS 3-4 EXERCISE (5 days per week)**

Treadmill 40 minutes, 5% to 6% incline, 3.5 to 4 miles per hour.

**Work up a sweat.**

## Weeks 5-6

| Time | Meal Options | |
|---|---|---|
| **5:30-6:00 am** | **Option 1:**<br>*Protein Shake:*<br>• 8 oz water<br>• 1 tsp flaxseed oil<br>• 6 frozen strawberries<br>• 2 scoops whey protein (1 scoop for females)<br>*Blend first three ingredients, add whey and blend again.* | **Option 2:**<br>You can use a different protein powder or choose a different fruit or choice of fruits up to ¾ cup. Fruit choices: strawberries, raspberries, mango, kiwi, papaya. |
| **8:30-9:00 am** | **Option 1:**<br>• 20 raw natural almonds (non-roasted, no added salt)<br><br>**Option 2:**<br>• 1 oz dry roasted soybeans or cashews | **Option 3:**<br>• 2 plain rice cakes, each with one slice tomato and one slice avocado |
| **11:30 am-12:00 pm** | **Option 1:**<br>• 7" whole wheat tortilla<br>• 4-6 oz grilled turkey or chicken<br>• Condiments (choose any or all): mustard, lettuce, tomato, peppers, hot peppers, cucumbers, tomatoes, onions<br><br>**Option 2:**<br>• 14-oz serving vegetable, beef vegetable or chicken vegetable soup with small whole grain roll or one slice whole grain bread | **Side options:**<br>• 1 oz bag of baked potato chips (about 15 chips) or 1 banana (choose one side for the entire two-week period.) |
| **2:30-3:00 pm** | **Option 1:**<br>• 6 oz nonfat, no-sugar-added yogurt<br><br>**Option 2:**<br>• 1 oz dry roasted soybeans or cashews | **Option 3:**<br>• 2 plain rice cakes, each with one slice tomato and one slice avocado |

## Weeks 5-6

| Time | Meal Options |
|------|--------------|

**5:30-6:00 pm**

**Option 1:**
- 6-8 oz fish, chicken breast or sirloin steak (steak a maximum of twice weekly), cooked without added fat or salt
- Large vegetable salad (Mix of greens and other raw vegetables. No cheese, croutons, carrots, cauliflower or olives.)
- 1 Tbsp sauce with your meat OR oil and vinegar dressing on salad – not both
- 2 cups one or a combination of: asparagus, shredded raw spinach, kale, broccoli, green cabbage, green beans

**Option 2:**
- 6-8 oz marinated tofu cooked without added fat or salt
- Large vegetable salad (Mix of greens and other raw vegetables. No cheese, croutons, carrots, cauliflower or olives.)
- Oil and vinegar dressing
- 2 cups one or a combination of: asparagus, shredded raw spinach, kale, broccoli, green cabbage

**Option 3:**
- 1½ cups lentils or beans cooked without added fat or salt
- Large vegetable salad (Mix of greens and other raw vegetables. No cheese, croutons, cauliflower or olives.)
- Oil and vinegar dressing
- 2 cups one or a combination of: asparagus, shredded raw spinach, kale, broccoli, green cabbage

**9:00 pm**

**Option 1:**
- 1 or 2 all-natural no-sugar-added frozen fruit bars

**Option 2:**
Choose any one of the following and stick with that choice throughout the two-week period:
- ½ apple
- ½ pear
- 1 peach
- 1 clementine
- 1 mango

Drink only zero-calorie beverages

→ **Saturday Dinner:** Refuel Meal

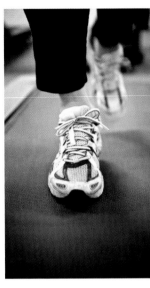

## Step It Up

Cardio getting too easy? Bump up that incline or speed and get the sweat dripping again! Most treadmill inclines go up to 15% – start working your way up to it. If you're on a bike, increase the number of miles you're getting in over the duration.

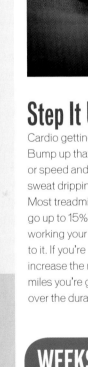

## WEEKS 5-6 EXERCISE
### (5 days per week)

Treadmill 45 minutes, 5% to 6% incline, 3.5 to 4 miles per hour.

**Work up a sweat.**

## Turkey

### 5 Reasons to Gobble It Up

→ This low-fat super-food is high in protein (34 g per 4-oz serving), which helps maintain muscle mass and keeps you full.

→ It is an excellent source of selenium, an immune-boosting antioxidant that can also help regulate thyroid function.

→ Turkey contains niacin, which helps lower cholesterol levels and helps the body turn food into fuel.

→ It's also a good source of vitamin B6, which helps keep blood sugar levels steady.

→ This versatile bird can be prepared in a number of healthy ways (roasted, grilled, stir-fried, on salads and more!).

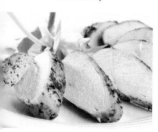

| | Weeks 7-8 | |
|---|---|---|
| **Time** | **Meal Options** | |
| 5:30-6:00 am | **Option 1:**<br>*Protein Shake:*<br>• 8 oz water<br>• 1 tsp flaxseed oil<br>• 6 frozen strawberries<br>• 2 scoops whey protein (1 scoop for females)<br>*Blend first three ingredients, add whey and blend again.* | **Option 2:**<br>You can use a different protein powder or choose a different fruit or choice of fruits up to ¾ cup. Fruit choices: strawberries, raspberries, mango, kiwi, papaya. |
| 8:30-9:00 am | **Option 1:**<br>• 20 raw natural almonds (non-roasted, no added salt)<br><br>**Option 2:**<br>• 1 oz dry roasted soybeans or cashews | **Option 3:**<br>• 2 plain rice cakes, each with one slice tomato and one slice avocado |
| 11:30 am-12:00 pm | **Option 1:**<br>• 7" whole wheat tortilla<br>• 6 oz grilled turkey or chicken<br>• Condiments (choose any or all): mustard, lettuce, tomato, peppers, hot peppers, cucumbers, tomatoes, onions<br>• 1 Tbsp of sauce<br>• No chips or banana | **Option 2:**<br>• 14-oz serving vegetable, beef vegetable or chicken vegetable soup with small whole grain roll or one slice whole grain bread |
| 2:30-3:00 pm | **Option 1:**<br>• 6 oz nonfat, no-sugar-added yogurt<br><br>**Option 2:**<br>• 1 oz dry roasted soybeans or cashews | **Option 3:**<br>• 2 plain rice cakes, each with one slice tomato and one slice avocado |

## Weeks 7-8

| Time | Meal Options |
|---|---|
| **5:30-6:00 pm** | **Option 1:** <br>• 6-8 oz fish, chicken breast or sirloin steak (steak a maximum of twice weekly), cooked without added fat or salt <br>• Large vegetable salad (Mix of greens and other raw vegetables. No cheese, croutons, carrots, cauliflower or olives.) <br>• Oil and vinegar dressing <br>• 2 cups of one or a combination of: asparagus, shredded raw spinach, kale, broccoli, green cabbage, green beans <br><br>**Option 2:** <br>• 6-8 oz marinated tofu cooked without added fat or salt <br>• Large vegetable salad (Mix of greens and other raw vegetables. No cheese, croutons, carrots, cauliflower or olives.) <br>• Oil and vinegar dressing <br>• 2 cups of one or a combination of: asparagus, shredded raw spinach, kale, broccoli, green cabbage <br><br>**Option 3:** <br>• 1½ cups lentils or beans cooked without added fat or salt <br>• Large vegetable salad (Mix of greens and other raw vegetables. No cheese, croutons, carrots, cauliflower or olives.) <br>• Oil and vinegar dressing <br>• 2 cups of one or a combination of: asparagus, shredded raw spinach, kale, broccoli, green cabbage |
| **9:00 pm** | **Option 1:** <br>• 1 or 2 all-natural no-sugar-added frozen fruit bars <br><br>**Option 2:** <br>Choose any one of the following and stick with that choice throughout the two-week period: <br><br>• ½ apple <br>• ½ pear <br>• 1 peach <br>• 1 clementine <br>• 1 mango |

Still only zero-calorie beverages – and yes, still no alcohol!

➜ **Saturday Dinner:** Refuel Meal

"The ultimate measure of a man is not where he stands in moments of comfort and convenience, but where he stands at times of challenge and controversy."

– Martin Luther King, Jr.

## WEEKS 7-8 EXERCISE
### (5 days per week)

Treadmill 50 minutes, 5% to 6% incline, 3.5 to 4 miles per hour.

**Work up a sweat.**

## No Popeye Jokes, Please

If just the mention of spinach brings back traumatic childhood memories, I'm sorry for what I'm about to say: It's time to turn over a new leaf and start a fresh relationship with this superfood. Spinach is jam-packed with vitamins, minerals and antioxidants, which can help prevent cardiovascular and inflammatory diseases as well several types of cancer. The fiber in spinach will help fill you up and improve your digestion, and the lutein it contains can help lower cholesterol and prevent age-related blindness. Spinach is also rich in folic acid, which can reduce the risk of heart disease, Alzheimer's and birth defects.

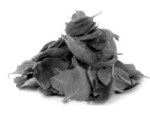

| Weeks 9-10 | | |
|---|---|---|
| Time | Meal Options | |
| 5:30-6:00 am | **Option 1:**<br>***Protein Shake:***<br>• 8 oz water<br>• 1 tsp flaxseed oil<br>• 6 frozen strawberries<br>• 2 scoops whey protein (1 scoop for females)<br>*Blend first three ingredients, add whey and blend again.* | **Option 2:**<br>You can use a different protein powder or choose a different fruit or choice of fruits up to ¾ cup. Fruit choices: strawberries, raspberries, mango, kiwi, papaya. |
| 8:30-9:00 am | **Option 1:**<br>• 20 raw natural almonds (non-roasted, no added salt)<br>**Option 2:**<br>• 1 oz dry roasted soybeans or cashews | **Option 3:**<br>• 2 plain rice cakes, each with one slice tomato and one slice avocado |
| 11:30 am-12:00 pm | **Option 1:**<br>• Grilled chicken or turkey salad: (Mix of greens and other raw vegetables. No cheese, carrots, cauliflower or olives.)<br>• Oil and vinegar dressing<br>**Option 2:**<br>• 14-oz serving vegetable, beef vegetable or chicken vegetable soup with small whole grain roll or one slice whole grain bread | **Side options:**<br>• 1 oz bag of baked potato chips (about 15 chips) or 1 banana (choose one side for the entire two-week period.) |
| 2:30-3:00 pm | **Option 1:**<br>• 6 oz nonfat, no-sugar-added yogurt<br>**Option 2:**<br>• 1 oz dry roasted soybeans or cashews | **Option 3:**<br>• 2 plain rice cakes, each with one slice tomato and one slice avocado |

| Time | Meal Options |
|------|--------------|

## Weeks 9-10

**5:30-6:00 pm**

**Option 1:**
- 6-8 oz fish, chicken breast or sirloin steak (steak a maximum of twice weekly), cooked without added fat or salt
- Large vegetable salad (Mix of greens and other raw vegetables. No cheese, carrots, cauliflower or olives.)
- 1 Tbsp sauce for your meat OR oil and vinegar dressing – not both
- 2 cups of one or a combination of: asparagus, shredded raw spinach, kale, broccoli, green cabbage, green beans

**Option 2:**
- 6-8 oz fish, chicken breast or sirloin steak (steak a maximum of twice weekly), cooked without added fat or salt
- Large vegetable salad (Mix of greens and other raw vegetables. No cheese, carrots, cauliflower or olives.)
- 1 Tbsp sauce for your meat OR oil and vinegar dressing – not both
- 2 cups of one or a combination of: asparagus, shredded raw spinach, kale, broccoli, green cabbage, green beans

**Option 3:**
- 1½ cups lentils or beans cooked without added fat or salt
- Large vegetable salad (Mix of greens and other raw vegetables. No cheese, carrots, cauliflower or olives.)
- Oil and vinegar dressing
- 2 cups of one or a combination of: asparagus, shredded raw spinach, kale, broccoli, green cabbage

**9:00 pm**

**Option 1:**
- 1 or 2 all-natural no sugar added frozen fruit bars

**Option 2:**
Choose any one of the following and stick with that choice throughout the two-week period:
- ½ apple
- ½ pear
- 1 peach
- 1 clementine
- 1 mango

Drink only zero-calorie beverages

➔ **Saturday Dinner:** Refuel Meal

"Do or do not; there is no try."
– Yoda

## WEEKS 9-10 EXERCISE
### (5 days per week)
Treadmill 55 minutes now (Wow, you're getting up there!), 5% to 6% incline, 3.5 to 4 miles per hour.
**Work up a sweat.**

## Weeks 11-12

| Time | Meal Options |
|------|--------------|
| **5:30-6:00 am** | **Option 1:**<br>***Protein Shake:***<br>• 8 oz water<br>• 1 tsp flaxseed oil<br>• 6 frozen strawberries<br>• 2 scoops whey protein (1 scoop for females)<br>*Blend first three ingredients, add whey and blend again.*<br><br>**Option 2:**<br>You can use a different protein powder or choose a different fruit or choice of fruits up to ¾ cup. Fruit choices: strawberries, raspberries, mango, kiwi, papaya. |
| **8:30-9:00 am** | **Option 1:**<br>• 20 raw natural almonds (non-roasted, no added salt)<br><br>**Option 2:**<br>• 1oz dry roasted soybeans or cashews<br><br>**Option 3:**<br>• 2 plain rice cakes, each with one slice tomato and one slice avocado |
| **11:30 am-12:00 pm** | **Option 1:**<br>• Grilled chicken or turkey salad: (3-6 cups of mixed greens and other raw vegetables. 4-6 oz grilled chicken or turkey breast. No cheese, croutons carrots, cauliflower or olives<br>• Oil and vinegar dressing<br><br>**Option 2:**<br>• 14-oz serving vegetable, beef vegetable or chicken vegetable soup with small whole grain roll or one slice whole grain bread<br><br>**Side options:**<br>• 1 oz bag of baked potato chips (about 15 chips) or 1 banana (choose one side for the entire two-week period.) |
| **2:30-3:00 pm** | **Option 1:**<br>• 6 oz nonfat, no-sugar-added yogurt<br><br>**Option 2:**<br>• 1 oz dry roasted soybeans or cashews<br><br>**Option 3:**<br>• 2 plain rice cakes, each with one slice tomato and one slice avocado |

## Weeks 11-12

| Time | Meal Options | |
|------|--------------|--|
| 5:30-6:00 pm | **Option 1:**<br>• 6-8 oz fish, chicken breast or sirloin steak (steak a maximum of twice weekly), cooked without added fat or salt<br>• Large vegetable salad (Mix of greens and other raw vegetables. No cheese, croutons, carrots, cauliflower or olives.)<br>• Oil and vinegar dressing<br>• 2 cups one or a combination of: asparagus, shredded raw spinach, kale, broccoli, green cabbage, green beans | **Option 2:**<br>• 6-8 oz marinated tofu cooked without added fat or salt<br>• Large vegetable salad (Mix of greens and other raw vegetables. No cheese, croutons, carrots, cauliflower or olives.)<br>• Oil and vinegar dressing<br>• 2 cups one or a combination of: asparagus, shredded raw spinach, kale, broccoli, green cabbage<br><br>**Option 3:**<br>• 1½ cups lentils or beans cooked without added fat or salt<br>• Large vegetable salad (Mix of greens and other raw vegetables. No cheese, carrots, cauliflower or olives.)<br>• Oil and vinegar dressing<br>• 2 cups one or a combination of: asparagus, shredded raw spinach, kale, broccoli, green cabbage |
| 9:00 pm | **Option 1:**<br>• 1 or 2 all-natural no sugar added frozen fruit bars | **Option 2:**<br>Choose any one of the following and stick with that choice throughout the two-week period:<br>• ½ apple<br>• ½ pear<br>• 1 peach<br>• 1 clementine<br>• 1 mango |

Drink only zero-calorie beverages

➔ **Saturday Dinner:** Refuel Meal

**AFTER THIS PHASE,** in weeks 13-14, simply drop out the chips at lunch. Continue with this diet and exercise phase until you are losing one pound or less a week and then start the whole process over, adding all the foods back in that were there in the beginning, and reduce the cardio back down to just 35 minutes to stimulate your metabolism again. Repeat this cycle until you reach your goal weight and then head over to the maintenance plan on page 166!

# Perfect to the Core

Delicious, portable, inexpensive and good for you – it's no wonder Thoreau called it "the noblest of fruits." One medium-sized apple contains 17% of your daily fiber and 14% of your vitamin C, and is loaded with free-radical-fighting antioxidants. Just make sure you wash it well and leave the skin on, as that's where most of the fiber and nutrients are found.

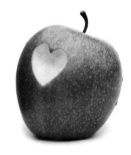

# WEEKS 11-12 EXERCISE
## (5 days per week)
Treadmill for 60 minutes! You're at an hour a day – bravo!

# Charles D'Angelo's Scary-Easy 12-Week Plan to Lose 50 Pounds or More

This plan is broken down into six two-week sections. For the duration of each section, you will eat the same foods each day, at the same times each day. If the times don't work for you, you can readjust them as I instructed on page 136. I offer a couple of options for each meal, but this does not mean you can make a different choice at each mealtime! **You must choose one of the options before beginning the program and then stick to that choice for the duration of each section.**

**NOTE:** *For the entire duration of this plan, drink only zero-calorie beverages such as water, black coffee or tea, herbal teas, unsweetened iced tea, sparkling water, zero-calorie diet sodas, zero-calorie sports drinks or zero-calorie enhanced waters.*

"The greatest danger for most of us is not that our aim is too high and we miss it, but that it is too low and we reach it."

– Michelangelo

## Weeks 1-2

| Time | Meal Options |
|---|---|
| 5:30-6:00 am | **Option 1:**<br>***Protein Shake:***<br>• 8 oz water<br>• 1 tsp flaxseed oil<br>• 6 frozen strawberries (see sidebar page 138)<br>• 2 scoops whey protein (1 scoop for females) (see sidebars, pages 139, 152)<br>*Blend first three ingredients, add whey and blend again.*<br>• 1⅓ cups lightly sweetened all-natural whole grain cereal. Eat the cereal dry without any milk (similar to eating trail mix).<br><br>**Option 2:**<br>You can use a different protein powder or choose a different fruit or choice of fruits up to 1 cup. Fruit choices: blackberries, blueberries, raspberries, mango, kiwi, papaya.<br><br>**\*Note:** If you have an allergy to whey protein, you may elect to have a two-egg white omelet. |
| 8:30-9:00 am | **Option 1:**<br>• One piece of fresh fruit (e.g., one apple, one orange, one pear, one mango) |
| 11:30 am-12:00 pm | **Option 1:**<br>• Using 3 pieces of whole grain bread, make a double-layer grilled turkey or chicken sandwich, each layer with 3-4 oz meat, mustard, dark green lettuce, tomato and onion.<br><br>**Option 2:**<br>• 12" turkey breast sub on whole wheat, double meat<br>***Optional Toppings:*** *lettuce (romaine preferred), tomato, onion, sprouts, spinach, mustard, vinegar and pepper only*<br><br>**Option 3:**<br>• 4-oz serving vegetable, beef vegetable or chicken vegetable soup with a large whole grain roll or two slices whole grain bread<br><br>**Side options:**<br>• 1 oz bag of baked potato chips (about 15 chips) or 1 banana (choose one side for the entire two-week period.) |

## Weeks 1-2

| Time | Meal Options | |
|---|---|---|
| **2:30-3:00 pm** | **Option 1:**<br>• 6 oz nonfat, no-sugar-added yogurt<br><br>**Option 2:**<br>• 1 oz dry roasted soybeans or cashews | **Option 3:**<br>• 2 plain rice cakes, each with one slice tomato and one slice avocado |
| **5:30-6:00 pm** | **Option 1:**<br>• 8-10 oz boneless, skinless chicken or turkey breast, cooked without added fat or salt<br>• 1 Tbsp nonfat sauce, if desired (throughout the program at dinner)<br>• 2 cups one or a combination of: asparagus, shredded raw spinach, kale, broccoli, green cabbage<br>• 1 cup brown or long grain wild rice.<br><br>**Option 2:**<br>• 8-10 oz white fish, cooked without added fat or salt<br>• 1 Tbsp nonfat sauce, if desired<br>• 2 cups one or a combination of: asparagus, shredded raw spinach, kale, broccoli, green cabbage<br>• 1 cup brown or long grain wild rice | **Option 3:**<br>• 8-10 oz marinated tofu cooked without added fat or salt<br>• 1 Tbsp nonfat sauce, if desired<br>• 2 cups one or a combination of: asparagus, shredded raw spinach, kale, broccoli, green cabbage<br>• 1 cup brown or long grain wild rice<br><br>**Option 4:**<br>• 2 cups lentils or beans cooked without added fat or salt<br>• 1 Tbsp nonfat sauce, if desired<br>• 2 cups one or a combination of: asparagus, shredded raw spinach, kale, broccoli, green cabbage<br>• 1 cup brown or long grain wild rice |
| **9:00 pm** | **Option 1:**<br>• 1 all-natural no-sugar-added frozen fruit bar | **Option 2:**<br>Choose any one of the following and stick with that choice throughout the two-week period:<br>• ½ apple<br>• ½ pear<br>• 1 peach<br>• 1 clementine |

Drink only zero-calorie beverages

➜ **Saturday Dinner:** Refuel Meal (See "What is a Refuel Meal?" on page 140.)

## Slow and Steady...

DON'T WORRY! When tackling the treadmill, if the incline or speed is too difficult at first, starting at a lower incline and slower speed isn't a problem, as long as you're working up a good sweat. The key is to start slowly and gradually increase your speed and incline.

## WEEKS 1-2 EXERCISE
### (5 days per week)

35 minutes on the treadmill, 3% to 6% incline, 2.8 to 3.5 mph.

**Work up a sweat.**

# Whey to Go!

Whey protein powder is the key ingredient of the breakfast shakes you will be drinking every day. Here's why it's so important to this plan:

- It's highly beneficial when losing weight or bodybuilding because it helps build muscle and burn fat.

- The whey in whey protein powder is a by-product of milk after it's been curdled and strained to make cheese. It supplies fat-fighting calcium as well as antioxidants that boost the immune system.

- Whey protein powder contains proteins that aid in muscle repair, making it perfect for a post-workout shake!

- If you're a vegan, there are plant-based protein powders available, including hemp, pea, soy and rice.

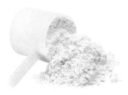

| Weeks 3-4 | |
|---|---|
| Time | Meal Options |
| 5:30-6:00 am | **Option 1:**<br>*Protein Shake:*<br>• 8 oz water<br>• 1 tsp flaxseed oil<br>• 6 frozen strawberries<br>• 2 scoops whey protein (1 scoop for females)<br>*Blend first three ingredients, add whey and blend again.*<br>• 1⅓ cups lightly sweetened, all-natural whole grain cereal, dry<br><br>**Option 2:**<br>You can use a different protein powder or choose a different fruit or choice of fruits up to ¾ cup. Fruit choices: blackberries, blueberries, raspberries, mango, kiwi, papaya. |
| 8:30-9:00 am | **Option 1:**<br>• One piece of fresh fruit (e.g., one apple, one orange, one pear, one mango) |
| 11:30 am-12:00 pm | **Option 1:**<br>• Using three pieces of whole grain bread, make a double-layer grilled turkey or chicken sandwich with 3-4 oz chicken or turkey on each layer, mustard and dark green lettuce, tomato and onion.<br><br>**Option 2:**<br>• 12" turkey breast sub on whole wheat, double meat<br>*Optional Toppings: lettuce, onion, tomato, spinach, sprouts, mustard, vinegar and pepper only*<br><br>**Option 3:**<br>• 4-oz serving vegetable, beef vegetable or chicken vegetable soup with large whole grain roll or two slices whole grain bread<br><br>**Side options:**<br>• 1 oz bag of baked potato chips (about 15 chips) or 1 banana (choose one side for the entire two-week period.) |

## Weeks 3-4

| Time | Meal Options |
|---|---|
| **2:30-3:00 pm** | **Option 1:**<br>• 8 oz nonfat, non-sugar-added yogurt<br><br>**Option 2:**<br>• 1 oz dry roasted soybeans or cashews | **Option 3:**<br>• 2 plain rice cakes, each with one slice tomato and one slice avocado |
| **5:30-6:00 pm** | **Option 1:**<br>• 8-10 oz of chicken, fish or sirloin steak (you may have steak a maximum of two times weekly)<br>• 1 Tbsp sauce<br>• 2 cups of one or a combination of: asparagus, shredded raw spinach, kale, broccoli, green cabbage | **Option 2:**<br>• 8-10 oz marinated tofu cooked without added fat or salt<br>• 2 cups of one or a combination of: asparagus, shredded raw spinach, kale, broccoli, green cabbage<br><br>**Option 3:**<br>• 2 cups lentils or beans cooked without added fat or salt<br>• 2 cups of one or a combination of: asparagus, shredded raw spinach, kale, broccoli, green cabbage |
| **9:00 pm** | **Option 1:**<br>• 1 all-natural no-sugar-added frozen fruit bar | **Option 2:**<br>Choose any one of the following and stick with that choice throughout the two-week period:<br>• 1 apple<br>• 1 pear<br>• 1 peach<br>• 1 clementine |

Drink only zero-calorie beverages

➜ **Saturday Dinner:** Refuel Meal

> "Be faithful in small things because it is in them that your strength lies."
> – Mother Teresa

## WEEKS 3-4 EXERCISE
### (5 days per week)
40 minutes on treadmill at 5% to 6% incline, 3.5 to 4 miles per hour.

**Work up a sweat.**

## Go Nuts!

When you're trying to lose weight, the humble almond can be your best friend. One serving of 20 almonds contains 5 g of protein and about 12% of your recommended daily fiber, both of which will help prevent cravings by keeping you full and satisfied. Almonds are also an excellent source of vitamin E and magnesium, and when eaten on a regular basis, they've been shown to reduce levels of "bad" cholesterol. It's no wonder Dr. Oz calls them "the best snack of all."

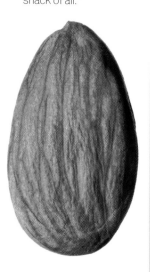

| | Weeks 5-6 | |
|---|---|---|
| **Time** | **Meal Options** | |
| **5:30-6:00 am** | **Option 1:**<br>***Protein Shake:***<br>• 8 oz water<br>• 1 tsp flaxseed oil<br>• 6 frozen strawberries<br>• 2 scoops whey protein (1 scoop for females)<br>*Blend first three ingredients, add whey and blend again.*<br>• 1⅓ cups lightly sweetened, all-natural cereal, dry | **Option 2:**<br>You can use a different protein powder or choose a different fruit or choice of fruits up to 1 cup. Fruit choices: strawberries, raspberries, mango, kiwi, papaya. |
| **8:30-9:00 am** | **Option 1:**<br>• 20 raw natural almonds (non-roasted, no added salt)<br><br>**Option 2:**<br>• 1 oz dry roasted soybeans | **Option 3:**<br>• 2 plain rice cakes, each with one slice tomato and one slice avocado |
| **11:30 am-12:00 pm** | **Option 1:**<br>• 1 x 9-12" whole wheat tortilla wrap<br>• 6 oz grilled turkey or chicken<br>• Condiments (choose any or all): mustard, lettuce, tomato, peppers, hot peppers, cucumbers, tomatoes, onions<br><br>**Option 2:**<br>• 14-oz serving vegetable, beef vegetable or chicken vegetable soup with small whole grain roll or one slice whole grain bread | **Side options:**<br>• 1 oz bag of baked potato chips (about 15 chips) or 1 banana (choose one side for the entire two-week period.) |

## Weeks 5-6

| Time | Meal Options |
|---|---|
| 2:30-3:00 pm | **Option 1:**<br>• 6 oz nonfat, no-sugar-added yogurt<br><br>**Option 2:**<br>• 1 oz dry roasted soybeans or cashews | **Option 3:**<br>• 2 plain rice cakes, each with one slice tomato and one slice avocado |
| 5:30-6:00 pm | **Option 1:**<br>• 6-8 oz fish, chicken breast or sirloin steak (steak a maximum of twice weekly), cooked without added fat or salt<br>• Large vegetable salad (Mix of greens and other raw vegetables. No cheese, croutons, carrots, cauliflower or olives.)<br>• 1 Tbsp sauce for your meat OR oil and vinegar dressing – not both.<br>• 2 cups of one or a combination of: asparagus, shredded raw spinach, kale, broccoli, green cabbage, green beans | **Option 2:**<br>• 8 oz tofu cooked without added fat or salt<br>• Large vegetable salad (Mix of greens and other raw vegetables. No cheese, croutons, carrots, cauliflower or olives.)<br>• Oil and vinegar dressing<br>• 2 cups of one or a combination of: asparagus, shredded raw spinach, kale, broccoli, green cabbage<br><br>**Option 3:**<br>• 1½ cups lentils or beans cooked without added fat or salt<br>• Large vegetable salad (Mix of greens and other raw vegetables. No cheese, croutons, carrots, cauliflower or olives.)<br>• Oil and vinegar dressing<br>• 2 cups of one or a combination of: asparagus, shredded raw spinach, kale, broccoli, green cabbage |
| 9:00 pm | **Option 1:**<br>• 1 all-natural no-sugar-added frozen fruit bar | **Option 2:**<br>Choose any one of the following and stick with that choice throughout the two-week period:<br>• 1 apple<br>• 1 pear<br>• 1 peach<br>• 1 clementine<br>• 1 mango |

Drink only zero-calorie beverages

➜ **Saturday Dinner:** Refuel Meal

"If one advances confidently in the direction of his dreams, and endeavors to live the life which he has imagined, he will meet with a success unexpected in common hours."

– Henry David Thoreau

## WEEKS 5-6 EXERCISE
### (5 days per week)

45 minutes on treadmill at 5% to 6% incline, 3.5 to 4 miles per hour.

**Work up a sweat.**

## Weeks 7-8

| Time | Meal Options | |
|---|---|---|
| **5:30- 6:00 am** | **Option 1:**<br>***Protein Shake:***<br>• 8 oz water<br>• 1 tsp flaxseed oil<br>• 6 frozen strawberries<br>• 2 scoops whey protein (1 scoop for females)<br>*Blend first three ingredients, add whey and blend again.*<br>• 1⅓ cups lightly sweetened, all-natural cereal with skim or 1% milk | **Option 2:**<br>You can use a different protein powder or choose a different fruit or choice of fruits up to ¾ cup. Fruit choices: strawberries, raspberries, mango, kiwi, papaya. |
| **8:30- 9:00 am** | **Option 1:**<br>• 20 raw natural almonds (non-roasted, no added salt)<br><br>**Option 2:**<br>• 1 oz dry roasted soybeans | **Option 3:**<br>• 2 plain rice cakes, each with one slice tomato and one slice avocado |
| **11:30 am- 12:00 pm** | **Option 1:**<br>• 1 x 9-12" whole wheat tortilla wrap<br>• 6 oz grilled turkey or chicken<br>• Condiments (choose any or all): mustard, lettuce, tomato, peppers, hot peppers, cucumbers, tomatoes, onions<br>• 1 Tbsp sauce, if desired (hot sauce, light ranch, etc.)<br>• No chips or banana | **Option 2:**<br>• 14-oz serving vegetable, beef vegetable or chicken vegetable soup with small whole grain roll or one slice whole grain bread |

| Time | Meal Options |
|------|--------------|

## Weeks 7-8

**2:30-3:00 pm**

**Option 1:**
- 6 oz nonfat, no-sugar-added yogurt

**Option 2:**
- ¼ cup dry roasted soybeans or cashews

**Option 3:**
- 2 plain rice cakes, each with one slice tomato and one slice avocado

**5:30-6:00 pm**

**Option 1:**
- 6-8 oz fish, chicken breast or sirloin steak (steak a maximum of twice weekly), cooked without added fat or salt
- Large vegetable salad (Mix of greens and other raw vegetables. No cheese, croutons, carrots, cauliflower or olives.)
- 1 Tbsp sauce for your meat OR oil and vinegar dressing – not both.
- 2 cups of one or a combination of: asparagus, shredded raw spinach, kale, broccoli, green cabbage, green beans

**Option 2:**
- 8 oz marinated tofu cooked without added fat or salt
- Large vegetable salad (Mix of greens and other raw vegetables. No cheese, croutons, carrots, cauliflower or olives.)
- Oil and vinegar dressing
- 2 cups of one or a combination of: asparagus, shredded raw spinach, kale, broccoli, green cabbage

**Option 3:**
- 1½ cups lentils or beans cooked without added fat or salt
- Large vegetable salad (Mix of greens and other raw vegetables. No cheese, croutons, carrots, cauliflower or olives.)
- Oil and vinegar dressing

  2 cups of one or a combination of: asparagus, shredded raw spinach, kale, broccoli, green cabbage

**9:00 pm**

**Option 1:**
- 1 all-natural no-sugar-added frozen fruit bar

**Option 2:**
Choose any one of the following and stick with that choice throughout the two-week period:
- ½ apple
- ½ pear
- 1 peach
- 1 clementine

Still only zero-calorie beverages – and yes, still no alcohol!

➔ **Saturday Dinner:** Refuel Meal

---

# Great Greens!

- Broccoli – This powerful source of vitamin C and fiber also helps your body's immune system fight disease.
- Kale – One cup of kale contains only 34 calories! Not only is it a satisfying part of any meal, but it lowers cholesterol, promotes good eyesight and helps fight off colds and the flu.
- Swiss chard – Along with protein, this leaf provides an abundance of vitamin K for healthy blood, bones and teeth. It also contains vitamins A, C and E.
- Asparagus – As an extremely nutrient-dense vegetable, asparagus has an amino acid named after it called asparagine. It contains no fat or cholesterol and is low in sodium.

# EXERCISE
### (5 days per week)

50 minutes on the treadmill now – great job! Still a 5% to 6% incline, 3.5 to 4 miles per hour.
**Work up a sweat.**

## Weeks 9-10

| Time | Meal Options | |
|------|-------------|---|
| 5:30-6:00 am | **Option 1:**<br>*Protein Shake:*<br>• 8 oz water<br>• 1 tsp flaxseed oil<br>• 6 frozen strawberries<br>• 2 scoops whey protein (1 scoop for females)<br>*Blend first three ingredients, add whey and blend again.*<br>• Cereal is now cut out. | **Option 2:**<br>You can use a different protein powder or choose a different fruit or choice of fruits up to ¾ cup. Fruit choices: strawberries, raspberries, mango, kiwi, papaya. |
| 8:30-9:00 am | **Option 1:**<br>• 20 raw natural almonds (non-roasted, no added salt)<br><br>**Option 2:**<br>• 1 oz dry roasted soybeans | **Option 3:**<br>• 2 plain rice cakes, each with one slice tomato and one slice avocado |
| 11:30 am-12:00 pm | **Option 1:**<br>• Grilled chicken or turkey salad: (3-6 cups of mixed greens and other raw vegetables. 4-6 oz grilled chicken or lean turkey breast. No cheese, croutons, carrots, cauliflower or olives.)<br>• Oil and vinegar dressing<br><br>**Option 2:**<br>• 14-oz serving vegetable, beef vegetable or chicken vegetable soup with small whole grain roll or one slice whole grain bread | **Side options:**<br>• 1 oz bag of baked potato chips (about 15 chips) or 1 banana (choose one side for the entire two-week period.) |

## Weeks 9-10

| Time | Meal Options | |
|---|---|---|
| **2:30- 3:00 pm** | **Option 1:**<br>• 6 oz nonfat, no-sugar-added yogurt<br><br>**Option 2:**<br>• 1 oz dry roasted soybeans or cashews | **Option 3:**<br>• 2 plain rice cakes, each with one slice tomato and one slice avocado |
| **5:30- 6:00 pm** | **Option 1:**<br>• 6-8 oz fish, chicken breast or sirloin steak (steak a maximum of twice weekly), cooked without added fat or salt<br>• Large vegetable salad (Mix of greens and other raw vegetables. No cheese, croutons, carrots, cauliflower or olives.)<br>• Oil and vinegar dressing<br>• 2 cups of one or a combination of: asparagus, shredded raw spinach, kale, broccoli, green cabbage, green beans | **Option 2:**<br>• 8 oz marinated tofu cooked without added fat or salt<br>• Large vegetable salad (Mix of greens and other raw vegetables. No cheese, croutons, carrots, cauliflower or olives.)<br>• 1 Tbsp sauce OR oil and vinegar dressing – not both.<br>• 2 cups of one or a combination of: asparagus, shredded raw spinach, kale, broccoli, green cabbage<br><br>**Option 3:**<br>• 1½ cups lentils or beans cooked without added fat or salt<br>• Large vegetable salad (Mix of greens and other raw vegetables. No cheese, croutons, carrots, cauliflower or olives.)<br>• Oil and vinegar dressing<br>• 2 cups of one or a combination of: asparagus, shredded raw spinach, kale, broccoli, green cabbage |
| **9:00 pm** | **Option 1:**<br>• 1 all-natural no-sugar-added frozen fruit bar | **Option 2:**<br>Choose any one of the following and stick with that choice throughout the two-week period:<br>• 1 apple<br>• 1 pear<br>• 1 peach<br>• 1 clementine<br>• 1 mango |

Drink only zero-calorie beverages

➜ **Saturday Dinner:** Refuel Meal

## "T" Time

Many serious symptoms of obesity go unnoticed because people attribute them to weight and age. In men, these symptoms may include low testosterone. In fact, studies have found a link between obesity and reduced levels of this hormone. Therefore, many of my male clients had been diagnosed with lower than normal testosterone and prescribed testosterone replacement therapy. This hormone helps maintain muscle mass, fat distribution and even sex drive. A physician or endocrinologist (hormone specialist) can run tests on your hormone levels and offer treatment if needed.

## WEEKS 9-10 EXERCISE
### (5 days per week)

55 minutes on the treadmill (almost an hour!) at a 5% to 6% incline, 3.5 to 4 miles per hour.

**Work up a sweat.**

## "My thyroid's making me fat!"

I've often heard this excuse from people trying to stay on a healthy track. They've heard that your thyroid can become "shot" after years of failed dieting, making weight-loss impossible. NOT TRUE! Yes, hypothyroidism can cause metabolic challenges, but that doesn't mean you can't lose weight! Basically, your body is under-producing thyroid hormones, so it isn't processing energy effectively. You can easily have your doctor administer a test, and if you're diagnosed, your doctor will likely prescribe a hormone prescription to remedy it.

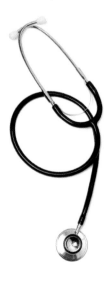

| Weeks 11-12 | |
|---|---|
| Time | Meal Options |
| 5:30-6:00 am | **Option 1:**<br>***Protein Shake:***<br>• 8 oz water<br>• 1 tsp flaxseed oil<br>• 6 frozen strawberries<br>• 2 scoops whey protein<br>*Blend first three ingredients, add whey and blend again.*<br>• Cereal is now cut out. | **Option 2:**<br>You can use a different protein powder or choose a different fruit or choice of fruits up to ¾ cup. Fruit choices: strawberries, raspberries, mango, kiwi, papaya. |
| 8:30-9:00 am | **Option 1:**<br>• 20 raw natural almonds (non-roasted, no added salt) | **Option 2:**<br>• 1 oz dry roasted soybeans<br>• 2 plain rice cakes, each with one slice tomato and one slice avocado |
| 11:30 am-12:00 pm | **Option 1:**<br>• Grilled chicken or turkey salad: (3-6 cups of mixed greens and other raw vegetables. 4-6 oz grilled chicken or turkey breast. No cheese, croutons, carrots, cauliflower or olives.)<br>• Oil and vinegar dressing (not too much oil!)<br>• No chips or banana. | **Option 2:**<br>• 14-oz serving vegetable, beef vegetable or chicken vegetable soup with small whole grain roll or one slice whole grain bread |
| 2:30-3:00 pm | **Option 1:**<br>• 6 oz nonfat, no-sugar-added yogurt<br>**Option 2:**<br>• 1 oz dry roasted soybeans or cashews | **Option 3:**<br>• 2 plain rice cakes, each with one slice tomato and one slice avocado |

## Weeks 11-12

| Time | Meal Options |
|------|--------------|
| **5:30- 6:00 pm** | **Option 1:**<br>• 6-8 oz fish, chicken breast or sirloin steak (steak a maximum of twice weekly), cooked without added fat or salt<br>• Large vegetable salad (Mix of greens and other raw vegetables. No cheese, croutons, carrots, cauliflower or olives.)<br>• Oil and vinegar dressing<br>• 2 cups of one or a combination of: asparagus, shredded raw spinach, kale, broccoli, green cabbage, green beans<br><br>**Option 2:**<br>• 8 oz marinated tofu cooked without added fat or salt<br>• Large vegetable salad (Mix of greens and other raw vegetables. No cheese, croutons, carrots, cauliflower or olives.)<br>• Oil and vinegar dressing<br>• 2 cups of one or a combination of: asparagus, shredded raw spinach, kale, broccoli, green cabbage<br><br>**Option 3:**<br>• 1½ cups lentils or beans cooked without added fat or salt<br>• Large vegetable salad (Mix of greens and other raw vegetables. No cheese, croutons, carrots, cauliflower or olives.)<br>• 1 Tbsp sauce for your meat OR oil and vinegar dressing – not both.<br>• 2 cups of one or a combination of: asparagus, shredded raw spinach, kale, broccoli, green cabbage |
| **9:00 pm** | **Option 1:**<br>• 1 all-natural no-sugar-added frozen fruit bar<br><br>**Option 2:**<br>Choose any one of the following and stick with that choice throughout the two-week period:<br>• 1 apple<br>• 1 pear<br>• 1 peach<br>• 1 clementine<br>• 1 mango |

Drink only zero-calorie beverages

➜ **Saturday Dinner:** Refuel Meal

> "We cannot solve our problems with the same thinking we used when we created them."
>
> – Albert Einstein

## WEEKS 11-12 EXERCISE
**(5 days per week)**

60 minutes on the treadmill! Still 5% to 6% incline or higher, 3.5 to 4 miles per hour. **Work up a sweat.**

**CONTINUE WITH THIS PHASE** until you are losing one pound or less a week. At that point, start the whole process over, including going all the way back down to just 35 minutes of cardio. Once you have lost enough weight that you have fewer than 50 pounds to lose and have finished at least one full cycle on this plan, you may use the plan on page 138.

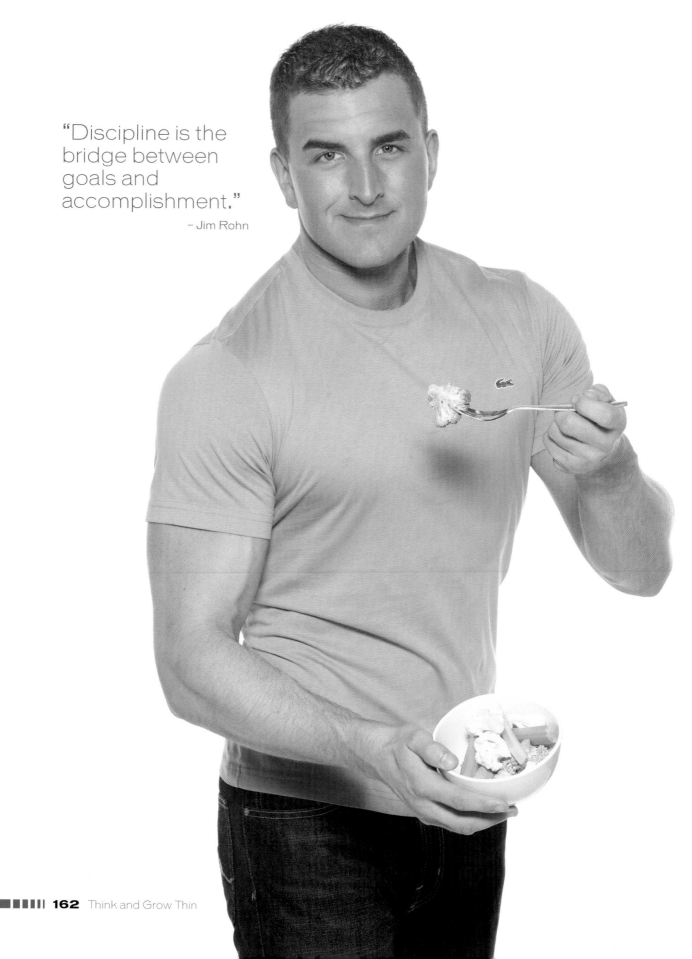

"Discipline is the bridge between goals and accomplishment."

– Jim Rohn

## *Putting the "Vitali" back in vitality!*

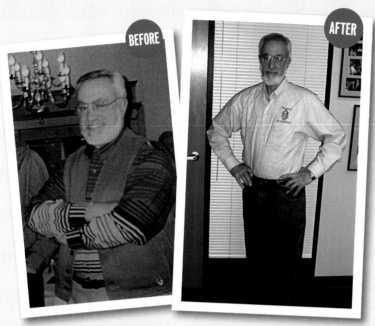

**NAME: Father Ted Vitali**
**AGE: 70**
**HEIGHT: 6'**
**WEIGHT BEFORE: 244 lbs**
**WEIGHT AFTER: 169 lbs**
**WEIGHT LOSS: 75 lbs**

is so fit that every morning he wakes up at 3:00 AM to do cardio and 800 crunches before heading out the door to the university where he teaches!

> *"He now treats unhealthy foods as a recovering alcoholic treats alcohol – calling them 'fatally dangerous.'"*

**CARELESSNESS IN DIET AND EXERCISE LEFT FATHER TED VITALI STRUGGLING WITH HIS WEIGHT. HE HAD DEVELOPED A REGULAR HABIT OF NOSHING ON LARGE AMOUNTS OF PASTA, FATTY FOODS AND FRUIT.** As his weight grew to its peak of 244 pounds, Father Vitali's interest in physical activity decreased. He gradually began to accept his weight and gave up on trying to change. But after some time, Father Vitali started feeling uncomfortable. He noticed a persistent ache in his knees and legs, as well as nagging negative feelings about himself. To top it all off, his doctor placed him on medication for high blood pressure. It was then that he decided something needed to be done!

In his previous efforts to lose weight, Father Vitali had purchased an exercise bike and had even incorporated it into his regular routine. Unfortunately, however, he neglected to clean up his

diet. "Ignorance of what was 'good' food versus 'bad' food kept me from losing weight," he says. But Charles D'Angelo changed all that. He provided Father Vitali with a framework of knowledge to guide him on a path to good health. Just the simple presence of Charles in his life encouraged the naturally disciplined Father Vitali to stick to the plan. Whenever he was tempted, repeating the mantra "Charlie says 'no'" would help Father Vitali overcome his food cravings.

With this marvelous combination of knowledge and discipline, Father Vitali was able to lose 75 pounds in less than one year. This amazing accomplishment was accompanied by the news that he would no longer need his blood pressure medication. Furthermore, his knees and legs no longer ached from all of the excess weight he was carrying. Father Vitali believes he is stronger and healthier now than he was in his 20s. In fact, he

"Charles' mentoring skills are incomparable," Father Vitali says. "I now know what I am doing, and I do it with both knowledge and discipline. I rarely, if ever, 'cheat.'" This decision is partly because his fear of regaining the weight outweighs his desire to eat poorly. He has also had a drastic change in mindset: He now treats unhealthy foods as a recovering alcoholic treats alcohol – calling them "fatally dangerous." Father Vitali's incredible efforts along with Charles' no-fail plan have given Father Vitali his life back – and for that he is immensely grateful.

# BOOST YOUR BONES
## (And More!)
# WITH CALCIUM

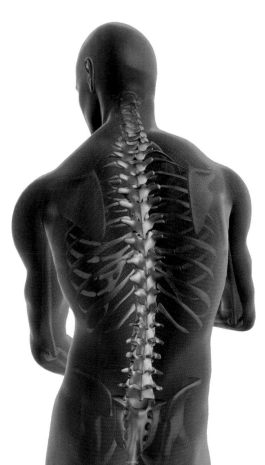

### What is Calcium?

We've all been told that drinking milk will help us grow up strong. That's because milk contains calcium, one of the most important nutrients your body needs. Calcium is necessary to maintain the strength of your bones and teeth, of course, but it also helps regulate nerve and muscle functions, and it allows for blood clotting.

When you were a kid, you really were laying the foundation for the future health of your bones (so hopefully you listened when your parents told you to drink that milk!). In fact, some health professionals have called osteoporosis, a common older person's disease, "a pediatric disease with geriatric consequences." This is because the amount of bone mass that is built up during your childhood will determine how much your bones will weaken later in life. As you age, your body begins to absorb calcium less efficiently, which causes your bone density to decline. You can help prevent this bone loss by eating calcium-rich foods, exercising with weights on a regular basis and avoiding calcium-leaching products such as sodas.

### How Much Calcium Do I Need?

The amount of calcium you need really depends on your age and sex. I've included a chart (at right) so you can find out what's best for you.

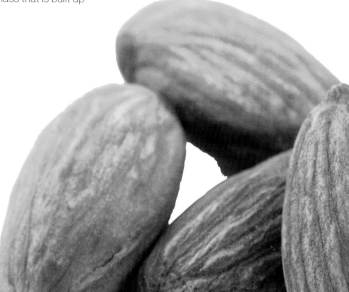

| The recommended daily amounts of calcium are: | | |
| --- | --- | --- |
| Age | RDA (Recommended Daily Allowance) | Daily Maximum |
| 9-18 years | 1,300mg | 3,000mg |
| 19-50 years | | |
| Men | 1,000mg | 2,000mg |
| Women | 1,000mg | 2,500mg |
| 51-70 years | | |
| Men | 1,000mg | 2,000mg |
| Women | 1,200mg | 2,000mg |
| >70 years | 1,200mg | 2,000mg |
| Pregnant &/or Lactating | | |
| 14-18 years | 1,300mg | 3,000mg |
| 19-50 years | 1,000mg | 3,000mg |

*Source: http://www.hc-sc.gc.ca/fn-an/nutrition/vitamin/vita-d-eng.php*

## Where Do I Find Calcium?

The best way to get your calcium and other vitamins and minerals (micronutrients), as well as your protein, carbs and healthy fats (macronutrients), is by eating a variety of whole, natural foods. Check out this list to find out how to add the most calcium to your diet.

## DAIRY PRODUCTS

**Milk:** 1 cup = 300mg
**Yogurt:** 1 cup = 400mg

**NOTE:** While you're on my Scary-Easy Weight-Loss Plan, you will find dairy to be limited. While following this plan or if you are sensitive to dairy or choose not to have it, there are plenty of high-calcium non-dairy choices. Some even contain as much calcium as a glass of milk!

## LEAFY GREENS

**Kale, cooked:** 1 cup = 200mg
**Spinach, cooked:** 1 cup = 250mg
**Broccoli, cooked:**
1 cup = 100mg

## SEAFOOD

**Salmon, bones in:**
6 oz = 300mg
**Seaweed, wakame:**
100g = 150mg

## NUTS/SEEDS

**Almonds:** ⅓ cup = 125mg
**Sesame seeds:** 1 Tbsp = 88mg

## How Do I Make Sure I'm Getting Enough?

If you are not getting enough calcium-rich foods in your diet at a given time, then you need to consider taking a calcium supplement. This may be the case if you're getting less than 1,000 to 1,200mg of calcium out of your food each day. You should also take calcium supplements if you're osteopenic/osteoporotic, postmenopausal, if you drink a lot of soda or coffee (four or more cups per day), if you don't exercise or if you smoke.

**Here are two popular calcium supplements:**

➔ Calcium citrate – doesn't need to be taken with food

➔ Calcium carbonate – needs to be taken with food

So which one should you take? Either supplement will give your body the calcium it needs, so it really depends on your preference. Calcium citrate is easier for the body to absorb because it's wrapped in citric acid, which means it doesn't require extra stomach acid to help it dissolve. On the other hand, calcium carbonate tends to be more commonly available and less expensive, but it may cause gas and bloating or leave you with a chalky taste in your mouth.

Generally, you should take one pill in the morning and one in the evening, and take the pill with vitamin D and magnesium for better absorption. Remember to avoid the foods and lifestyle choices that make it harder for your body to absorb calcium.

# CHAPTER TEN
## Maintenance: The Key to Lasting Results

"Patience and perseverance have a magical effect before which difficulties disappear and obstacles vanish."

– John Quincy Adams

You've made it! You're finally at your goal. You look great, you feel great and you can't go anywhere without everyone talking about your amazing transformation – you're on top of the world. Or maybe you're scared to death, fearing that all the weight you've lost could be regained just as quickly. Many of my clients feel fear or anxiety when they think about the amount of effort required to maintain what they've worked so hard to achieve. The reality is that, as with anything else you fear, once you confront your fear of weight maintenance you realize it's not insurmountable. Yes, you've only just begun your journey. Together we've corrected the mistakes you made in your past. Now it's time for you to embark on the lifestyle that will help you maintain your weight loss for the rest of your life.

You might be feeling invincible right now – and that's great – but before we proceed I would like to offer this word of warning: It's easy to fall back into bad habits. In fact, more than 90 percent of people who lose weight will have gained it all back within two years. But don't worry. Right now we're going to make sure you are part of the 10 percent that keeps it off. It's important to hold yourself accountable, especially if you haven't enlisted the help of a counselor or coach. Since structure works so well for those I personally coach, I am going to provide you with the exact maintenance plan I give to my clients. More rules and limits, you ask? You better believe it! Disci-pline equals freedom! If you stay disciplined and follow a structure that meets your needs, you will never have to be afraid of losing the body you've worked so hard to achieve. When you realize you have control over your food and your lifestyle, you'll continue to grow in ways you never thought possible. During the maintenance segment of my program, food isn't your enemy – spontaneity is! You must not abandon the structure that worked so well for you all along.

The reason 90 percent of people gain back their weight is that they have the idea that they can simply slide back into their old ways after reaching their goal. "Okay, I've lost 100 pounds, so it doesn't matter if I eat these cookies." DANGER! This type of internal dialogue will definitely result in damage to all you've accomplished. Slipping back into old habits is the worst thing you can do. A few cookies may seem harmless at first, but inside your brain those destructive mental associations – the ones that we worked so hard to short circuit – are quickly becoming reestablished. As soon as you begin to think that you're in control

"Many of my clients feel fear or anxiety when they think about the amount of effort required to maintain what they've worked so hard to achieve."

and "everything in moderation" becomes your mantra, you are on a dark path. Moderation is fine, as long as it's planned, followed and is truly moderate. If you walk by someone's desk and gobble down a handful of M&M's you could say, "Oh, it was just a handful and only one time." Wrong! You are veering away from the course and structure you've committed to, worked so hard on and succeeded at. One handful of M&M's eaten unconsciously is

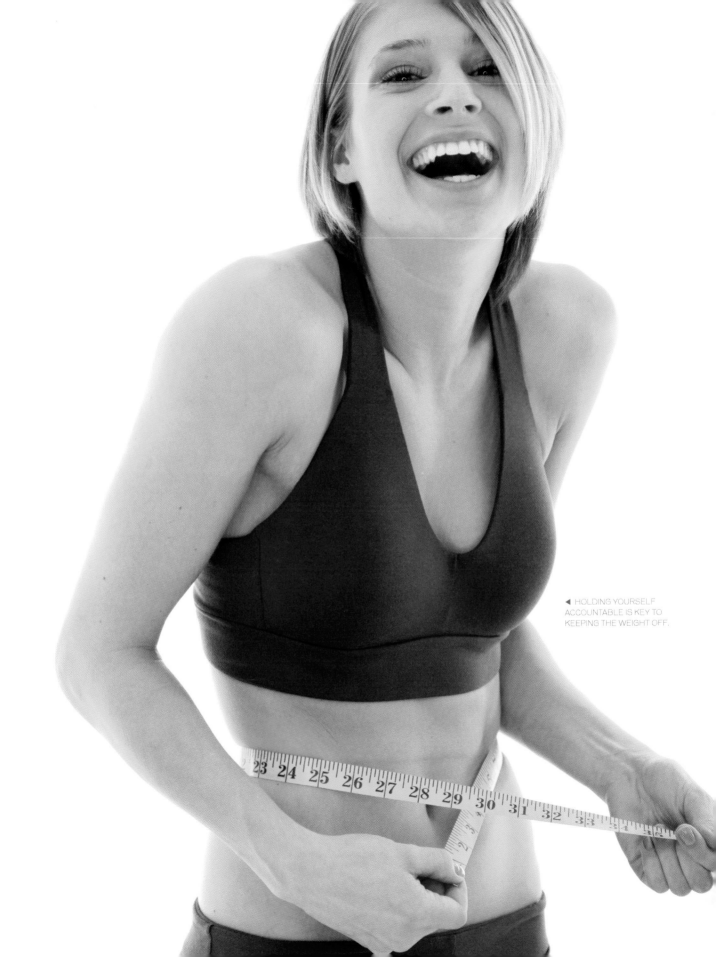

◄ HOLDING YOURSELF
ACCOUNTABLE IS KEY TO
KEEPING THE WEIGHT OFF.

extremely dangerous. It leads back to the place of no control, no plan and no discipline, which will then lead you back to the store to buy bigger clothes again!

If you are going to have something you wouldn't normally eat, such as a Refuel Meal, you need to plan for it. Spontaneously eating a handful of M&M's is the same to me as someone working hard to save money and then spontaneously spending $1,000 on a new outfit. Although that person may have the money to purchase the outfit, doing such a thing consistently – or unconsciously on a consistent basis – will ultimately result in the quick loss of all his or her hard-earned wealth.

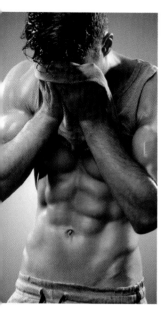

To maintain your ideal weight, you have to make wise choices and you have to make them count. All of the people I've coached to their goals have been able to maintain their success because they've learned how to make healthy eating and exercise fit into their lifestyle. If you've sought the help of a counselor or coach in reaching your goal, you need to strategi-

> "To maintain your ideal weight, you have to make wise choices and you have to make them count. All of the people I've coached to their goals have been able to maintain their success because they've learned how to make healthy eating and exercise fit into their lifestyle."

cally create a step-down plan of less frequent visits so you can become more accountable to yourself. This means it's time to invest in a home scale if you haven't already. I suggest coming up with a weight range in which you're comfortable – no more than three or four pounds above or below your ideal weight. I recommend weighing yourself the morning of your Refuel Meal so you can be certain the week has been a success and you've kept your-

self within the range you've specified. Weighing yourself once a week is enough. This will help you maintain control without becoming obsessed with the number on the scale. After all, ultimately it's your level of health and happiness that matters, not a number. Your weight can be misleading – certain times you may be retaining water, for example. Your energy level, how your clothes fit and your overall health are the best indicators of your physical condition. That being said, a weekly scale reading is very helpful in keeping you where you want to be.

When your weight is near the lower spectrum of your ideal range, you may be a bit more liberal when you have your Refuel Meal. This does not mean having a crazy pig-out; it means you can plan to have a few more carbs than you might otherwise have had. Conversely, if you had a week where you missed several workouts, were not as strict as you should have been on your food plan or weighed in near the high end of your weight range, then you should skip the Refuel Meal altogether that week. Stick to the maintenance plan over the next week and your weight will be back on target.

What is the maintenance plan, you ask? Eat according to the following recommendations 80 percent of the time. Make sure any deviation accounts for less than 20 percent of what you eat. As for exercise, it has to be 100 percent! While you were losing weight, your focus on the foods had to be 100 percent. Now, it's simple math. The amount of food going into your system has to be balanced with what you're expending each day. As we discussed in Chapter 8, your body requires a surprising amount of calories just to perform daily functions. To figure out just how many calories you need to maintain your current weight, see sidebar at right.

The best way to design a maintenance plan is by slowly introducing higher-energy foods such as healthy complex carbs and healthy fats back

# HOW TO CALCULATE YOUR DAILY CALORIE REQUIREMENTS

To find out how many calories you need in order to maintain your current weight, you first need to calculate your Basal Metabolic Rate (BMR) (Step 1). This will tell you approximately how many calories your body burns daily, not including physical activity. Then you need to multiply your BMR by the appropriate activity factor (Step 2). If this sounds like too much math, there are also several online calorie requirement calculators.

## STEP 1:
### Calculate your BMR

**Women**
BMR = 655 + (4.35 x weight in pounds) + (4.7 x height in inches) - (4.7 x age in years)

**Men**
BMR = 66 + (6.23 x weight in pounds) + (12.7 x height in inches) - (6.8 x age in years)

## STEP 2:
### Multiply your BMR by the appropriate activity factor

**Little or no exercise:** Daily calorie needs = BMR x 1.2

**Light exercise, 1-3 days/week:** Daily calorie needs = BMR x 1.375

**Moderate exercise, 3-5 days/week:** Daily calorie needs = BMR x 1.55

**Strenuous exercise, 6-7 days a week:** Daily calorie needs = BMR x 1.725

**Very strenuous exercise and a physical job:** Daily calorie needs = BMR x 1.9

### EXAMPLE:
If your BMR is 1,500 and you exercise moderately, your equation would be:

1,500 x 1.55 = 2,325

The answer (2,325 in this case) is the number of calories you need to eat daily to maintain your current weight.

---

into your diet. Most of us don't need as much energy in the evening, so start off by introducing small quantities of these items to the first three meals of the day, and eventually to all meals except dinner. For example, at breakfast you can now have some cereal with the protein shake that you had first thing every morning during the weight-loss plan. At this point, you can also choose from more options for each meal (You might find it helpful to refer to the list of foods in Chapter 8).

# MAINTENANCE DIET PLAN

### BREAKFAST
One serving of protein and one starchy complex carb
Examples:
• protein shake and a bowl of oatmeal
• eggs and a bowl of cereal
• marinated or scrambled tofu and a bowl of quinoa

### MID-MORNING SNACK
One serving of fruit, healthy fats or high-protein carbs
Examples:
• 1 serving of fruit
• 1 serving of almonds, cashews or dry roasted soybeans
• ½ protein bar
• ⅓ cup cottage cheese with two slices of apple
• Low-fat string cheese stick
• 1 serving of soy yogurt

### LUNCH
One to two servings of starchy complex carbohydrates, one serving of lean protein and one

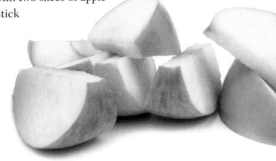

to two servings of non-starchy complex carbs
**Examples:**
- Grilled chicken, turkey or salmon on a salad plus a bag of baked chips or one cup whole grain rice or one serving of roasted sweet potatoes
- Turkey, tuna or chicken sandwich on whole-grain bread
- Black beans, green veggies and avocado on a brown rice wrap
- Tofu or chicken stir-fry on buckwheat soba noodles

### AFTERNOON SNACK
One serving of fruit, healthy fats or high-protein carbs
**Examples:**
- 1 serving of fruit
- 1 serving of almonds or cashews
- ½ protein bar
- ⅓ cup cottage cheese with two slices of apple
- Low-fat string cheese stick
- 1 serving of soy yogurt

### DINNER
One serving of lean protein and two or three servings of non-starchy complex carbs
**Examples:**
- Lean protein (meat, poultry, fish, eggs, tofu, quinoa) with green veggies or salad

### AFTER DINNER
One serving of fruit or high-protein carbs
**Examples:**
- Protein shake
- No-sugar-added fruit popsicle
- Low-fat or Greek yogurt

After two months of maintaining your weight successfully, you can introduce one more Re-fuel Meal to your weekly schedule. This Refuel Meal can be for breakfast, lunch or dinner, but it needs to be scheduled in such a way that your Saturday dinner Refuel Meal (which you've been having all along) is at least two nights after that meal. This means you should have your second weekly Refuel Meal on a

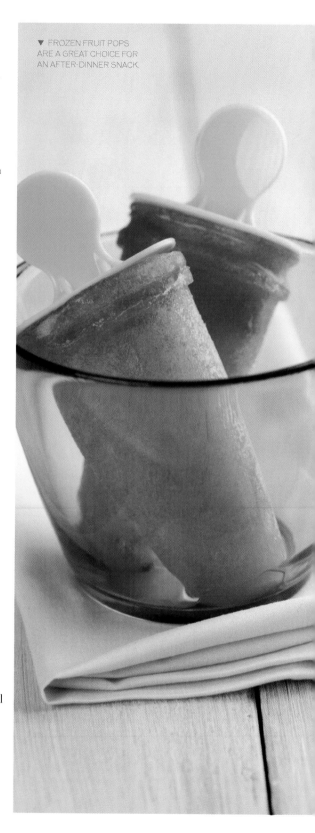

▼ FROZEN FRUIT POPS ARE A GREAT CHOICE FOR AN AFTER-DINNER SNACK.

Tuesday or Wednesday to make sure that it is not too close to your Saturday Refuel Meal.

## MASTERY LEVEL: CREATING A "TEST" DAY

**Note:** The following is a step in mastery. I wouldn't recommend taking this test until you've maintained your weight loss for at least one year. This is an advanced way of testing your commitment to your new way of life. It is not for someone who is fresh to this lifestyle or who believes that straying from the diet, even in a planned way, could trigger a relapse into old habits.

If you've maintained your weight constantly for at least a year, and the thought of eating something you haven't allowed yourself on this weight-loss journey inspires fear in your very core, I understand. When we've achieved tremendous success by following a specific course of action, changing course, even slightly, can seem daunting. But becoming a master of your mind and body requires that you continue to grow and test yourself. In my practice I have encountered clients who fear the idea of having a bowl of ice cream or piece of cake so much that they avoid any socializing where they might have to make a choice about eating or not eating these items. This behavior can eventually lead down a dangerous path toward eating disorders and other psychological issues.

You're bigger than the food! You need to know that you can control yourself. If you will be at a holiday gathering or celebration that is meaningful to someone who would like you to celebrate with them (and to them celebration is equivalent to bad foods) you need to thoroughly think out what you are going to eat during the event, and label that day far in advance as a "test day." This will be a day where you go off-course in a planned way. You will maintain control by having only a small

amount of the food in question, and by resuming your program 100 percent the next day, as planned. By doing so, you've proven to yourself that you are in control. I recommend that you do this only once or twice a year at the most. If your test-day experience is anything like those of my clients, you'll indulge in something rich only to find that it makes you ill – and you won't want to be repeating that incident again, anyway.

I remember days right after reaching my goal weight, when the thought of having one little Hershey's Kiss disturbed me to the point where I thought I could totally mess up everything I'd worked for if it even entered my system! Crazy, right? I've been where you are. I get it. The point is that the food won't

> **"By testing yourself in such a way, you have demonstrated that even though you've consumed a food item that once was a factor in your becoming overweight, that food no longer controls you – you control it."**

screw you up irreversibly – but getting back into the mindset you once had certainly will. While I don't find sweets appealing anymore, I know that if I have them, I am in control and have made a conscious decision to eat them. Although I hate the way these "un-clean" foods make me feel, I know that by taking this test and having them, nothing is lost. I know my mindset about those unhealthy foods hasn't changed in the slightest. I am on target, and the test was a part of the plan. By testing yourself in such a way, you have demonstrated that even though you've consumed a food item

| M | T | W | T | F | S | S |
|---|---|---|---|---|---|---|
|  | 1 | 2 | 3 | 4 | 5 |
| 6 | 7 | 8 | 9 | 10 | 11 | 12 |
| 13 | 14 | 15 | 16 | 17 | 18 | 19 |
| 20 | 21 | 22 | 23 | 24 | 25 | 26 |
| 27 | 28 | 29 | 30 | 31 |  |  |

that once was a factor in your becoming over-weight, that food no longer controls you – you control it. This reality banishes the fear that plagued you when you were overweight. You face it, confront it, test yourself, pass the test and move on. Most of the people I've coached in this step have reported that they actually feel disgusted eating the foods they once believed they couldn't live without! They have to forcefully eat the junk they once craved. They test themselves as rarely as possible because

they know how wonderful their healthy new diet makes them feel and they don't want to go back to feeling lousy and eating the foods that were at the core of their original problem.

What a great revelation! Don't fear food. You are in control. As with a Jedi, this is just another step in mastering yourself, proving that you're bigger than anything you've ever faced or ever will face. You are in control, so long as you choose to be.

▼ YOU WILL BE AMAZED AT HOW WONDERFUL YOUR HEALTHY NEW DIET MAKES YOU FEEL!

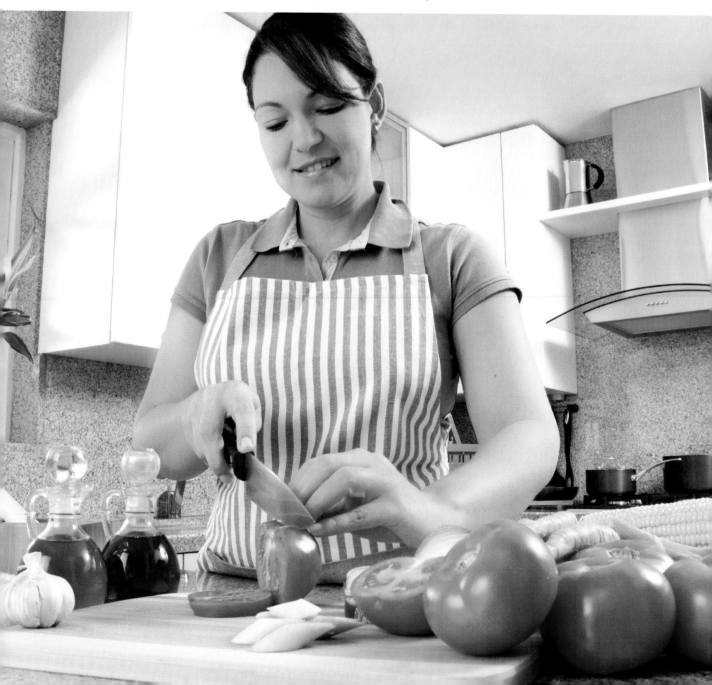

## *"A better, more productive, happier person."*

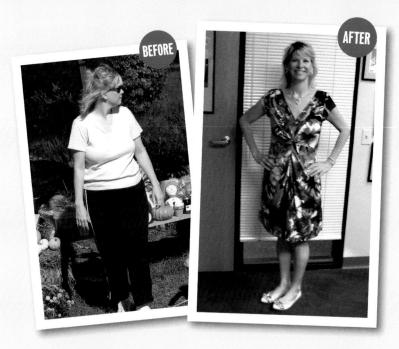

BEFORE

AFTER

**NAME: Cheree Daven**
**AGE: 43**
**HEIGHT: 5'6"**
**WEIGHT BEFORE: 183 lbs**
**WEIGHT AFTER: 135 lbs**
**WEIGHT LOSS: 48 lbs**

**AS A REGISTERED NURSE, CHEREE DAVEN KNEW THE IMPORTANCE OF HEALTHY EATING AND EXERCISE;** unfortunately she didn't make them a part of her lifestyle – at least until she met Charles. Her weight gain had started slowly during high school and increased steadily, year after year, until she was a 183-pound size 18 – numbers Cheree never thought she would see.

Cheree had her "Aha!" moment when she was going through family photos and discovered very few pictures of herself. When she finally came across one, she was horrified. Although her weight had not yet caused any health issues, Cheree knew that they would be lurking around the corner if she didn't make a change – immediately. She didn't want to risk losing out on creating happy memories with her children.

Cheree had tried fad diets before, to no avail, and this time she knew she needed something different. That difference was Charles D'Angelo. Cheree appreciated his passion, confidence and down-to-earth manner, and she felt comfortable knowing that Charles had experienced the same struggles with weight. Cheree had finally found the motivation to begin her journey.

Within days of starting the program, Cheree's weight began to drop. In fact, she says she had never experienced an easier, more healthful form of weight loss than she had on Charles' plan. Cheree's initial goal was to lose 30 pounds, but Charles convinced her she could go for more. Cheree ended up dropping 48 pounds in six months and now wears a flattering size eight! She says she feels better than ever and has ex-

ceeded her wildest dreams. She now has the energy to play with her kids and the confidence to take photos with her children. Oh, and she loves it when her husband calls her "skinny, sexy and hot"!

Best of all, Cheree has realized how important it is to make the time to take care of herself. She forces herself to set aside one hour each day for her workouts so she can be "a better, more productive, happier person." She has also come to terms with her poor eating habits. No longer does she rely on drive-thru meals to get her through the day. She now chooses restaurants where she can order healthy fare that will properly nourish her body.

Cheree is very grateful for Charles and his program. His guidance and support have led her to an incredible weight-loss experience. She relishes the memory of the day she went below 140 pounds, saying she was so thrilled that she grabbed Charles and gave him a massive hug!

# TAKE THE POWER BACK!
## 4 Ways to Combat Emotional Eating

*You've committed to the* **Think and Grow Thin** *program, you've gone shopping for all the right foods and you've bought a treadmill or joined the gym, but you still have to go out and face the world each day, and you're taking "you" with you wherever you go. As I've demonstrated throughout this book, success is more mindset than mechanics. In order for the physical diet and exercise program to work, you need to go on a mental diet. Take the following steps to get your head where it needs to be!*

How many times have you caught yourself opening the fridge after a yelling match with your spouse or children, even though you weren't hungry? How many times have you been sitting in front of the TV, poking your finger around for crumbs at the bottom of the bag of potato chips you'd just opened, telling yourself you'd have only a few? How many times have you dipped a spoon into a container of ice cream for a tiny taste, and then kept going back for more and more?

For a person who struggles with weight, there is almost always an emotional component tied to food. Mindfulness, a technique that involves paying attention to the present moment in a nonjudgmental manner, is a helpful way to reduce the impulsivity associated with emotional eating. Here are some mindfulness techniques that, if practiced consistently, will help you find the power to harness the emotions that sometimes drive your eating behavior.

### 1 Be aware of your "state."

Ask yourself how you're feeling when you feel compelled to eat and it's not time to, especially if you know you cannot logically be hungry. Are you stressed, angry, fearful, bored or excited? Interrupt yourself before you start shoving food in your mouth, take a deep breath and count to 10. With a little forethought, you can halt a mistake that could cost you a whole day or week's worth of great behavior!

### 2 Respond to events instead of reacting to them.

You might think these words mean the same thing, but there is a big difference between responding and reacting, and you need to start being very conscious of this distinction. When we respond to a situation, we look at it carefully and make decisions based on this careful consideration. When we react to a situation, our emotions cause us to act, and do so immediately and unconsciously.

This principle is often taught to those with anger management issues. I believe it is just as appropriate for those who react to their emotions or environment by eating as it is for those

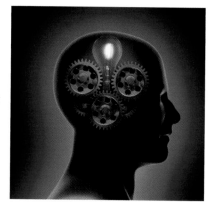

who lose their cool and erupt angrily at those they love. When we react instead of responding, we aren't even reacting to the current situation in reality; we're reacting to our interpretation of the event in the context of a past

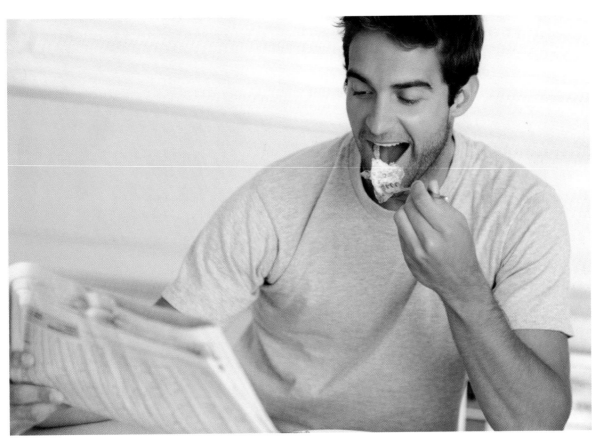

experience. Making quick and irrational decisions based upon something that's not real is never a good idea. As Austrian psychiatrist Viktor Frankl said, "Between stimulus and response there is a space. In that space is our power to choose our response. In our response lies our growth and our freedom."

## 3 Slow down!

The first step to stopping the process of behaving unconsciously is to go about your day in a slower, more planned way. That's one of the reasons you have to decide on just one food choice for each meal in my Scary-Easy Weight-Loss Plan. Forcing yourself to make the decision ahead of time will help to train you to think before you eat. By not allowing options initially, you'll learn to make eating much like getting dressed in the morning – a necessity without much emotionality tied in.

## 4 Savor each bite.

If you've ever polished off a bag of chips in front of the TV, I'm willing to bet that that bag was gone before you knew it! This lack of awareness of hunger and satisfaction is one of the main causes of overeating. If we slow down and pay full attention to the smells, textures and flavors of each bite, as well as our thoughts and the messages our bodies are sending us, we will avoid overeating, enjoy our food more and our digestion will improve.

Here are some tips to help you practice mindful eating:

• Before eating, take note of your emotions and how hungry you are

▲ ELIMINATING DISTRACTIONS IS ONE WAY TO HELP YOU AVOID OVEREATING.

• Sit down and eat at a table – eliminate distractions such as TV, cell phones, etc.
• Take a moment to be grateful for your meal
• Appreciate the way the food looks and smells
• Focus on each mouthful and chew slowly
• Listen to your body and stop eating when you feel 80 percent full (at this point you are actually full; your body just takes a little while to recognize it)
• Pay attention to how you feel when you've finished eating

# CHAPTER ELEVEN
## Cardio: The Key to Fitness

"If you always put a limit on everything you do, physical or anything else, it will spread into your work and into your life. There are no limits. There are only plateaus, and you must not stay there, you must go beyond them."

– Bruce Lee

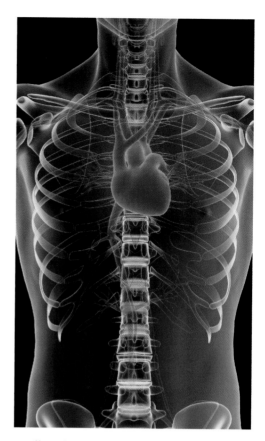

When we picture a fit person, we usually imagine someone who is quite thin. But this isn't necessarily always the case. A thin person can be completely unfit, and a person with a few extra pounds can be very fit. This is because the term "fitness" doesn't specifically refer to weight.

The generally accepted definition of fitness is: the condition of being physically strong and healthy. A person cannot be fit if he or she is very overweight, because excess fat wreaks havoc on the body and prevents a person from being able to properly perform cardiovascular activities. However, all is not lost. Even a severely overweight person can start the process of getting fit simply by slowly and patiently introducing cardiovascular exercise into his or her life.

## CARDIO

Also referred to as aerobic exercise, cardio is the name generally used because this type of exercise stresses, and therefore strengthens, the cardiovascular system. The cardiovascular system is made up of the heart (a muscle) and blood vessels (including arteries, veins and capillaries) with some help from the lungs. Here's how it works: Blood is constantly circulating throughout your body. When you take a breath, blood vessels in your lungs absorb the oxygen, making your blood oxygen rich. Your heart contracts and pushes the oxygenated blood through the arteries. This blood then picks up nutrients from the digestive system and carries the oxygen and nutrients to every tiny cell in your body.

I'm sure you can see that if this system is not functioning properly, you will have serious – and possibly life-threatening – problems. If you have any overweight individuals in your family, you may have heard of the terms atherosclerosis (hardening of the arteries), hypertension (high blood pressure), stroke and heart disease. In fact, if obesity is a problem in your family, there is a good chance your relatives may have suffered from these problems, meaning you should be especially concerned with keeping your cardiovascular system in tip-top shape.

If you want to keep your cardiovascular system in optimal condition (and after what you've just read, who wouldn't?), you have to develop and maintain good habits in the following two aspects of your life. First, a healthy diet is important. In particular, you should eliminate trans fats altogether and substantially decrease your consumption of saturated fats and salt. You should also increase your consumption of omega-3 fatty acids and your consumption of vegetables, especially high-fiber vegetables. Second, you need to get regular, consistent cardiovascular exercise.

## THE HEART IS A MUSCLE

Now it's time to get to the heart of the matter. Yes, there's a reason the word "heart" is used to describe not only the organ we've been discussing but also the central or most vital part of something. The heart is the director, master and governor of the cardiovascular system. If the heart can't pump, the whole system shuts down. And like any other muscle, the heart has to be challenged in order to improve. If you want the muscles in your legs to be stronger, you have to exercise them, right? If you sit on your tush all day, your legs will get weaker. The same is true for your heart. If you are overweight and sedentary, you are putting your heart under severe pressure every day. You are not strengthening your heart with exercise, yet you are asking it to pump blood over ever-increasing distances. That is like asking someone to run a marathon without any training. Your weak heart has to try to pump faster and faster just to get the blood where it's got to go. Conversely, a strong heart is normally a slow heart, because it gives a good, strong contraction that pushes the blood forcefully on its route.

Here's a story to illustrate this concept: Imagine there's a contest between someone who is very strong and healthy and someone who is weak and sickly. They each have to move a rock to a target that is 100 yards away. The strong person takes the rock and hurls it as far as possible. In two or three throws, the rock meets its target and the strong person has barely put forth any effort. The weak person throws the rock but it doesn't go very far. He throws it again, but it barely moves. After a number of throws, this person is too tired to throw and now has to push the rock to the finish line. The weak person has to work far

> "If you are overweight and sedentary, you are putting your heart under severe pressure every day. You are not strengthening your heart with exercise, yet you are asking it to pump blood over ever-increasing distances. That is like asking someone to run a marathon without any training."

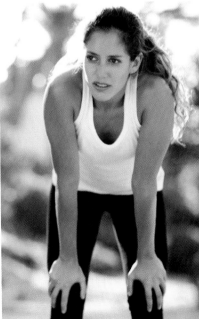

harder than the strong person to get the same result. The same can be said for a weak heart muscle. If you are overweight and in poor cardiovascular condition, you are asking your weak heart to pump blood over far greater distances than the average person. In effect, by being overweight and sedentary you are asking your heart to do far more than the average heart, with far less strength. Your poor heart! It can't talk to you, but if you notice yourself panting after climbing a few stairs, you'll now know that it's trying to tell you something!

So how do you turn your heart into a well-oiled machine that can effortlessly push your blood (and thus oxygen and nutrients) everywhere it needs to go? Simple: cardiovascular exercise.

If you are healthy and between the ages of 18 and 65, The American Heart Association recommends you get 30 minutes of moderate-intensity aerobic exercise at least five times a week, or 20 minutes of vigorous activity at least three times a week to keep your heart functioning at a healthy level. Remember, these are the minimum requirements. To achieve superior cardiovascular fitness you will have to do more than this. In fact, the *Journal of the American Medical Association* states that cardiovascular health is improved when aerobic exercise is performed five times each week.

> ## "Aerobic exercise is any exercise that raises your heart rate over an extended period of time."

Aerobic exercise is any exercise that raises your heart rate over an extended period of time. The word aerobic literally means "with oxygen," and refers to the fact that during aerobic exercise your body uses oxygen to convert fats and carbohydrates into energy. You breathe faster and deeper to bring more oxygen into the lungs, and your heart beats faster and harder to get that oxygen to the cells that need it. These extended exercise sessions increase your lung capacity and your heart strength, both of which improve your cardiovascular fitness.

## MUSCULAR FITNESS AND WEIGHT LOSS

Although knowing that cardiovascular exercise reduces the risk of heart disease and stroke – the most common causes of death – is a great motivator, the benefits of cardio aren't limited to a healthier, more efficient cardiovascular system. According to the Exercise is Medicine program developed by the American College of Sports Medicine, exercise can also decrease depression, reduce the incidence of high blood pressure and diabetes by almost 50 percent and lower the risk of developing Alzheimer's disease by one-third and colon and breast cancer by 60 percent and almost 50 percent, respectively. Of course, exercise also increases your muscular endurance and burns energy (aka calories), which helps you get or stay lean.

In Chapter 8, we explored how exercise itself doesn't make a huge difference in weight loss. That is true to a degree, but the more exercise you get, the more calories you burn, so you certainly can improve your rate of weight loss by increasing the frequency and intensity of the exercise you do. If you were to run at 6 mph, for example, you would burn twice as many calories in the same amount of time as if you were to walk at 3 mph. If you were to run at 6 mph for one hour, you would burn four times the energy that you would by walking at 3 mph for 30 minutes. So, as you can see, weight loss and weight maintenance certainly are improved with an increase in cardio exercise and with an increase in the intensity of that exercise. (Just as long as you don't use your workout as a reason to justify having that big bowl of ice cream or an extra serving at dinner!)

One of the great side effects of regular cardiovascular exercise is the strength it builds in your muscles, specifically endurance strength. Why is this important? Because it means you can enjoy your life a lot more. If your cardiovascular system and your muscles are stronger, you will have more energy and you will be able to sustain that energy for longer periods of time without getting tired. That means you can go dancing. It means on a beautiful summer evening when your husband suggests you go for a walk, it will sound wonderful instead of painful. It means you can play with your kids at the park. It means when your friends are going on a walking tour of Rome you can go too.

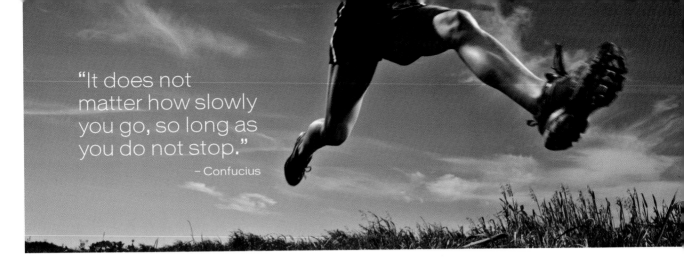

> "It does not matter how slowly you go, so long as you do not stop."
> – Confucius

If you carry a great deal of extra fat, then you know how tiring it is to perform the simplest of tasks. A mere 20 or 25 extra pounds can make going up a flight of stairs exhausting. In fact, most activities that are fun for those who are physically fit do not sound at all fun to you, and the more fat you accumulate, the less enjoyable these activities become. In addition, your fat cells release chemicals called interleukins that can make you feel even more tired and in pain. The vicious cycle continues. But all of this can change once you begin improving your weight and exercising regularly.

Adding regular cardio exercise to your life can seem a bit intimidating at the outset, but so do many other activities that result in positive gains. (Think of home renovation projects, learning a new computer program, etc.) The key is to start slowly and improve consistently. People who are out of shape are often hesitant to begin an exercise program because they feel embarrassed about their lack of ability. In reality, no one can do anything very well when they first begin. Most of the people you see at gyms or running outdoors began as adults, and most of them looked awkward and unskilled when they first started. You assume they were good at it right away because you didn't see them at the beginning! They got to an advanced level of ability by being consistent with their efforts and by challenging themselves to do a little more each time.

It makes no sense to expect yourself to be able to run a marathon, for example, when you are just beginning to exercise. If you decided to play the piano would you expect to just sit down and start banging out a Rachmaninoff concerto? Of course not. You would expect to learn a little this week, a little more next week and so on, slowly progressing to the point where you have the skills to play the more complicated pieces.

There is nothing wrong with a slow progression, as long as you are progressing. Confucius said, "It does not matter how slowly you go, so long as you do not stop." Some very overweight people might find their first attempt at cardio consists of simply lacing up their shoes and walking to the front door. That's fine, as long as the next attempt includes walking to the front door plus five more steps. When developing a cardio routine, the keys to success are to do it at least three times a week, but preferably five (and make sure the two days off are never taken in succession), to do it consistently every week and to give yourself small, achievable goals so your system is always being challenged to reach a higher level of fitness. The starting point will be different for everyone because each individual has his or her own distinct abilities and handicaps. One of the worst things you can do is compare yourself to others. Instead, compare yourself with the "you" of last week or last month. Are you walking further than you did last week? Are you biking faster than you did last week? If you've started a walk/jog program, then are you jogging for longer periods of time than you were last week? If the answer is yes, then you are improving your cardiovascular strength and your muscular endurance. Congratulations!

# INTENSITY

I've mentioned intensity a few times now, and I'd like to go into a little more detail about exercise intensity and aerobic conditioning. Here is a heart-rate chart.

▼ TO FIGURE OUT YOUR HEART RATE, TAKE YOUR PULSE FOR 10 SECONDS AND MULTIPLY BY 6.

## TARGET HEART-RATE ZONES
*Beats Per Minute*

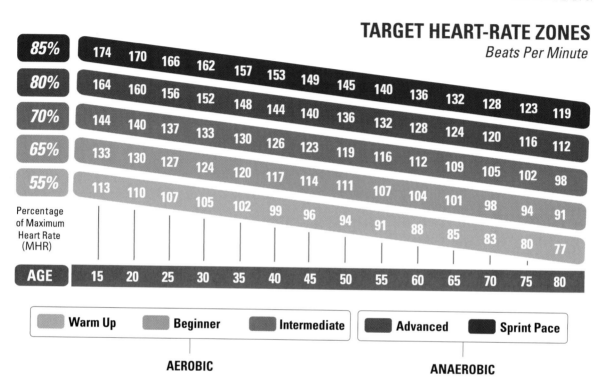

| Percentage of Maximum Heart Rate (MHR) | 15 | 20 | 25 | 30 | 35 | 40 | 45 | 50 | 55 | 60 | 65 | 70 | 75 | 80 |
|---|---|---|---|---|---|---|---|---|---|---|---|---|---|---|
| 85% | 174 | 170 | 166 | 162 | 157 | 153 | 149 | 145 | 140 | 136 | 132 | 128 | 123 | 119 |
| 80% | 164 | 160 | 156 | 152 | 148 | 144 | 140 | 136 | 132 | 128 | 124 | 120 | 116 | 112 |
| 70% | 144 | 140 | 137 | 133 | 130 | 126 | 123 | 119 | 116 | 112 | 109 | 105 | 102 | 98 |
| 65% | 133 | 130 | 127 | 124 | 120 | 117 | 114 | 111 | 107 | 104 | 101 | 98 | 94 | 91 |
| 55% | 113 | 110 | 107 | 105 | 102 | 99 | 96 | 94 | 91 | 88 | 85 | 83 | 80 | 77 |

**AGE**

Warm Up   Beginner   Intermediate    Advanced   Sprint Pace

**AEROBIC**    **ANAEROBIC**

To improve your cardiovascular system through exercise, you must get your heart rate up to at least 55 percent of your maximum heart rate. The basic formula for figuring out your maximum heart rate is 220 minus your age. If you are 40 years old, for example, your maximum heart rate will be 220 minus 40, or 180 beats per minute (bpm). Multiply 180 by 0.55 to figure out the minimum rate at which your heart has to beat during your exercise session in order to be beneficial. In this case, the answer is 99 bpm.

If you are a real beginner and have not been doing any cardio exercise then you will want to keep your heart rate in the 55 to 65 percent range. As you progress, you can challenge yourself up into the 65 to 75 percent range. When your heart rate goes above 80 percent of your maximum, then you are working in the anaerobic range, which is beyond where we want to be right now. Once you have gotten into fairly good shape, you can push yourself into this level in short bursts during your aerobic activity in order to greatly improve your fitness level and calorie burning. Getting to this level takes time and hard work, so this type of training should not be done by anyone in the beginner to intermediate phases of fitness.

# FAT-BURNING MYTH

You will often hear people talk about staying in the "fat-burning" heart-rate zone. You'll even see this on charts on cardio machines and in the machines' preset programs. Many people and even uninformed trainers believe the best way to achieve weight loss is to stay inside the fat-burning zone, but this is simply not reality.

The fat-burning zone simply means that when you exercise within that range, your body uses a higher percentage of fat for energy as opposed to using glucose. The lower your intensity level, the higher the percentage of fat used for energy. This absolutely does not mean that this is the best range for overall fat loss! Your fat loss is determined by the amount of energy you use, not by the percentage of fat versus glucose used. If you increase the intensity of your workout, the total number of calories burned is higher.

Look at it this way: Let's say you run at 6 mph for 30 minutes. During that time you burn 300 calories, 70 percent of which is glucose and 30 percent of which is fat. Then the 100 calories or so of fat you burn comes right out of your fat cells. Great! But the other 200 calories have to come from somewhere, right? They come from the food you eat. If you did not burn those 200 calories of glucose, then that energy might very well become fat. Conversely, if you are losing weight and thus consuming fewer calories than you are burning each day, those 200 calories will have to be replenished by something other than food – and that something is your fat stores. Either way, you end up burning 300 extra calories of energy which will now not be stored as fat on your body.

Now let's compare that to walking at 3 mph for 30 minutes. During that time you burn 150 calories, 60 percent of which is fat. You're in the so-called fat-burning zone, because you are burning a higher percentage of energy as fat. However, you are burning only 90 calories of fat, because you have used less energy

overall. And the other 60 calories you burn come from glucose, which again must be made up somewhere. If you are trying to lose weight by consuming fewer calories than you need for your activities, then these 60 calories of glucose will have to be replenished from your fat stores.

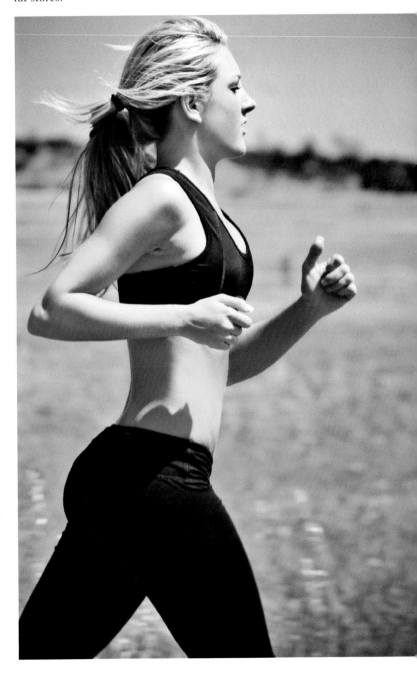

| HIGH-INTENSITY WORKOUT 75-85% of MHR | VS | FAT-BURNING WORKOUT 60-65% of MHR |
|---|---|---|
| Running Speed **6 mph** | | Running Speed **3 mph** |
| Duration **30 minutes** | | Duration **30 minutes** |
| Total Fat Calories Expended **100** | | Total Fat Calories Expended **90** |
| Total Glucose Calories Expended (from food) **200** | | Total Glucose Calories Expended (from food) **60** |
| Total Calories Expended **300** | | Total Calories Expended **150** |

## THE WINNER!

**Remember:** The more energy (calories) you use, the more fat you will lose.

"Cardiovascular exercise will benefit you in so many ways."

In the end, the percentage of calories being used from fat itself or from glucose is completely irrelevant. The goal is to use more energy than you are consuming if you are trying to lose fat. And the more energy you use during your workouts, the more fat you will lose. So the more intense the workout, the more weight you'll lose. But remember, don't increase the intensity until your body is ready for it.

Cardiovascular exercise will benefit you in so many ways. It helps you lose weight, especially when paired with a healthy diet. It benefits your health in extraordinary ways, such as preventing the most common causes of death, including heart disease and stroke. And while it may be tough to get started, you will soon find that regular cardiovascular exercise will lift your spirits and fill you with a vibrancy, energy and confidence you could never have imagined. Instead of reaching for a sugar-loaded snack to boost your energy at the end of the day, you'll be going for a walk or a run because that will boost your energy tenfold (without the horrible sugar crash at the end). In addition, your stronger muscles will help you to engage in all sorts of fun activities that will make your life a true pleasure.

## "*Bursting with newfound energy!*"

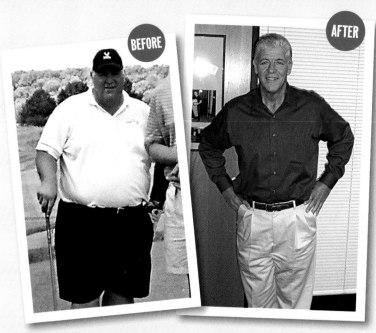

**NAME:** Bruce Baggio
**AGE:** 56
**HEIGHT:** 6'
**WEIGHT BEFORE:** 389 lbs
**WEIGHT AFTER:** 215 lbs
**WEIGHT LOSS:** 174 lbs

**AT A STAGGERING 389 POUNDS, BRUCE BAGGIO WAS PLAGUED BY A SERIES OF WEIGHT-RELATED HEALTH ISSUES.** He was suffering from constant lower-back pain, he relied on hypertension medications to get through each day and he was told he would soon need medication to help control his blood-sugar levels. Bruce also lacked the energy and self-confidence to participate in activities outside of the home, so he chose to hide away indoors. This, in combination with his poor health, meant Bruce was letting his life pass him by. The gravity of the situation finally clicked for him when he realized that he might not live to see his two grandchildren grow up.

Their young spirits were motivation enough for Bruce to finally change his ways. But how would he reach his goals? Bruce thought he had tried every weight-loss program out there – but then he found Charles D'Angelo.

With great compassion and sensitivity, Charles taught Bruce what not to eat (and why) and then gave Bruce a framework laying out exactly which foods he should eat (and when). Bruce especially liked that he didn't have to record his food intake each and every day. The fact that this was a simple program to follow amounted to great success for Bruce.

*"Bruce thought he had tried every weight-loss program out there — but that was before he found out about Charles D'Angelo."*

Eleven months after he began working with Charles, Bruce weighed in at 215 pounds – an incredible loss of 174 pounds! This weight loss resulted in a huge improvement to his health. He was able to significantly reduce the amount of medication he was taking for hypertension while also completely relieving his lower back of pain. Bruce is bursting with newfound energy, which he uses in both his professional and personal lives – especially with his two grandchildren. He says he feels at least 10 years younger!

How does Bruce stay on top of his weight-loss success? He often looks at pictures of himself from when he was obese to remind him of the many challenges he faced during that time. Charles' guidance and support also help keep Bruce on track. He speaks very highly of Charles and his no-nonsense manner. In fact, of the impact Charles has made on his life, Bruce says, "You helped me achieve a goal and a change in my life that I doubted was ever possible."

# BE FIT AND FEARLESS!

## Conquering Your Fear of Joining a Gym

*It's funny to think that the Woody Allen quip – "Eighty percent of life is just showing up." – also applies to working out at the gym. This would explain all of those unused gym memberships, right? It's easy to not go. We can come up with a million excuses: "There aren't enough hours in the day," "I'm not a morning person," "It's too far," "Gas is too expensive," blah, blah, blah! When we start coming up with excuses such as these, normally an underlying fear is the reason. Don't let this fear prevent you from reaching your goals! I'm going to help you beat these feelings by reminding you of the amazing pros of gym membership and then blasting all those flimsy "cons"!*

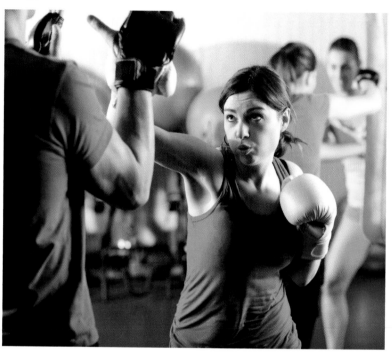

## Pros:

### Camaraderie

Being in the presence of fit, healthy people who are working toward similar goals is a huge motivator. Chances are, you will find you have more in common with your fellow gym-goers than you might have thought, and you may even find yourself making friends with the very people you feared would be judging you! People who go to fitness centers are goal-oriented, which can be very energizing and inspiring for you. Remember that many people join gyms because they need to lose weight, just like you. Just because you're seeing them after they've accomplished that goal doesn't mean they can't relate to you.

### Support

Most good fitness centers make a real effort to hire positive, friendly and supportive staff. These people can help you understand how to use the various machines and weights and will offer words of encouragement, especially when they start to notice that you're coming in on a regular basis. At a good fitness center, staff members keep tabs on who is actually coming to the gym and working out, who shows up but spends the workout time chatting and who doesn't show up at all. What a great way to keep you honest!

### Resources

Once you start to feel comfortable at the gym, you may find that you want to take your training to a new level. If so, one of the ways you can mix things up is by trying a group fitness class. Many gyms offer everything from martial arts to Pilates to water workouts. You can also pick up lots of valuable tips from the trainers. In fact, if you find you are stuck in a rut or trying to break through a plateau, you might want to hire a personal trainer to recharge your routine, stretch your limits and help fire up your motivation.

## Environment

Once you're at the gym (Congratulations! You're one of that 20 percent!), you have no excuse not to work out. At home, temptation abounds and it can be very easy to cut your workout short to check out what's in the fridge, do laundry, answer the phone or catch up on the latest Hollywood gossip. Speaking of excuses, unlike exercising outdoors, working out at the gym also means that neither rain, nor sleet nor snow will hamper your workouts.

# Cons:

## People

You may fear going to a gym because it's full of gorgeous fitness models and cocky beefcakes, and you feel like you don't belong. But step back for a moment and take your personal history and emotion out of the equation. Does this preconception still seem realistic? Remember this: Gyms are for people who want to improve their health and fitness. Does this sound like you? Yes it does! You might be surprised to find out how ordinary the gym-goers actually are. And remember this, too: Most people at the gym are completely focused on themselves and what they are doing. They are paying attention to the muscles they're working on, not you.

## Fee

You will have to pay a monthly or yearly fee to join, and there may be a cost to driving there. But think of this: How much will your weight-related health

issues cost you? How much did it cost you to buy fast food, sodas and the other junk that made you overweight? When I was fat, I spent a lot more money on junk food than I have since spent on my gym membership! And how much will diabetes and heart medications cost you? How much will you have to pay for your future health care when you've been refused insurance because of a preexisting condition? According to one study, obese Americans spend approximately 36 percent more on health care services and 77 percent more on medications than average-sized Americans.[1]

## Distance

Getting to the gym uses too much gas, you have to wake up earlier or come home later, it's out of the way ... all of these are excuses that you can use to convince yourself not to go, and there is some validity to them. Yes, you will have to go out of your way, or use up gas, or get up earlier or stay out later to get to the gym. You will have to change your habits. But this is good! Your habits brought you to where you are now, which is not where you want to be. Once you get used to your new habits, you will have taken a giant leap in the right direction. (And I'm willing to bet that you won't even notice the drive!)

## Fear

Your mind can paint a dreadfully dark picture of something you fear. You might be afraid of trying something new, you might be afraid of failure, you might be afraid that being in a gym environment will bring out your feelings of inferiority. Whatever your fear, you are now in a place where you can combat it. You know you have to try something new because doing the same things you've been doing will not bring you where you want to be. You may feel out of place at first – I sure did – but once you've gone a few times you won't feel that way anymore. And if the gym brings out feelings of inferiority, then use those feelings to spur yourself on. Tell yourself you will succeed at this so you never have to feel that way again!

1. Roland Strum et al. "Obesity and Disability: The Shape of Things to Come." Online Research Brief RB-9043-1, Rand Corporation, 2007.

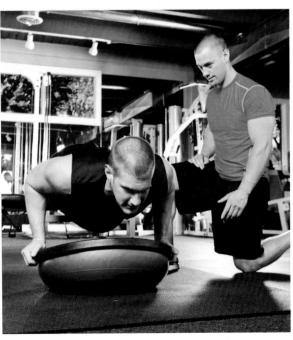

## CHAPTER TWELVE
## Weight Training:
## The Key to Your Dream Body

> "Make the most of yourself,
> for that is all there is of you."
>
> – Ralph Waldo Emerson

We've all seen people we might describe as "too skinny" or "shapeless." While these people are far from overweight, they don't have attractive-looking bodies. Some of them look weak and almost wasted, as if they've had a disease. And in fact, many of these small people are what we call "skinny-fat." This means they have a fairly high body-fat percentage even though they are not technically overweight. A person becomes skinny-fat because he or she does not have very much muscle mass.

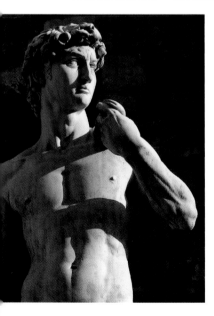

▼ AS MICHELANGELO CARVED BODIES USING CHISEL AND FILE, YOU CAN CARVE YOUR BODY USING FOOD AND EXERCISE.

Have you ever seen a slim-looking woman on the beach with jiggly, cottage-cheese thighs and an upper arm that keeps waving long after she's stopped? You can diet till all your excess weight is gone and you can do cardio till your ticker is stronger than an ox's, but you won't get the shape you desire until you pick up some weights. And there's good reason for this.

The shape you associate with a body is created, for the most part, by muscle. Sure, your skeleton plays a role as well, but attached to those bones are muscles. With the exception of a woman's breasts (made mostly of fat), the curves and angles that together formulate what we think of as an attractive body, whether that body is male or female, are made up of muscle. This is great news for you! It means you don't have to settle with the shape you think you're stuck with! You can decide what shape you want that muscle, and by extension your body, to be, and you can create it.

## BODY SCULPTING

The concept behind sculpting your body is just that. To start off with, your body is whatever shape it is right now, just like a block of marble. And just as a sculptor uses a chisel, hammer and file to shape this block of marble into a masterpiece, you can use food, cardio and weights to shape your body into a masterpiece of your very own.

## MISCONCEPTIONS

There are so many misconceptions about weight training that I hardly know where to begin, but let's start with the idea that women who train with weights will end up looking like Arnold Schwarzenegger circa 1975. Yes, there are female bodybuilders who end up looking like very muscular men. But these women a) eat, breathe, sleep and dream about building muscle and b) may take steroids. The reality is that, with very few exceptions, women have a difficult time building muscle. Those who work hard and persevere are rewarded with beautiful strong curves, not grotesquely bulging muscles.

Women are also often under the mistaken belief that if they do train with weights, these weights should be very light and the repetitions, or reps (the number of times you complete a specific move), should be endless. This belief stems from the misconception above. The theory is that women will get "toned" from using light weights, whereas they get "bulky" from using heavier weights. The reality is that the toned look women seek comes from building muscle and losing fat, and the best way to build that muscle is to use substantial weights.

I can hardly believe that some people still think training with weights will make them muscle bound, but yes some do indeed believe this. The term "muscle bound" means that you have a hard time functioning, moving gracefully or even moving normally because your muscle size restricts you from doing so. While some enormous competitive bodybuilders with great slabs of muscle do reach this point, getting there means basing your whole life around building muscle. These bodybuilders are made up of 250 pounds of solid muscle and practically no fat. Their lifestyles revolve completely around muscle building, with some of them even setting their alarms to wake up every two or three hours through the night in order to drink protein shakes. In addition, yes, some probably do use steroids. People who train with weights as a regular part of their exercise program look great. Those without the goal of becoming enormous with muscle simply do not get that way. Bodybuilders work very hard

to look the way they do – so don't worry! After a few months of weight training, chances are you will start to look and feel amazing, but you won't suddenly wake up looking like Mr. or Ms. Olympia!

You may have heard that if you stop training all of your muscle will turn to fat. This is simply not true. Muscle is muscle and fat is fat. If you stop training then you will lose your muscle. If you continue to eat as much as you did when you were training, you will gain fat. If you stop training and also decrease your calories to compensate, you will not gain fat; you will just decrease your muscle. A better option is to keep training! Conversely, fat does not "turn into" muscle when you begin training. Building muscle increases your metabolism, and if your diet stays the same or if you eat more carefully, you will burn some fat at the same time.

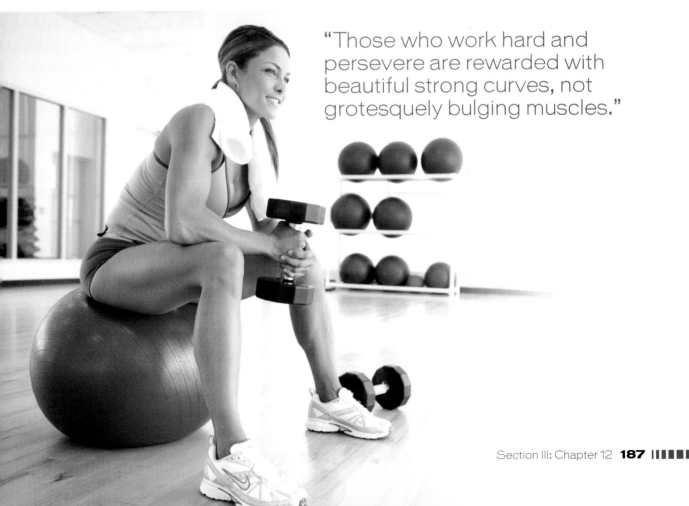

"Those who work hard and persevere are rewarded with beautiful strong curves, not grotesquely bulging muscles."

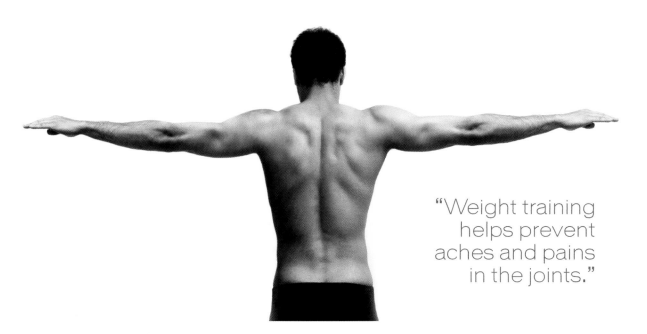

"Weight training helps prevent aches and pains in the joints."

# BENEFITS OF WEIGHT TRAINING

Training with weights builds a beautiful body, sure, but it has many other benefits too.

**1** Building muscle increases your metabolism, even while you sleep. Fat is meant to be stored. That's the whole point of it – to be there in case of starvation. By definition it cannot take much energy to keep fat, because that would defeat its purpose. Muscle, on the other hand, is metabolically active. It takes lots of energy, i.e., calories, to maintain. This means muscle helps you lose fat, and helps prevent you from gaining fat once you've lost it. This doesn't mean once you build some muscle you can eat whatever you want and not gain fat. But, in combination with a good diet, muscle does make keeping your fat off a lot easier.

**2** Weight training helps prevent aches and pains in the joints. Progressive weight training strengthens not only your muscles, but also your tendons and ligaments, making your joints stronger.

**3** More muscle makes you better able to do everyday tasks. Everything from carrying in the groceries to gardening to rearranging the furniture is easier when you've built some muscle.

**4** Weight training strengthens your bones. Women especially need to be concerned about osteoporosis, and training with weights helps prevent it.

**5** Building muscle helps keep you mobile as you age. I'm sure you've seen people who have a hard time getting in and out of chairs. They start to sit and sort of fall the rest of the way. When they're trying to get up they have to push themselves up with their arms, and get to their feet with difficulty. Perhaps you have trouble with this yourself. This is caused by lack of muscle, pure and simple. Lack of muscle also makes us more likely to fall. And if you think it's too late to start training once you're already at that point, think again. Studies show that people in their 90s and even over 100 years old benefit from weight training. Several studies in nursing homes have demonstrated enormous gains in strength, mobility, activity levels and even sleep when elderly residents embarked on a 12-week strength training program.[1]

# BALANCE

Men in particular like to pick and choose which muscles they train and which never get worked. Men are far more likely to work the "mirror muscles" – the ones they see when they look in the mirror. They forget they have a whole other side to them! Typically men like to train their chests and biceps, and then their backs and triceps end up underdeveloped. A guy looks pretty funny when he's developed on one half of his body and undeveloped on the other half. But more than looking funny, he puts himself in danger of injury by having an unbalanced body.

To create a body that is at its best, both functionally and aesthetically, you need to build balance. That means you train your legs as well as your upper body. It means you train both your back and chest. It means whatever muscle you're developing, you need to think of the opposing muscle and develop that too.

# MACHINES VS. FREE WEIGHTS

Many trainers swear you can't get a great body unless you use free weights almost exclusively. A few work mainly with machines. In general, free weights definitely give a better workout, but machines are great for certain exercises, and they are especially useful for beginners.

# HOW OFTEN?

To reap the most benefits from weight training you have to understand that the training session itself stresses the muscle, but muscle growth occurs at rest. If you work the same muscle too often without giving it enough rest between workouts, you will not gain the benefits you think you should from all that effort. The amount of rest you need depends on the effort put forth during the workouts.

Real heavy-duty bodybuilders split their training up, working only one muscle group per workout and sometimes giving it an entire week's rest before working that muscle group again. Beginners will find best results from doing whole-body workouts three times per week. And there are many variations between these extremes. Most people do really well with three or four weight-training sessions per week. I have provided three training programs at the end of this chapter. Once you've been following the beginner program for about six to eight weeks, you can progress to the intermediate training program. Reading as much as you can about weight training and muscle building will help you make the most of your sessions. It's also a great idea to hire a personal trainer to help you reach your goals.

# PROGRESSION!

Just as with cardio, the key to success with weight training is to progress regularly. That's why you will often hear the term "progressive resistance training" being thrown around in the gym. The concept, which originated in ancient Greece, refers to developing strength by progressively increasing resistance (aka the amount of weight you are lifting). No one starts a cardio program able to run a marathon, and no one starts a weight-training program able to lift massive weights. The key in both areas is to challenge yourself every week.

On the next few pages you will find some of the best exercises for working each body part, or muscle group. Explanations of each exercise can be found in the section that follows.

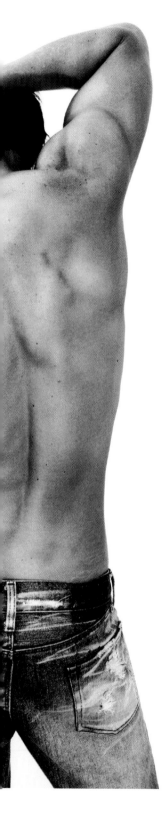

## Gluteals

The gluteus maximus is the largest and most powerful muscle in the body. If you're like most people, you don't think of your butt as being a muscle (it's actually made up of a few muscles, but the gluteus maximus, as its name suggests, is the biggest). Lots of people seem to think a lovely roundness on the buttocks comes from fat, but believe me, when it's made of fat it is not a lovely roundness; instead it looks like a blob that's flat on the top and droopy at the bottom. Unfortunately lots of people do have butts that look like that, and you might be one of them. To get that nice attractive roundness, you need muscle.

**Best exercises for gluteals:** lunges (standing and walking), squats (various forms), cable kickbacks and stiff-leg deadlifts

## Legs

Shapely legs with narrow ankles gracefully sweeping into well-proportioned calves and thighs – weight training can make these yours. If you're a man, you might want solid, masculine legs that look as if you could hold the weight of the world. If you're a woman you may want legs that are sleek and toned. Both of these come from training with weights.

**Best exercises for legs:** squats (various forms), lunges (standing and walking), deadlifts, hamstring curls, stiff-leg deadlifts, standing and seated calf raises

## Back

The back is very complex, with a number of both large and small muscles. The main large muscles are the latissimus dorsi (lats) and the trapezius (traps). Working your back not only helps with everyday strength for carrying things, it also helps keep the back healthy and prevents back pain. Men normally want a V-taper – broad shoulders and lats that taper down into a narrow waist and hips. This comes partly from back training. Women want a toned back without bulges, so they feel comfortable wearing backless dresses, tank tops and swimsuits. Most back exercises also work the biceps and the shoulder muscles.

**Best back exercises:** chin-ups (these are difficult for most people to do, but they are very effective), lat pulldowns, rows (various types), deadlifts and hyperextensions

## Chest

Men normally love working the chest. Women tend to fall into one of two camps – either they avoid chest work altogether or they mistakenly believe chest training will give them larger breasts. Training the chest will never give a woman larger breasts, but it does make the entire chest area look attractive, on a man or a woman. Chest training also benefits the triceps and shoulders, helps with posture and makes you look more confident.

**Best chest exercises:** push-ups, bench presses with a barbell or dumbbells, incline presses, flyes and cable crossovers

## Shoulders

Broad, toned shoulders look fantastic on a man or a woman. Clothes hang nicely on a strong set of shoulders, and they make your waist look extra small in comparison. We can't do much about our bone structure, which affects how broad our shoulders are by nature, but we can definitely build up our shoulder muscles to make them look broad and toned.

"Broad, toned shoulders look fantastic on a man or a woman."

**Best shoulder exercises:** military presses, dumbbell presses (standing or seated), laterals with a dumbbell or cable, upright rows and reverse flyes

# Arms

When you talk about training arms, most people just think "biceps," but in truth this muscle makes up only a third of your upper arm mass, whereas the triceps makes up two thirds. Men are more likely to spend time working the biceps and forgetting about triceps because they associate strength and masculinity with bulging biceps. Women are more likely to train triceps and skip biceps because they are trying to get rid of the upper-arm jiggle. Men and women both need to remember balance – to look your best you need to work both opposing muscles … in this case, triceps and biceps.

**Best arm exercises:** This may sound crazy, but some of the best exercises for your arms are actually exercises for your back and chest.

Chin-ups or lat pulldowns and rows are great for biceps and push-ups and bench presses are great for triceps. An especially good part about these exercises is that they train the whole area, so you get an attractive flow from one muscle into the next. To isolate the biceps, you will want to do biceps curls with a barbell, EZ-curl bar, dumbbells or cables. You can sit or stand for some of these, and there are many slight variations. For triceps, the best exercises are dips, either on a parallel dip apparatus or on benches or even a chair. Other good triceps exercises are lying extensions with a barbell, triceps pressdowns and kickbacks.

# Abs

Before we continue, I want to convince you that doing ab exercises will never give you beautiful abs. Countless people seem to believe that doing hundreds of reps of ab exercises will magically transform their midsections, when the reality is that diet is by far the most important and effective way to an attractive middle. You can do thousands of crunches, but if you have extra fat on top of your abdominal

## Opposing Muscles

To get the idea of opposing muscles, it's helpful to think of the task muscles perform in your body. Muscles are attached to two bones, over a joint (or sometimes more than one joint). The one bone is the stabilizer, and the muscle pulls on the other bone in order to move that part of your body.

For example, your biceps muscle's origin is at the scapula (in the shoulder area). That is the stabilizing bone. The biceps muscle is attached to the radius and ulna – your forearm bones. When you contract your muscle it pulls on your forearm to bring this body part closer to your upper arm. In other words, it bends your arm. So the opposing muscle would be the muscle that pulls your forearm away from your upper arm – in other words, the muscle that straightens your arm. This is the triceps.

### OPPOSING MUSCLES/MUSCLE GROUPS:
**Chest / back**
**Anterior deltoid / posterior deltoid**
**Biceps / triceps**
**Abs / Erector spinae (lower back)**
**Quadriceps / hamstrings**

There are others of course, but these are the main opposing muscle groups for weight-training purposes.

muscles, then your stomach will look as pudgy as ever. For a good-looking middle you have to lose your excess fat. That's the most important step. Then you have to do cardio and weight training in general – this does plenty to tone your middle and make it stronger, because you use your abdominal muscles (as part of your core) to support you in almost any exercise you do. However, you can certainly improve both the look of your midsection and the strength of that area, which will help you prevent lower back strain, by doing ab exercises.

**Best ab exercises:** reverse crunches, hanging leg raises or captain's chair leg raises, bicycle crunches and regular crunches (especially on an exercise ball)

> "As you learn more about training, you will begin to notice which muscles are being worked in each exercise as well as what works best for you."

If you are a beginner, you will want to get set up with a basic program at your gym or use the beginner program later in this chapter. Do it regularly until you're feeling comfortable. Then you can start adding new exercises, doing different rep ranges in order to stimulate the muscle fibers differently, and changing your routine around. As you learn more about training, you will begin to notice which muscles are being worked in each exercise as well as what works best for you. You will also start to feel excitement and exhilaration as your very own masterpiece begins to take shape right before your eyes!

---

1. "Strong Medicine," David Pacchioli, Research/Penn State, Vol. 16, no. 2 (June, 1995)

# Muscle Groups

Unless you are using the intensity technique known as "pre-fatiguing" your muscles, which you will certainly not be doing unless you decide to become a bodybuilder, always start with large muscles/muscle groups at the beginning of the workout and then work your way to smaller muscles/muscle groups. Working smaller muscle groups first makes you unable to effectively work the larger muscle groups. If you were to work your biceps, for example (a smaller muscle), and then work your back (a larger muscle group), then your fatigued biceps, which help you in all back exercises, will be a weak link and prevent you from doing as much as you could for your back. This means your back will not be worked adequately.

**HERE IS THE ORDER YOU SHOULD DO YOUR TRAINING IN:**

**LOWER BODY**

➡ **Glutes**

➡ **Quadriceps**

➡ **Hamstrings**

➡ **Adductor muscles**

➡ **Calves**

**UPPER BODY**

➡ **Back**

➡ **Chest**

➡ **Shoulders**

➡ **Triceps**

➡ **Biceps**

➡ **Forearms**

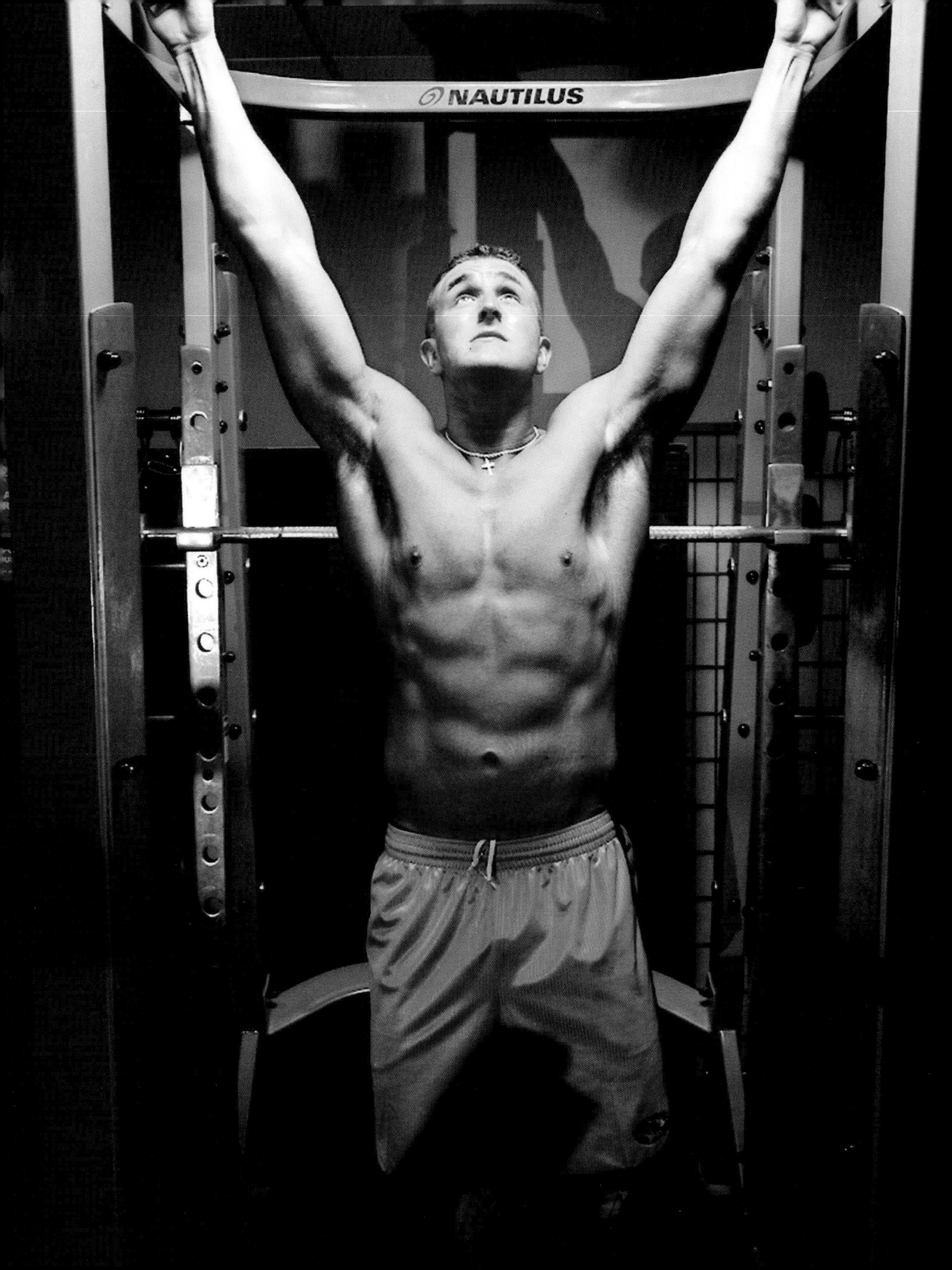
NAUTILUS

# Weight-Training Routines

**NOTE:** Always start by warming up on cardio equipment for five minutes. Your muscles should be warm when you start training with weights to help prevent injury.

## Beginner ▪▪▪▪▪

### Full-Body Workout

Do this workout 3 days per week. For each of the following moves, you should perform 2 sets of 15 reps. This means you will complete an entire movement from start to finish (e.g., bending and then extending your leg in the leg press) 15 times for 1 set, rest for 20 to 30 seconds and then complete the second set by doing the exercise another 15 times.

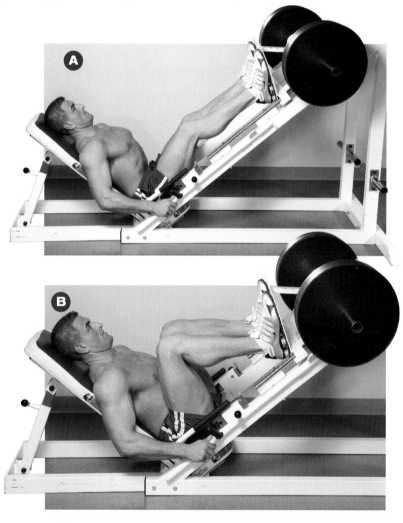

**THIGHS AND BUTTOCKS**

## Leg Press

**TARGET MUSCLES:**
Quadriceps, Glutes and Hamstrings

**SET UP:** Set the machine to an appropriate weight for you. Lie on the machine and place your feet on the footrest, hip-width apart. Push the footrest off the rack and unlock the machine by twisting the handles outward.

**ACTION:** Lower the weight until your legs are bent at a 90° angle, with your knees in line with your ankles. Extend your legs back to the starting position and repeat.

## HAMSTRINGS
# Lying Hamstring Curl

**TARGET MUSCLES:**
Hamstrings

**SET UP:** Adjust the weight on the machine to one that allows you do to 15 reps. Adjust the footrest so that it will fall just above your ankles when you are lying down. Climb into the machine face down, putting your lower legs underneath the footrest.

**ACTION:** Curl the footrest up toward the back of your legs and then return to the starting position with control. Repeat this action.

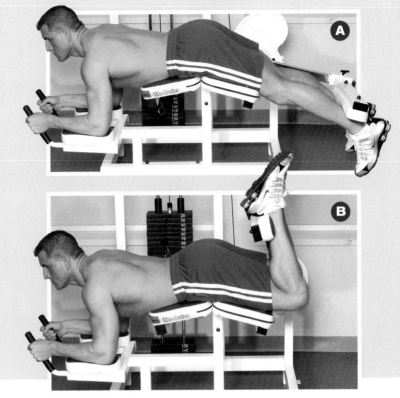

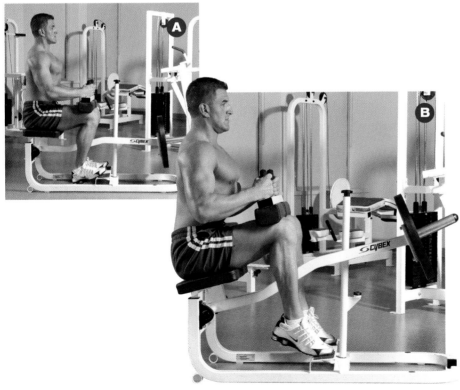

## CALVES
# Seated Calf Raise

**TARGET MUSCLES:**
Soleus

**SET UP:** Adjust the height of the kneepad so it rests lightly on your knees. The balls of your feet should be resting lightly on footrest with your heels extending downward off the footrest to enable a stretch in your calf area.

**ACTION:** Press up onto the balls of your toes to lift the weight. Return to the starting position and repeat this action.

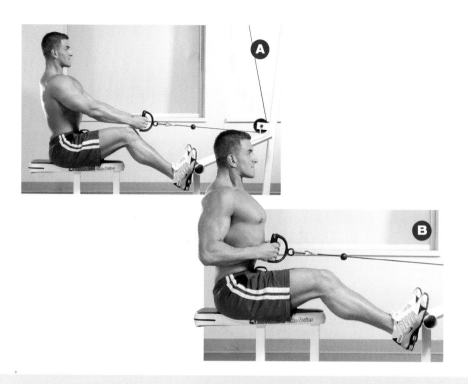

## BACK
# Cable Row

**TARGET MUSCLES:**
Rhomboids, Latissimus Dorsi and Trapezius

**SET UP:** Select an appropriate weight that will allow you to do 15 reps. Select the double-D grip. Bend forward and grasp the handle, and then carefully sit back on the bench with your back upright and a slight bend in your knees. Hold the grip with your arms extended.

**ACTION:** Pull the grip into your midsection, keeping your elbows close to the sides of your body. Return to the starting position. Repeat this action.

## CHEST
# Incline Dumbbell Press

**TARGET MUSCLES:**
Pectoralis Major and Minor

**SET UP:** Adjust the back of an adjustable bench to a 30° – 45° angle, and adjust the seat up to a slight angle. Lie back on the bench with your feet flat on the floor. Hold a dumbbell in each hand with your arms bent, your elbows straight out to the sides and your hands in line with your shoulders.

**ACTION:** Extend your arms so the dumbbells meet above your chest. Lower back to the starting position, keeping your elbows straight out to the side and feeling a stretch in your chest. Repeat this action.

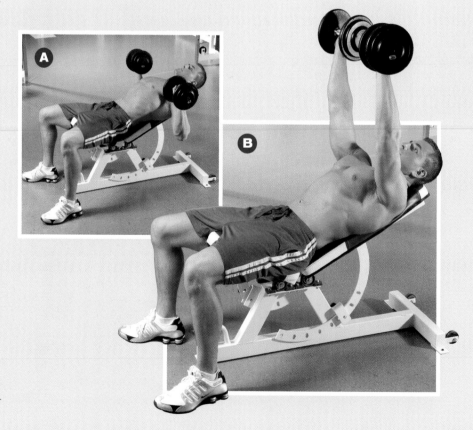

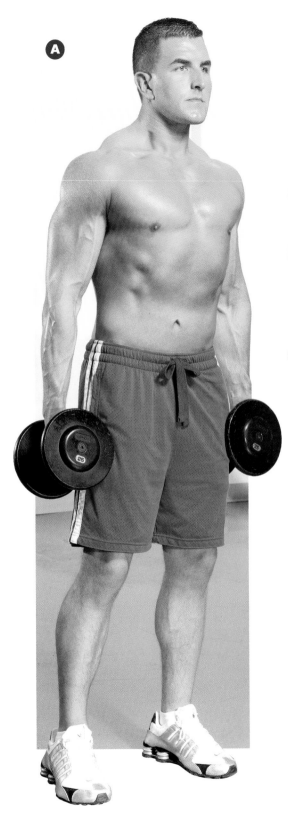

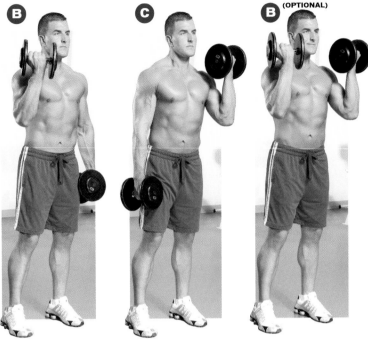

## BICEPS

# Alternating Dumbbell Curl

**TARGET MUSCLES:**
Biceps

**SET UP:** Hold a dumbbell in each hand. Place your arms down at your sides.

**ACTION:** Curl the right dumbbell with an underhand grip to nearly touch your shoulder. While lowering the right arm down to the starting position, curl the left dumbbell up as you did with the right, keeping your body still and your elbows at your sides. Do not swing your body. Repeat this action. If you prefer, you can lift both arms at the same time.

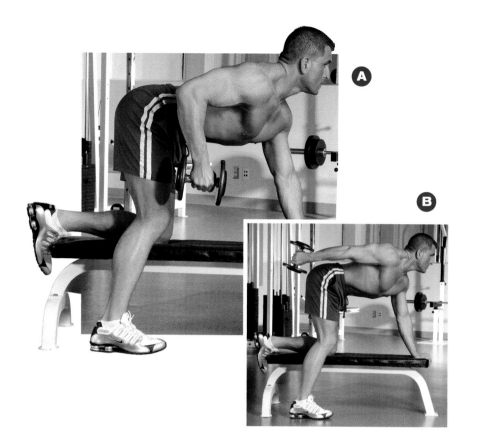

## TRICEPS
# Triceps Kickback

**TARGET MUSCLES:**
Triceps

**SET UP:** Hold a dumbbell in your right hand. Kneel on a flat bench with your left knee and place your right foot flat on the floor. Support your upper body with your left hand. Your back should be flat, your right arm tucked in close to your side, elbow at a 90° angle.

**ACTION:** Extend your right arm back until it is straight, without moving it away from your body. Keep your upper arm tucked in close to your torso. Return to the starting position. Repeat this action until you have completed all repetitions, and then switch your body position to repeat the movement with the left arm.

## ABS
# Crunch

**TARGET MUSCLES:**
Abdominals

**SET UP:** Lie on a mat with your knees bent and your feet flat on the floor. Hold your hands crossed over your chest.

**ACTION:** Use your abdominals to lift your shoulder blades up off the mat then lower back down to the starting position. Keep your gaze fixed on a point on the ceiling throughout the movement. Repeat this action. Once you have developed some abdominal strength you can do this movement with your hands at your head.

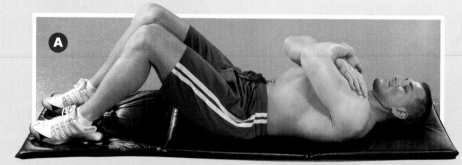

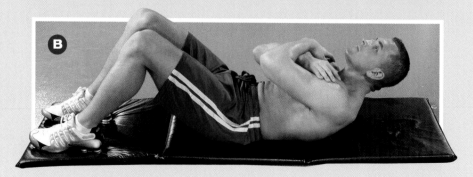

# Intermediate

## Split Routine: Upper Body and Lower Body
2 times each week for each body part, 3 sets of 12 reps

Now that you've been working out for a few months, you can try a split routine. This means that you'll train your lower body and abs on days 1 and 4, and your upper body on days 2 and 5.

## Lower Body and Abs - Days 1 and 4

**THIGHS AND BUTTOCKS**

## Lunge

**TARGET MUSCLES:**
Quadriceps, Glutes and Hamstrings

**SET UP:** Stand with feet together holding a dumbbell at arms' length in each hand with an overhand grip.

**ACTION:** Step forward with your left foot and lunge down until your right knee nearly touches the ground. Make sure your left knee is in line with your left ankle. Keep your back straight. Push off your left foot to return to the starting position. Then repeat the action with your right leg.

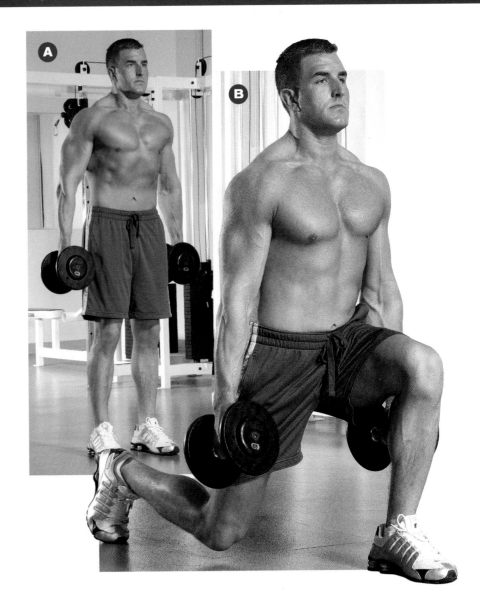

## THIGHS AND BUTTOCKS
# Smith Machine Squat

**TARGET MUSCLES:**
Quadriceps, Glutes and
Hamstrings

**SET UP:** Adjust the height of
the barbell so when you climb
underneath it and stand up, it
will come off its supports. Place
weight plates on both sides to
total desired weight. Stand with
your feet hip-width apart under the
barbell and lift off the supports.

**ACTION:** Holding the barbell
lightly, bend your knees and hips
as if you were sitting in a chair.
Come down as far as you can,
making sure your knees don't jut
out beyond your toes. Return to
the starting position and repeat.

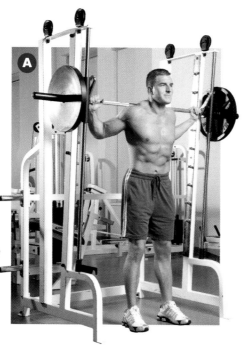

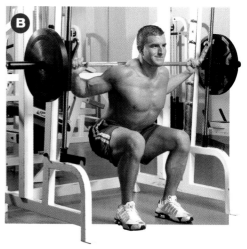

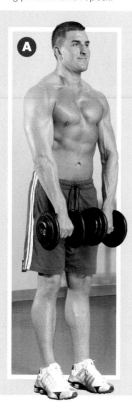

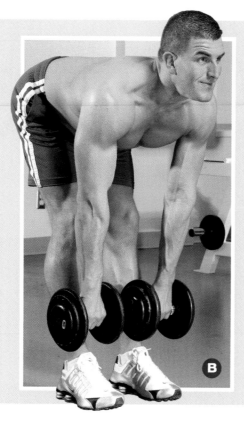

## HAMSTRINGS
# Stiff-Leg Deadlift

**TARGET MUSCLES:**
Hamstrings and Glutes

**SET UP:** Hold a dumbbell at
arms' length in each hand, resting
your hands lightly on your thighs.
Place your feet hip-width apart
with knees very slightly bent.

**ACTION:** Flex your hips so the
dumbbells travel down toward the
floor. Keep a slight bend in your
knees and your back flat. Staring
straight ahead at a spot on the wall
or at yourself in the mirror will help
you keep your back from round-
ing. Return to the starting position,
keeping the weight of your body
on your heels. Repeat.

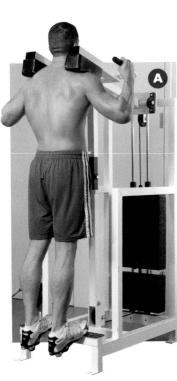

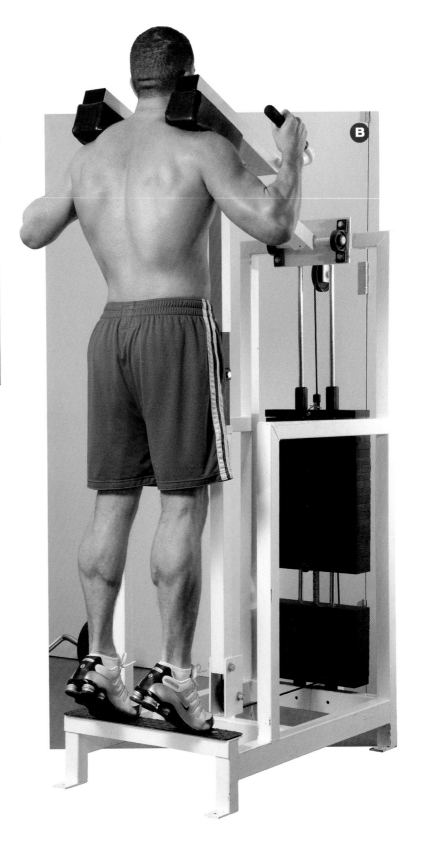

## CALVES
# Standing Calf Raise

**TARGET MUSCLES:**
Gastrocnemius and Soleus

**SET UP:** Set an appropriate weight. If necessary, adjust the shoulder pads so when you climb underneath them and stand up, they are resting securely on your shoulders. This may feel heavy on your shoulders. Stand with your feet hip-width apart, the balls of your feet resting lightly on the footrest and your heels extending down off the footrest until you feel a stretch in your calves. Hold the grips with your hands.

**ACTION:** Press upward onto the balls of your feet. Then return to the starting position with control. Repeat this action.

## ABS
# Ball Crunch

**TARGET MUSCLES:**
Abdominals

**SET UP:** Lie back on an exercise ball with it resting under your upper back. Hold your hands under your head with your elbows bent and out to the sides. Conversely, you can cross your arms over your chest. Keep your knees bent and close together to form a tabletop position. Keep your abs tight. Keep your eyes fixed to one spot on the ceiling.

**ACTION:** Lift your head and shoulder blades off the ball using your abs and without yanking on your neck. Keep your eyes fixed to the ceiling. Return to the starting position and repeat.

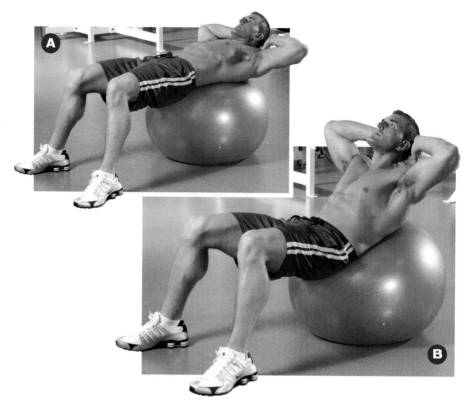

## CORE
# Plank

**TARGET MUSCLES:**
Abdominals and Erector Spinae

**SET UP:** Lie on your stomach on a mat. Position your elbows underneath your shoulders.

**ACTION:** Press up onto your forearms and toes. Keep your body in a straight line. Hold this position for as long as you can. Each time you do it, try to hold a little longer.

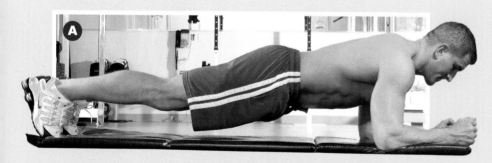

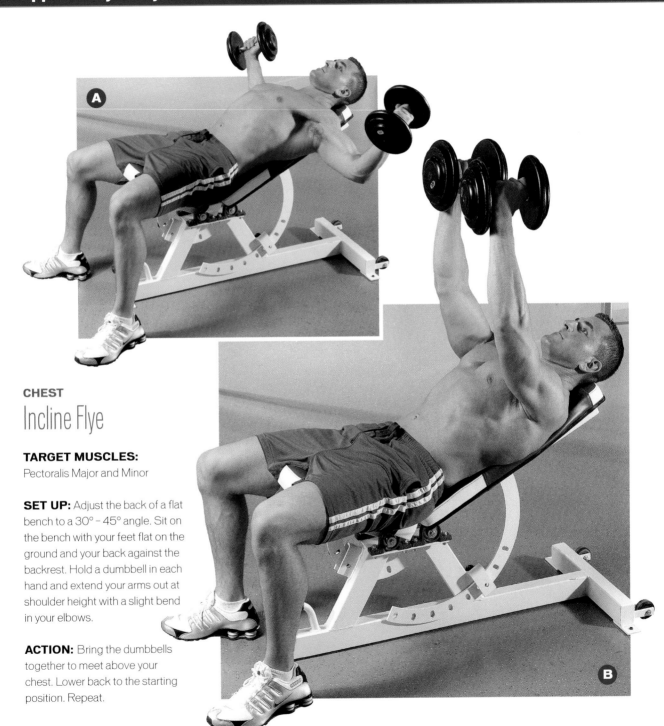

## CHEST
# Incline Flye

**TARGET MUSCLES:**
Pectoralis Major and Minor

**SET UP:** Adjust the back of a flat bench to a 30° – 45° angle. Sit on the bench with your feet flat on the ground and your back against the backrest. Hold a dumbbell in each hand and extend your arms out at shoulder height with a slight bend in your elbows.

**ACTION:** Bring the dumbbells together to meet above your chest. Lower back to the starting position. Repeat.

# Bent-Over Barbell Row

**TARGET MUSCLES:**
Trapezius, Rhomboids, Latissimus Dorsi, Posterior Deltoids and Erector Spinae

**SET UP:** Set a loaded barbell on the floor and stand behind it, feet hip-width apart. Squat down and, using your legs and with your back flat, stand up with the barbell. Have a slight bend in your knees and flex your hips so that your upper body is tilted forward. Looking straight ahead at yourself in the mirror or at a spot on the wall will help you keep your back in the correct position.

**ACTION:** Using your back muscles and without yanking your neck, pull the barbell into your upper abdominal area. Keep your abdominals tight and your back flat or arched – never rounded! Return to the starting position and repeat the movement.

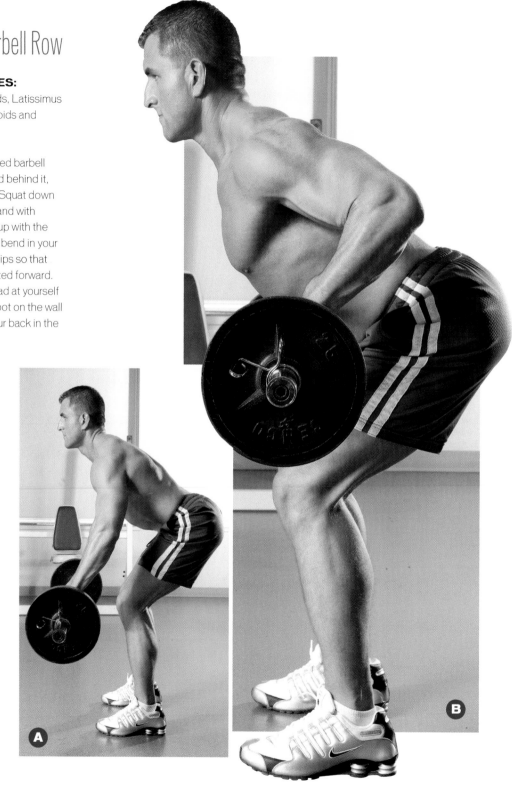

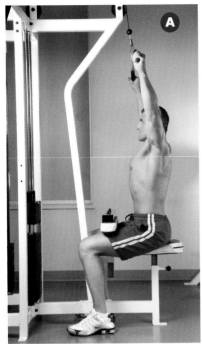
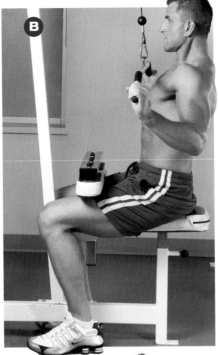

## LATS
# Lat Pulldown

**TARGET MUSCLES:**
Latissimus Dorsi, Trapezius, Posterior Deltoids and Rhomboids

**SET UP:** Adjust the weight on the machine. Make sure the bar is in place. Adjust the kneepad to rest lightly on your knees. Your feet should be flat on the floor with your back straight and your hands holding either side of the bar. You will have to stand up slightly to grasp the bar.

**ACTION:** Keeping your back arched and sitting up straight, pull the bar down in front of you until it reaches just above your chest bone. Return to the starting position and repeat.

## SHOULDERS
# Side Lateral

**TARGET MUSCLES:**
Lateral Deltoids

**SET UP:** Stand with feet hip-width apart. Hold a dumbbell in each hand at arms' length in front of your thighs.

**ACTION:** Lift the dumbbells out to your sides until they reach slightly above shoulder height, maintaining a bend in your arms. Tilt your thumbs down at the top of this exercise, as if you were pouring from a pitcher. Return to the starting position and repeat.

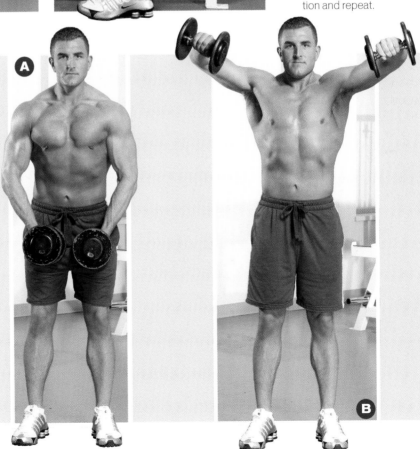

## BICEPS
# EZ-Bar Curl

**TARGET MUSCLES:**
Biceps

**SET UP:** Stand with feet hip-width apart. Hold an EZ-curl bar at arms' length with an underhand grip, resting lightly on your thighs.

**ACTION:** Bend your elbows, curling the bar upward to almost touch your shoulders. Lower back to the starting position with control and repeat.

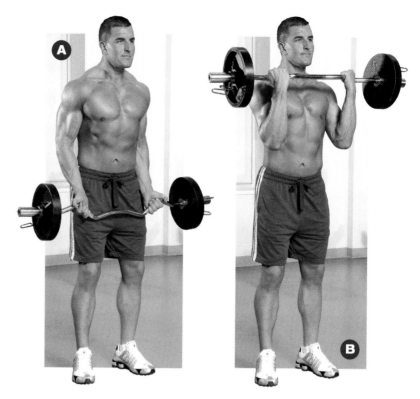

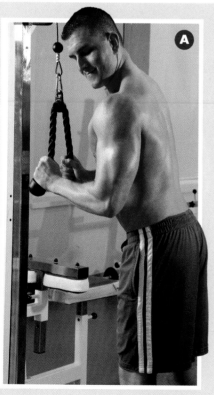

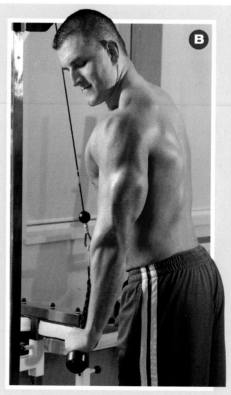

## TRICEPS
# Triceps Pressdown

**TARGET MUSCLES:**
Triceps

**SET UP:** Adjust the weight on the machine and connect the rope attachment. Stand facing the machine with feet hip-width apart. Hold the rope, keeping your elbows bent and tucked closely next to your body.

**ACTION:** Pull down on the rope to straighten your elbows. Make sure your arms stay tucked in and stable at the sides of your body. Return to the starting position and repeat.

# Advanced ▐▐▐▐▐ ▬▬▬▬▬▬▬▬▬▬▬▬▬▬▬▬▬▬▬▬▬▬▬

## Split Routine: Back, Biceps, Abs; Chest, Shoulders, Triceps; Legs
2 times each week for each body part, 3 sets of 8 reps

## Back, Biceps and Abs - Days 1 and 5

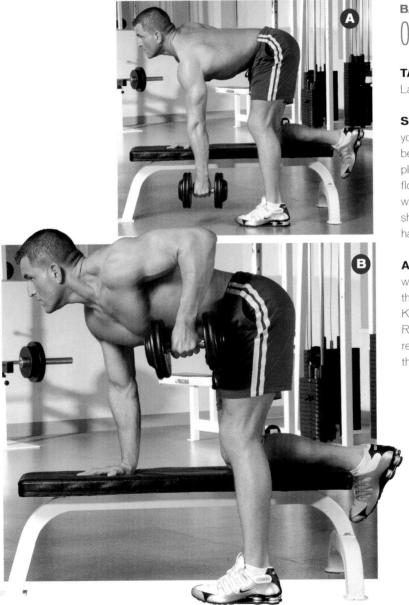

**BACK**
## One-Arm Row

**TARGET MUSCLES:**
Latissimus Dorsi and Trapezius

**SET UP:** Hold a dumbbell in your left hand. Kneel on a flat bench with your right knee and place the other foot flat on the floor. Support your upper body with your right hand. Your back should be flat and your left arm hanging toward the floor.

**ACTION:** Using your lat, and without twisting your body, hoist the dumbbell up to your side. Keep your arm close to your body. Return to the starting position and repeat. Switch your position to do the action with the right arm.

## LATS
# Lat Pulldown

**TARGET MUSCLES:**
Latissimus Dorsi, Trapezius, Posterior Deltoids and Rhomboids

**SET UP:** Adjust the weight on the machine. Make sure the bar is in place. Adjust the kneepad to rest lightly on your knees. Your feet should be flat on the floor with your back straight and your hands holding either side of the bar. You will have to stand up slightly to grasp the bar.

**ACTION:** Keeping your back arched and sitting up straight, pull the bar down in front of you until it reaches just above your chest bone. Return to the starting position and repeat.

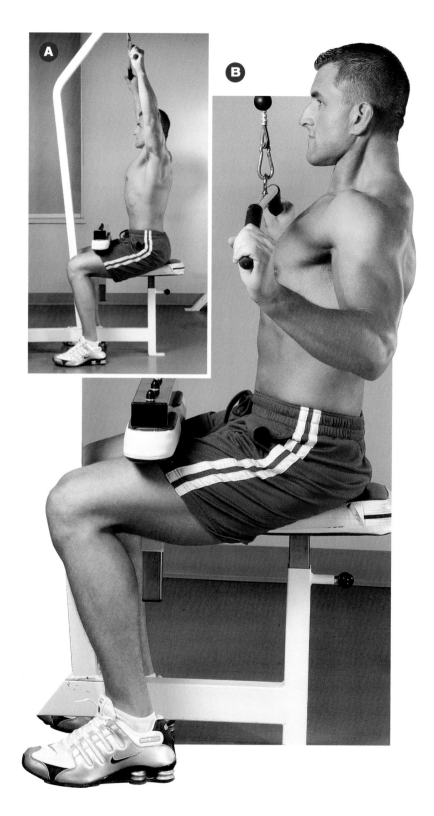

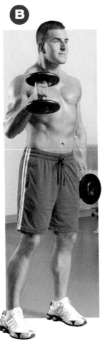

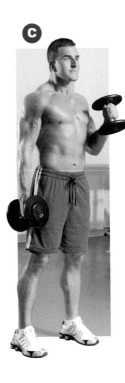

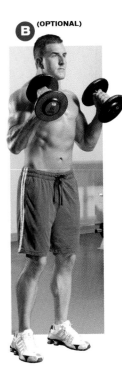

**A**

**B**

**C**

**B** (OPTIONAL)

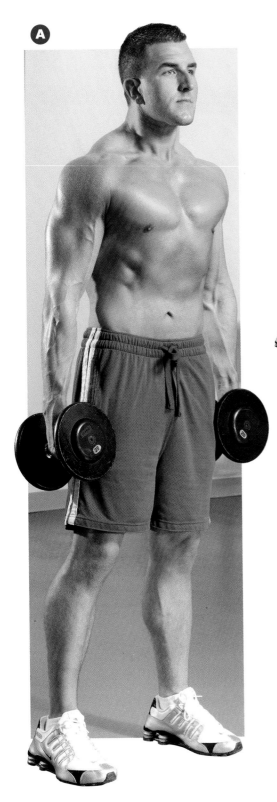

## BICEPS
# Hammer Curl

**TARGET MUSCLES:**
Biceps and Brachialis

**SET UP:** Stand with feet hip-width apart. Hold a dumbbell in each hand at arms' length. Your palms will be facing in.

**ACTION:** Curl the dumbbells up to nearly touch your shoulders while keeping your palms facing inward. Keep your elbows tucked in close to your body. Return to the starting position and repeat. Option: Curl both hands at the same time.

## BICEPS
# Preacher Curl

**TARGET MUSCLES:**
Biceps, Brachialis and Brachioradialis

**SET UP:** Select a barbell with appropriate weight for you. Sit or stand at a preacher bench with the back of your upper arms resting on the pad. Hold the barbell or EZ-curl bar with an underhand grip.

**ACTION:** Curl the barbell up to almost meet your upper arms. Return to the starting position and repeat.

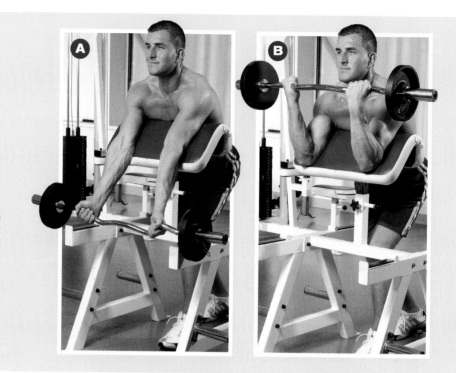

## ABS
# Reverse Crunch

**TARGET MUSCLES:**
Abdominals

**SET UP:** Lie on a mat with your knees bent and your feet off the floor. Hold your arms down at your sides resting lightly on the mat.

**ACTION:** Lift your backside off the mat by curling your knees in toward your chest. Return to the starting position and repeat. You can also do this exercise on a bench: Lie supine on a bench with your butt just starting to creep past the end. Hold the bench above your head. Extend your legs with a slight bend. Lift up, using your abdominals, until your toes point to the ceiling. With control, bring your legs back down until your toes almost touch the floor and repeat.

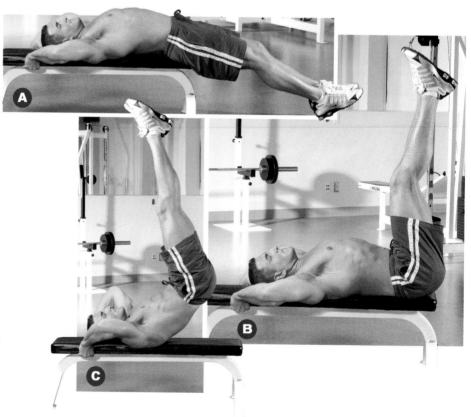

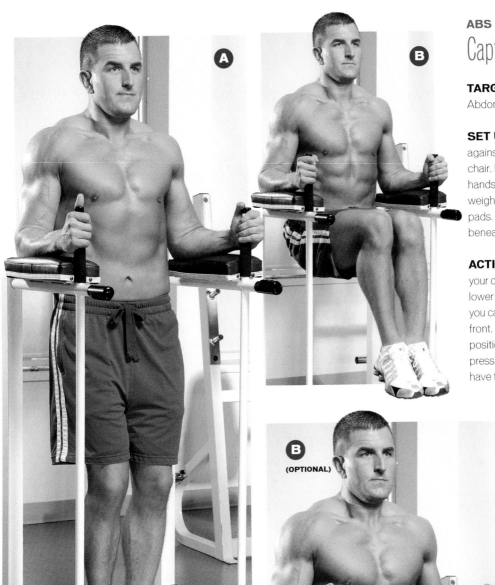

# Captain's Chair

**TARGET MUSCLES:**
Abdominals

**SET UP:** Place your back firmly against the back support of the chair. Hold the rails with your hands, supporting your body weight with your forearms on the pads. Keep your legs extended beneath you.

**ACTION:** Lift your knees to your chest with control and then lower them slowly. Conversely, you can lift your legs straight in front. This is a more difficult position and it's easy to take the pressure off the abs, so you will have to do it very consciously.

## ABS
# Knee In

**TARGET MUSCLES:**
Abdominals

**SET UP:** Sit sideways on a bench, placing your hands on either side of your body for support. You should be leaning backward slightly. Lift your feet slightly from the floor.

**ACTION:** Using your abdominal muscles, bring your knees in close to your chest. Extend back to the starting position and repeat.

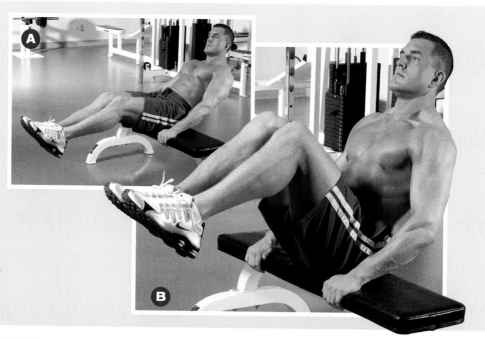

# Legs - Days 2 and 6

## QUADS, HAMSTRINGS AND GLUTES
# Smith Machine Squat

**TARGET MUSCLES:**
Quadriceps, Glutes and Hamstrings

**SET UP:** Adjust the height of the barbell so when you climb underneath it and stand up, it will come off its supports. Place weight plates on both sides to total desired weight. Stand with your feet hip-width apart under the barbell and lift off the supports.

**ACTION:** Holding the barbell lightly, bend your knees and hips as if you were sitting in a chair. Come down as far as you can, making sure your knees don't jut out beyond your toes. Return to the starting position and repeat.

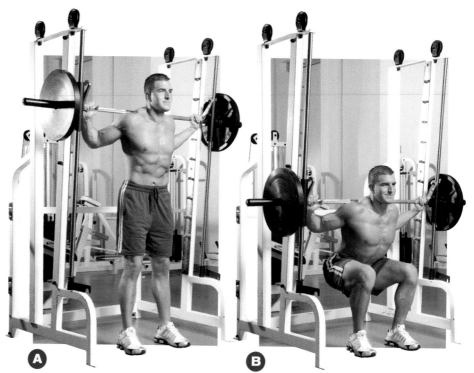

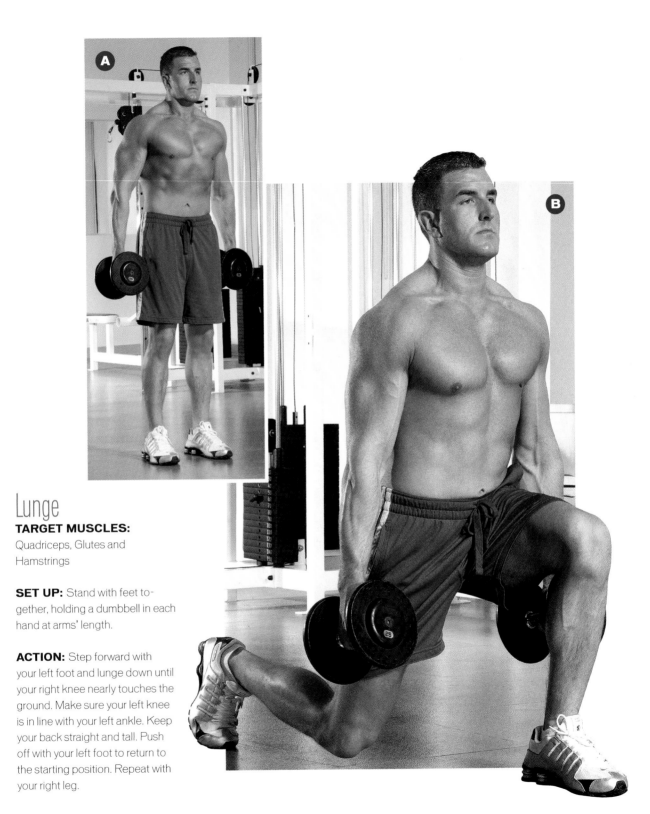

# Lunge

**TARGET MUSCLES:**

Quadriceps, Glutes and Hamstrings

**SET UP:** Stand with feet together, holding a dumbbell in each hand at arms' length.

**ACTION:** Step forward with your left foot and lunge down until your right knee nearly touches the ground. Make sure your left knee is in line with your left ankle. Keep your back straight and tall. Push off with your left foot to return to the starting position. Repeat with your right leg.

# Lying Hamstring Curl

**TARGET MUSCLES:**

Hamstrings

**SET UP:** Adjust the weight on the machine to one that allows you to do 8 reps but no more. Adjust the footrest so that it will fall just above your ankles when you are lying down. Climb into the machine facedown, putting your lower legs underneath the footrest.

**ACTION:** Curl the footrest up toward the back of your legs and then return to the starting position with control. Repeat this action.

## CALVES
# Standing Calf Raise

**TARGET MUSCLES:**

Gastrocnemius and Soleus

**SET UP:** Set an appropriate weight. If necessary, adjust the shoulder pads so when you climb underneath them and stand up, they are resting securely on your shoulders. This may feel heavy on your shoulders. Stand with your feet hip-width apart, the balls of your feet resting lightly on the footrest and your heels extending down off the footrest until you feel a stretch in your calves. Hold the grips with your hands.

**ACTION:** Press upward onto the balls of your feet. Then return to the starting position with control. Repeat this action.

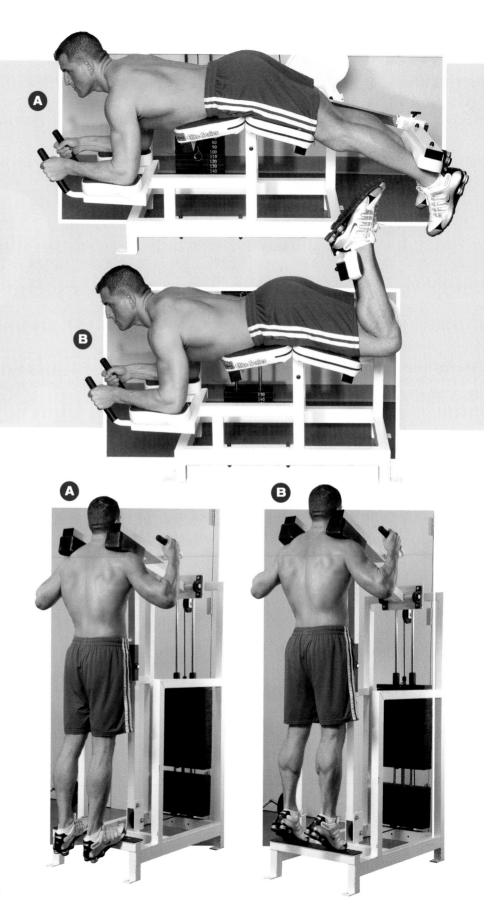

## CHEST
# Bench Press

**TARGET MUSCLES:**
Pectoralis Major and Minor,
Triceps and Anterior Deltoids

**SET UP:** Select or load a
barbell with an appropriate
weight for you. Rest the barbell
on the rack. Lie on the bench
underneath the rack, with your
feet flat on the ground. Lift the
barbell off the rack and hold it
up straight above your chest.

**ACTION:** Bring the bar to
your chest and immediately but
smoothly push back up to the
starting position. Repeat for desired number of reps, and
put barbell back on the rack
between sets. You may need
someone to help you with this
exercise, especially if you are
using challenging weights.

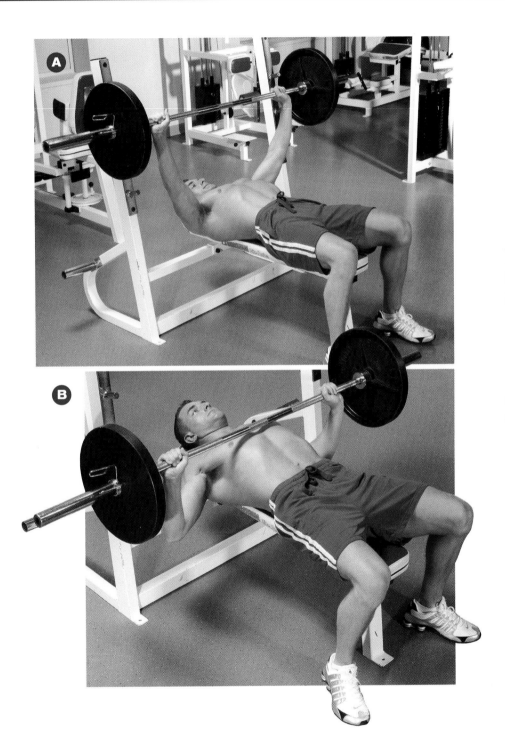

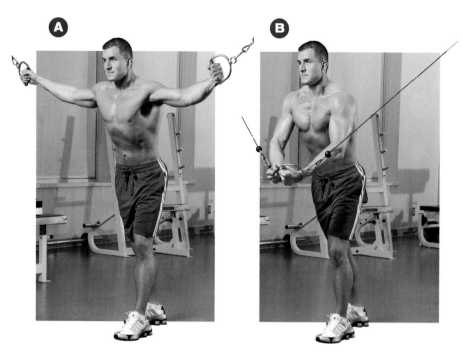

# Cable Crossover

**TARGET MUSCLES:**

Pectoralis Major

**SET UP:** Adjust the height of the cables so they are at the top of the machine. Select an appropriate weight. Make sure the single-grip handles are in place. Hold the handles with arms extended at shoulder height and a slight bend in the elbows. Stand between the cables with knees slightly bent for support. You can place one foot in front of the other for added stability if you like.

**ACTION:** Bring the cables to meet in front of your chest in a hugging motion. Return to the starting position and repeat.

**SHOULDERS**

# Seated Shoulder Press

**TARGET MUSCLES:**

Deltoids, Trapezius and Rotator Cuff

**SET UP:** Sit on a bench with your feet flat on the floor. Hold a dumbbell in each hand at your shoulders with your elbows bent and tucked in close to your body.

**ACTION:** Extend the dumbbells overhead until your arms are nearly straight. Return to the starting position and repeat.

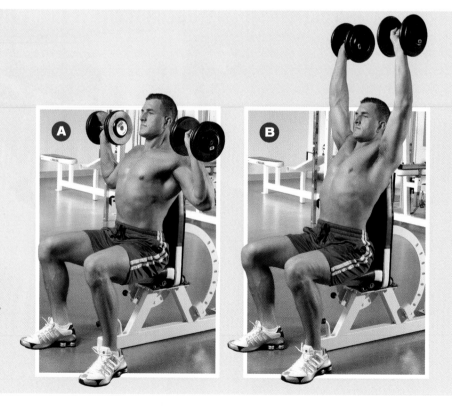

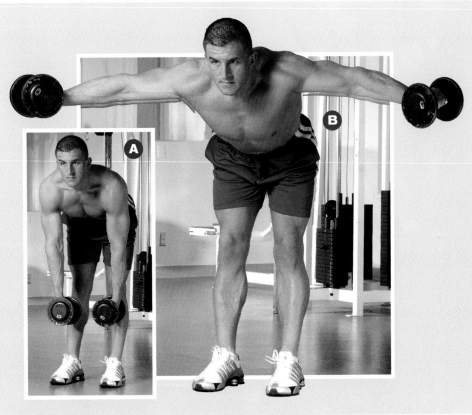

# Bent-Over Lateral

**TARGET MUSCLES:**
Posterior Deltoids

**SET UP:** Stand with feet hip-width apart. Bend at the hips so your upper body is tilted forward. Maintain a flat back and a slight bend in your knees. Hold a dumbbell in each hand, hanging in front of your legs, your palms facing each other. Maintain a slight bend in your elbows.

**ACTION:** Keeping your elbows slightly bent, bring your arms back until they are in line with your shoulders. Return to the starting position and repeat.

## TRICEPS
# Lying Triceps Extension/Skullcrusher
**TARGET MUSCLES:**
Triceps

**SET UP:** Lie face up on a flat bench with your feet flat on the floor. Extend your arms out in front of you holding an appropriately weighted barbell with an overhand grip.

**ACTION:** Keeping your upper arms perpendicular to the floor, bend your elbows until the barbell nearly reaches your forehead. Return to the starting position with control by extending your elbows. Repeat this action. Do not allow your elbows to drift outward during this movement.

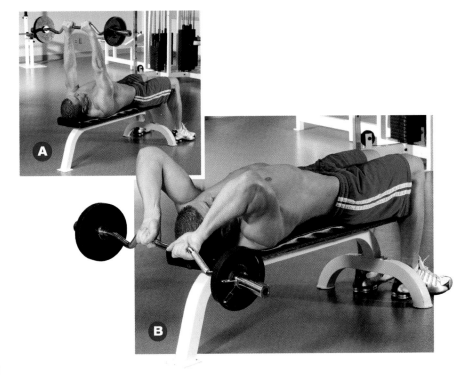

## TRICEPS
# Bench Dip

**TARGET MUSCLES:** Triceps

**SET UP:** Position two stable flat benches parallel to one another. Sit at the very edge of one bench, placing your heels on the opposite bench or on the floor. Place your hands close to your body on the bench. Lift your weight up on your hands and slip your buttocks just in front of the bench.

**ACTION:** Lower your buttocks down close to the floor by bending your elbows. Your elbows will want to flare out, but try to keep them close to your body. Push your body back up by straightening your arms.

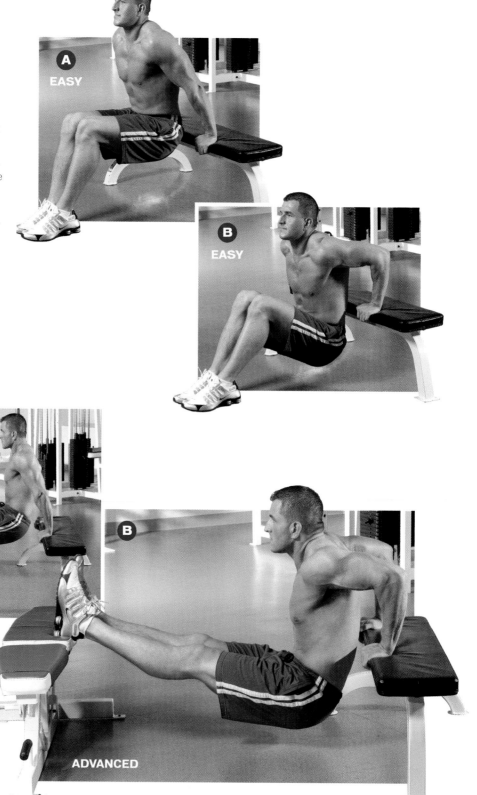

## *No longer the "fattest dad"!*

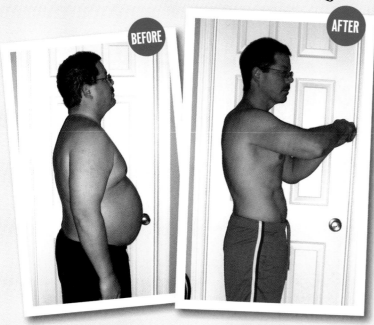

BEFORE

AFTER

**NAME:** Brent Ray
**AGE:** 43
**HEIGHT:** 5'8"
**WEIGHT BEFORE:** 245 lbs
**WEIGHT AFTER:** 175 lbs
**WEIGHT LOSS:** 70 lbs

**LIKE SO MANY AMERICANS, BRENT RAY HAS SUFFERED AT THE HANDS OF UNHEALTHY, PRE-PACKAGED FOODS AND A SEDENTARY LIFESTYLE.** Brent's wake-up call came when he realized he was no longer able to participate in sports with his two sons. Years of eating poorly and exercising very little, combined with several failed fad diets, had left him at an unhealthy 245 pounds.

With each failed attempt to lose weight, Brent grew more and more frustrated with his physical appearance. He always felt like the "fattest dad" at events, and eventually wound up avoiding them altogether. Not only were his family and social lives suffering, Brent was developing serious health issues. He discovered he had high cholesterol, he used a CPAP machine nightly to deal with his sleep apnea and he had prediabetes. Enter Charles D'Angelo.

Having gone through the same struggles with weight loss in his own life, Charles understood firsthand Brent's trials and tribulations. And when Brent learned about Charles' transformation, he realized that it was possible to overcome your demons

## *"Not only were his family and social lives suffering, Brent was developing serious health issues."*

and live a happy, fulfilled and confident life. This was pivotal for Brent, since he needed the motivation to know that he could do this. According to Charles, there was never any

doubt! Charles formed a plan for Brent that took the guesswork out of weight loss. Brent knew exactly what to eat and how to exercise. Best of all, he was accountable for his actions at every meeting. No excuses! This same attitude keeps Brent motivated to this day.

## *"Brent was able to drop the weight and keep it off."*

After working with Charles, Brent was able to drop the weight and keep it off. One of the strategies Brent uses to maintain his impressive weight loss is: No mindless eating! Instead, he thinks actively about every morsel that goes into his mouth. Brent says, "If I had done that before, I probably wouldn't have ended up that way in the first place."

Brent is grateful for his newfound attitude and skills, and, as he says, he owes it all to Charles. In fact, Brent would encourage anyone wanting a weight-loss plan that works to adopt Charles' teachings. "He will motivate, encourage, demonstrate and ultimately take you where you want to be." Which in Brent's case was back on the playing field with his sons!

# WORK IT!
## 8 Ways to Make the New You Look Even Better

*Don't you love the feeling you get when you put on something you haven't worn in a while, only to realize that it's several sizes too big? If you haven't experienced this yet, don't worry, you will! And if you have encountered this feeling, it means you've been working hard and burning fat, of course, but it also means something else – it's time to go shopping! Chances are, for the first time in a long time, or maybe for the first time ever, you're actually excited at the prospect of trying on clothes. Isn't it amazing? Here are some fashion secrets to help you look and feel your best when you come out of hiding and reveal the new you.*

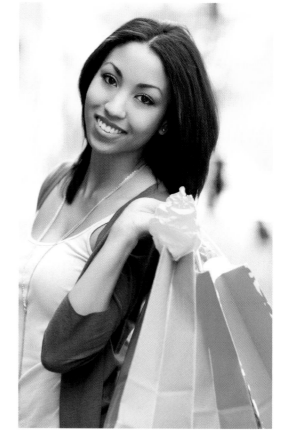

### 1 Ask for help.

Almost any celebrity you can name has a personal stylist – someone whose job is simply picking out the best outfits for his or her clients. It's unlikely that a stylist is within your budget, but some large department stores do offer a free personal shopper service to help you find the best clothes for your style and budget. If you prefer to shop at a variety of places, most stores have friendly, knowledgeable salespeople with a flair for fashion. (Just watch out for high-pressure sales tactics!) After my weight loss as a teen, I went to buy my very first pair of jeans. I couldn't believe there were so many to choose from! Luckily, the new me had the confidence to approach a very attractive salesgirl who was more than happy to help me choose a few pairs. Talk about a self-esteem booster! Another option is to ask an honest friend with a fashion sense you admire to join you on your shopping excursions.

### 2 Accentuate the positives.

If you genetically carry more weight in your lower half, for example, try to pick out outfits that will draw attention to your upper half, helping you appear as symmetrical as possible. Wear more vibrant colors, patterns and jewelry up top and more conservative dark colors down below. Conversely, if you're heavier up top and slimmer in the bottom, you can balance your body by wearing more flowing, light-colored pants and a darker blouse or tee. If this is something you are interested in, there are some great books out there about dressing for your body type. Pick one up and have some fun with your new shape!

### 3 Wear clothes that fit.

Clothes that are too big make you lose your shape and look bulky, and clothes that are too small pull, bunch up and cause rolls where there really aren't any. Once you're lean, toned and consider yourself to be a certain size, you may be shocked to find that sizes vary quite a bit from designer to designer. In one brand you may be a size four and in another you're a size six or eight! Don't worry about the number on the tag. Your health and the way you feel are the most important thing, not the size on the label.

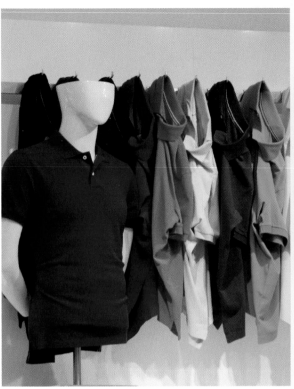

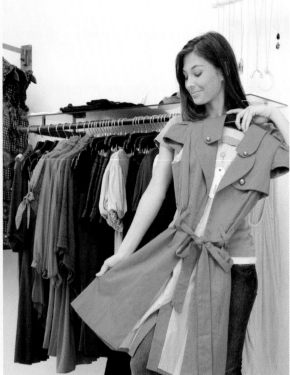

Trying to fit into a smaller size simply because of your attachment to the number can make you look bigger. Remember, no one can see the number on the tag, but everyone can see that your pants are stretched precariously across your rear end! Base your decision on how the outfit feels and looks, and keep in mind that a tailor can shape your clothes to make them quite flattering. This is one service that is definitely worth the fee.

 **Splurge a little.**
You deserve at least one well-made outfit, especially after all the work you've done. I know that it may be more expensive, but if you choose something classic that won't soon go out of style, it will last longer than something that's cheaper but poorly made. A well-made, well-cut article of clothing just feels better on, which can be a great confidence-booster. And as motivational

speaker Zig Ziglar said, "You cannot climb the ladder of success dressed in the costume of failure."

 **Wear solids, not stripes.**
No matter how lean and fit you are, horizontal stripes always make you look broader. Unless you're a guy who wants to appear as muscular and big as possible, avoid stripes and go for colorful solids.

6 **Pick comfortable fabrics.**
Avoid starched, stiff materials and look for shirts that fit to your form but are still loose enough to allow you to move comfortably.

7 **Go beyond basic black.**
In an effort to hide yourself when you were fat, you may have become used

to throwing on a dark suit jacket. It's time for it to go! Wear fitted and flowing shirts and blouses in vibrant colors. Try something sleeveless – you have been working on those arms after all. Stand out from the crowd and project the confidence you have in the new you. Be bold! You no longer need to fill your closet with black.

 **Accessorize!**
A pair of nice shoes, a nice watch and some carefully chosen jewelry will all work to accentuate your new outfit – and the new body underneath it. In my opinion, simple speaks louder than flashy. A girl I once dated said she would always put on all the jewelry she wanted to wear out, and then would take off one or two pieces before she left the house. Good rule of thumb!

IV

# section IV

## Recipes

# Beef Vegetable Soup

**Prep time:** 20 minutes
**Cooking time:** 2 hours 30 minutes
**Yield:** 4 x 2 cups

There's nothing like a healthy dose of lean protein and carbs all in one bowl! Use locally farmed and organic veggies along with beef from grass-fed cows for the freshest flavor and maximum health benefits.

## Ingredients

- 1 Tbsp extra virgin olive oil
- 1 lb flank steak, visible fat removed, cut into ½-inch pieces
- 1 medium cooking onion, chopped
- 4 ribs celery, chopped
- 2 cloves garlic, minced
- 2 cups button mushrooms, sliced
- 8 cups low-sodium beef or vegetable broth
- 2 cups diced tomatoes (fresh or canned)
- 2-3 bay leaves
- 2 cups green beans, topped, tailed and chopped (frozen is fine)
- Black pepper, to taste
- Tabasco or other hot sauce, to taste

## Method

1 In a soup pot, heat oil to medium-high. Add meat and brown on all sides. Remove meat and set aside.

2 Add onion and celery to pot, and sauté for about 5 minutes. Add garlic and mushrooms and sauté for another 3 to 4 minutes.

3 Return beef to pot, adding broth, tomatoes with juices and bay leaves.

4 Bring to a boil, reduce heat to simmer and cook, uncovered, for 1½ hours.

5 Add green beans, black pepper and hot sauce and cook for another ½ hour.

**TIP:** Meat from grass-fed animals is richer in antioxidants and has two to four times more heart-healthy omega-3s than meat from animals that are fed grains.

**Nutritional value per serving:**
Calories: 437 | Calories from Fat: 154 | Protein: 49 g |
Carbs: 23 g | Total Fat: 16 g | Saturated Fat: 5 g | Trans Fat: 0 g |
Fiber: 6 g | Sodium: 1082 mg | Cholesterol: 116 mg

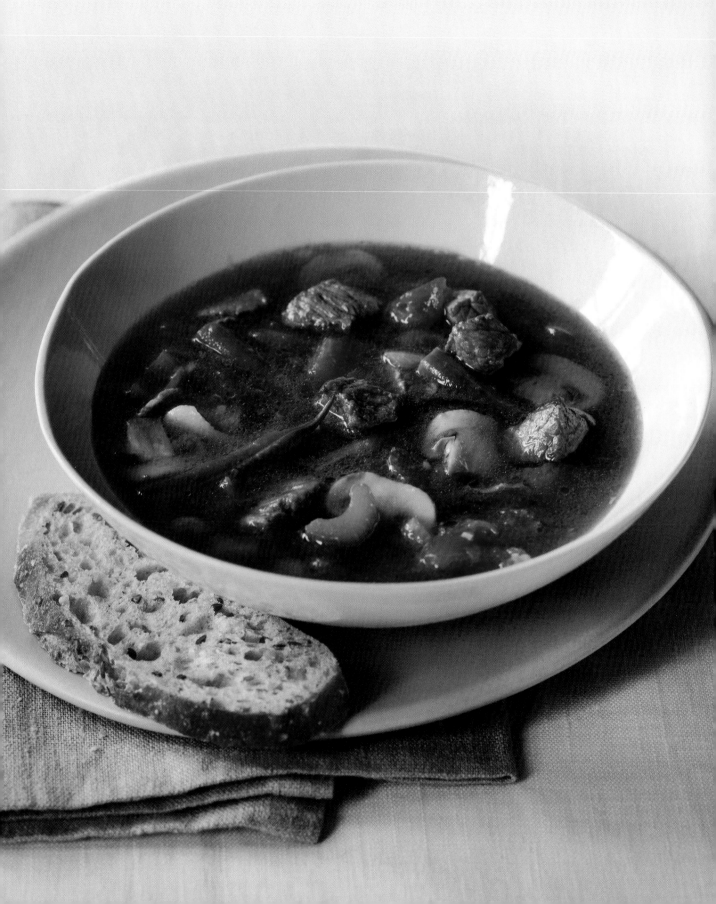

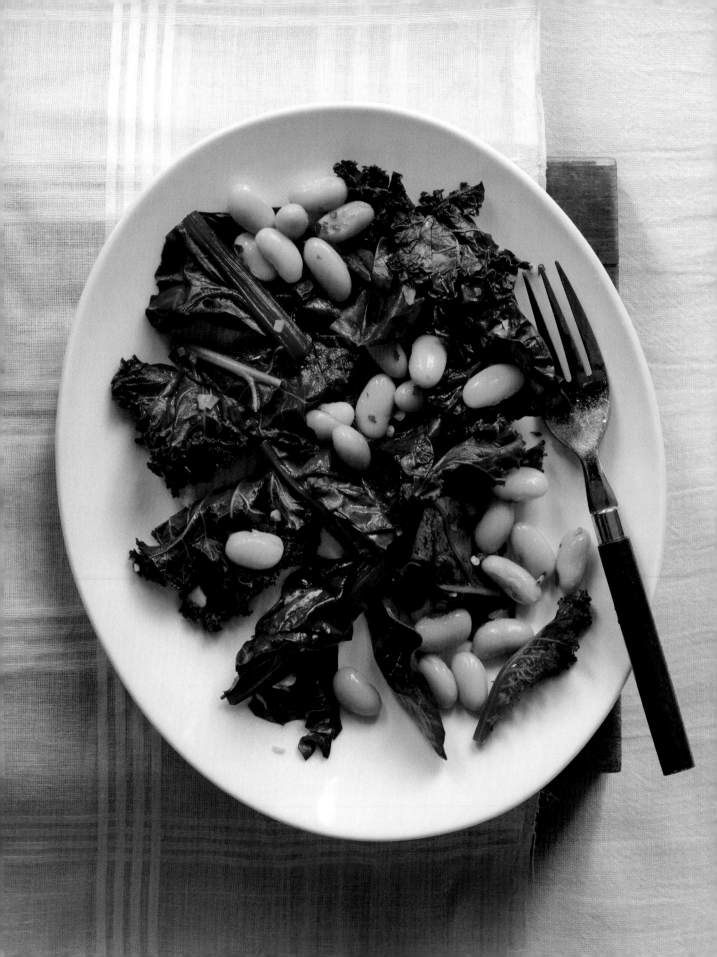

# Beans and Greens

**Prep time:** 12 minutes
**Cooking time:** 25 minutes
**Yield:** 2 x 2 cups as main course,
4 x 1 cup as side dish

Kale and other greens are packed with cancer-fighting antioxidants and dietary fiber. Paired with high-protein beans, this dish is sure to leave you satisfied and less likely to indulge in fatty foods.

## Ingredients

- 1 Tbsp extra virgin olive oil
- 1 small white onion, finely chopped
- 4 garlic cloves, minced
- ¼ to ½ tsp red pepper flakes, to taste
- 1 large bunch kale, collard greens, Swiss chard or a combination, chopped, toughest stems removed
- 1 cup low-sodium vegetable or chicken broth
- 2 cups cooked or 1 x 15-oz can cannellini beans, drained and rinsed
- 2 tsp red wine vinegar

## Method

1  Heat oil in large skillet over medium heat. Add onion and sauté until translucent, about 6 minutes. Add garlic and pepper flakes and sauté for 1 minute. Add greens, a handful at a time. As the first handful wilts, add the next.

2  Add broth, cover and simmer for about 5 to 8 minutes, stirring once or twice to ensure even cooking. Add beans and simmer, uncovered, until any excess liquid is gone. Stir in red wine vinegar.

> **TIP:** Turn to page 157 to get the scoop on the amazing health benefits of the greens used in this recipe.

**Nutritional value per serving (as a main dish):**
Calories: 352 | Calories from Fat: 71 | Protein: 19 g | Carbs: 53 g | Total Fat: 8 g | Saturated Fat: 1 g | Trans Fat: 0 g | Fiber: 14 g | Sodium: 916 mg | Cholesterol: 0 mg

**Nutritional value per serving (as a side dish):**
Calories: 176 | Calories from Fat: 36 | Protein: 10 g | Carbs: 27 g | Total Fat: 4 g | Saturated Fat: 0.5 g | Trans Fat: 0 g | Fiber: 7 g | Sodium: 458 mg | Cholesterol: 0 mg

# Chicken Okra Soup

**Prep time:** 20 minutes
**Cooking time:** 1 hour 30 minutes
**Yield:** 4 x 1 ½ cups

This spice-filled soup gives the chicken and okra pair a nice zing! Okra is full of antioxidants and lowers cholesterol, while promoting good eyesight. When paired with the lean protein of chicken, okra makes for a nutritious addition to any pot of soup.

## Ingredients

- 1½ pounds chicken breast, cut into ½-inch cubes
- 5 cups chicken broth
- 1 medium onion, chopped
- 2 stalks celery, chopped
- 2 cloves garlic, minced
- 2 bay leaves
- 1 tsp oregano
- 1 tsp thyme
- 1 tsp ground cumin
- ¼ tsp smoked paprika
- ¼-½ tsp cayenne pepper, to taste
- ¼ tsp black pepper
- 1 large green bell pepper, chopped
- 10 ounces okra, cut into ½ inch slices
- Tabasco or other hot sauce, to taste

## Method

1 Place all ingredients except green pepper and okra in a large pot or Dutch oven. Bring to a boil over medium-high heat. Reduce heat and simmer, uncovered, for 1 hour.

2 Add green pepper and okra and simmer for 15 minutes further. Stir in hot sauce or add at the table.

**TIP:** Okra is often used to thicken soups and stews because it releases pectins. Bonus! These pectins are heart-healthy forms of soluble fiber.

**Nutritional value per serving:**
Calories: 281 | Calories from Fat: 30 | Protein: 50 g | Carbs: 8 g | Total Fat: 3 g | Saturated Fat: 0 g | Trans Fat: 0 g | Fiber: 2 g | Sodium: 1159 mg | Cholesterol: 0 mg

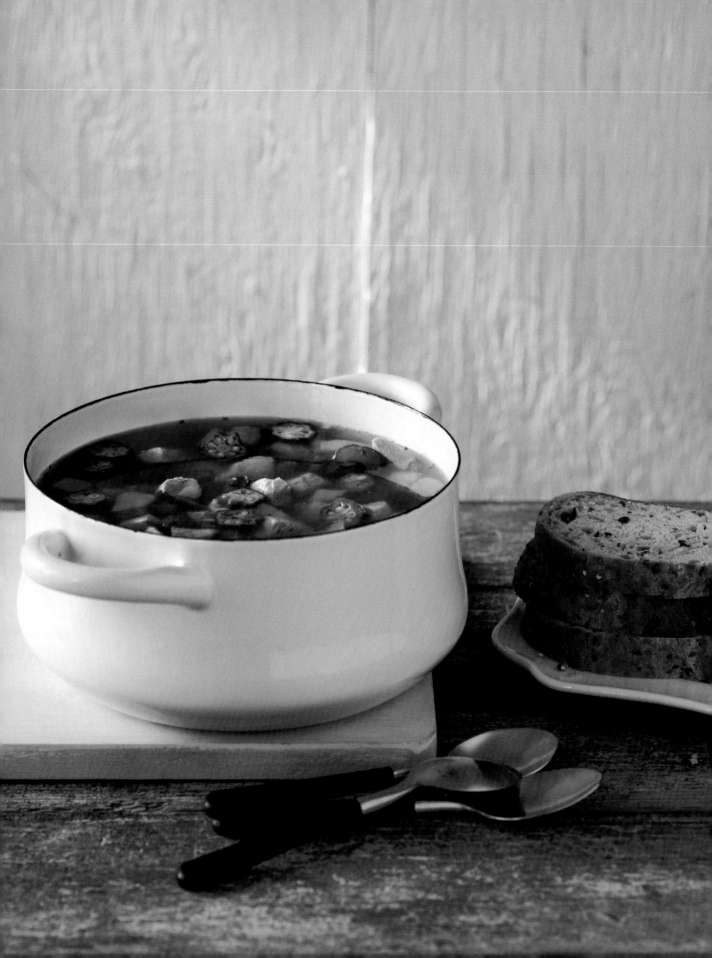

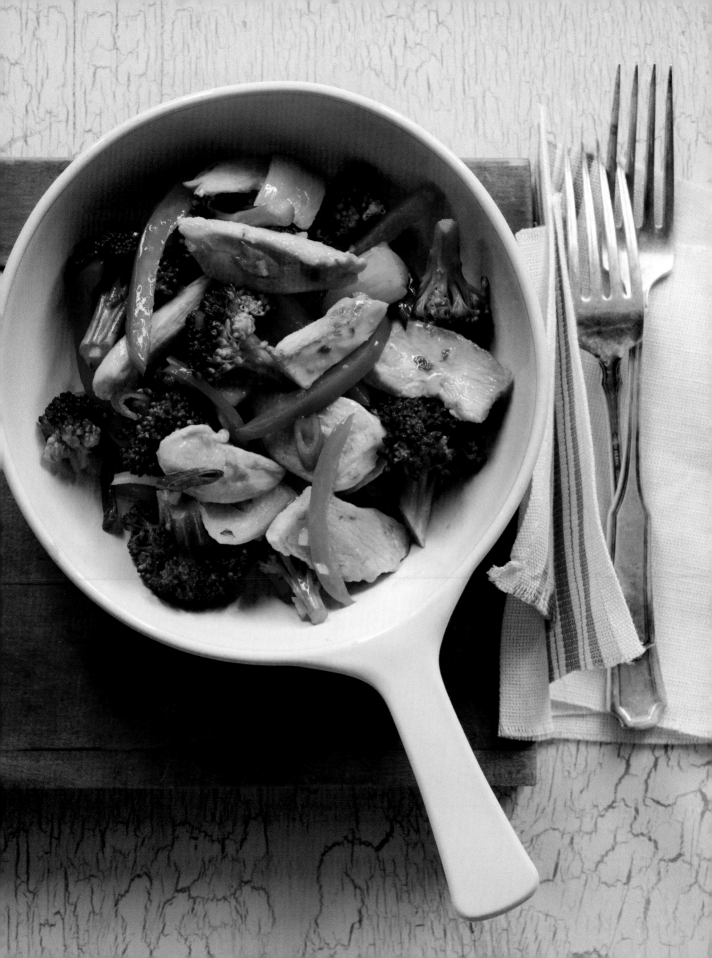

# Chicken Broccoli Stir-Fry

**Prep time:** 25 minutes
**Cooking time:** 45 minutes
**Yield:** 4 x 2 cups

Chicken and broccoli are powerful staples in a healthy diet. Broccoli is full of vitamin C and fiber that aids in digestion. Stir-frying both foods in a mix of spices and veggies makes this an easy-to-cook, gourmet meal.

## Ingredients

- Cooking spray
- 1 Tbsp coconut oil or butter
- 1 cooking onion, chopped
- 1-inch piece ginger, minced, divided
- 3 cloves garlic, minced, divided
- 1½ pounds boneless, skinless chicken breast, cut into bite-sized pieces
- 1 large or 2 small bunches broccoli, stem peeled and cut into small pieces, crown cut into small florets
- 1 red bell pepper, thinly sliced
- 1 cup green onions, chopped, divided
- Red pepper flakes
- Juice of 1 lime
- 1 Tbsp cornstarch
- 6 oz chicken broth, cold

## Method

1  Coat a large skillet or wok with cooking spray and heat on high. Add coconut oil or butter to hot pan, and immediately add chopped cooking onion. Cook, stirring, for 3 minutes. Add half of ginger and garlic along with all chicken. Cook, stirring constantly, for about 5 minutes. Remove chicken from pan and set aside.

2  Spray pan again, and add the rest of the ginger and garlic. Add broccoli in batches, removing to set aside as each batch cooks.

3  Add red pepper to pan and cook for 2 minutes, stirring often. Return chicken and broccoli to the pan. Add half of green onions, red pepper flakes and lime juice. Cook, stirring, until heated through.

4  In a small bowl, mix cornstarch with cold chicken broth. Stir into pan and bring to a boil. Reduce heat to low and simmer for 2 to 3 minutes. Sprinkle remaining green onions on top of each plate when serving.

**TIP:** Broccoli and chicken both contain powerful cancer-fighting components that become up to three times more beneficial when eaten together – like in this stir-fry!

**Nutritional value per serving:**
Calories: 397 | Calories from Fat: 72 | Protein: 56 g | Carbs: 25 g | Total Fat: 8 g | Saturated Fat: 3 g | Trans Fat: 0 g | Fiber: 7 g | Sodium: 502 mg | Cholesterol: 1.75 mg

# Colorful Salad
## with Grilled Chicken and Shrimp

**Prep time:** 15 minutes
**Cooking time:** 16 minutes
**Yield:** 4 servings

Throwing some fresh, natural color onto your plate guarantees you're eating a nutrient-rich meal. Whites and greens supply helpings of antioxidants and reds and yellows promote good cholesterol. The browns and oranges provide a lean source of delicious protein to complete the dish.

## Ingredients

- 2 Tbsp extra virgin olive oil, divided
- 2 x 5-ounce boneless, skinless chicken breasts
- 4 cloves garlic, minced
- 16 large shrimp
- Black pepper
- 2 cups red leaf lettuce
- 2 cups Boston lettuce
- ½ red pepper, sliced thin
- ½ orange pepper, sliced thin
- ½ yellow pepper, sliced thin
- 1 cup broccoli florets, cut small
- ½ purple onion, sliced thin
- 1 cup combination yellow and red grape tomatoes
- ¼ cup balsamic vinegar

## Method

1. In a large skillet, heat 1 Tbsp oil on medium high. Add chicken and garlic. Cook for about 4 minutes, uncovered. Flip chicken over and cook for 5 minutes more. Turn heat to medium-low and continue cooking for 3 minutes, again uncovered.

2. At this point, move the chicken breasts to the side and add shrimp to pan. Cook them for about 2 minutes on one side, then flip over and cook for about 2 minutes on other side. Crack black pepper over chicken and shrimp, to taste. At this time your chicken and shrimp should all be cooked. Set them aside.

3. Wash red leaf and Boston lettuce well, and spin in a salad spinner. Tear into small pieces and place in a decorative bowl. Add peppers, broccoli, onion and tomatoes. Toss just a little.

4. In a small bowl, whisk together balsamic vinegar and remaining Tbsp of olive oil. Drizzle overtop salad.

5. Slice chicken into strips and place on top of salad. Place shrimp overtop as well. Conversely, you can divide the salad among four plates and then place half of each chicken breast plus four shrimp on each plate.

**TIP:** If possible, try to use cold-pressed olive oil – it is the least processed and therefore contains the most nutrients.

**Nutritional value per serving:**
Calories: 303 | Calories from Fat: 103 | Protein: 36 g |
Carbs: 12 g | Total Fat: 11 g | Saturated Fat: 2 g | Trans Fat: 0 g |
Fiber: 3 g | Sodium:188 mg | Cholesterol: 121 mg

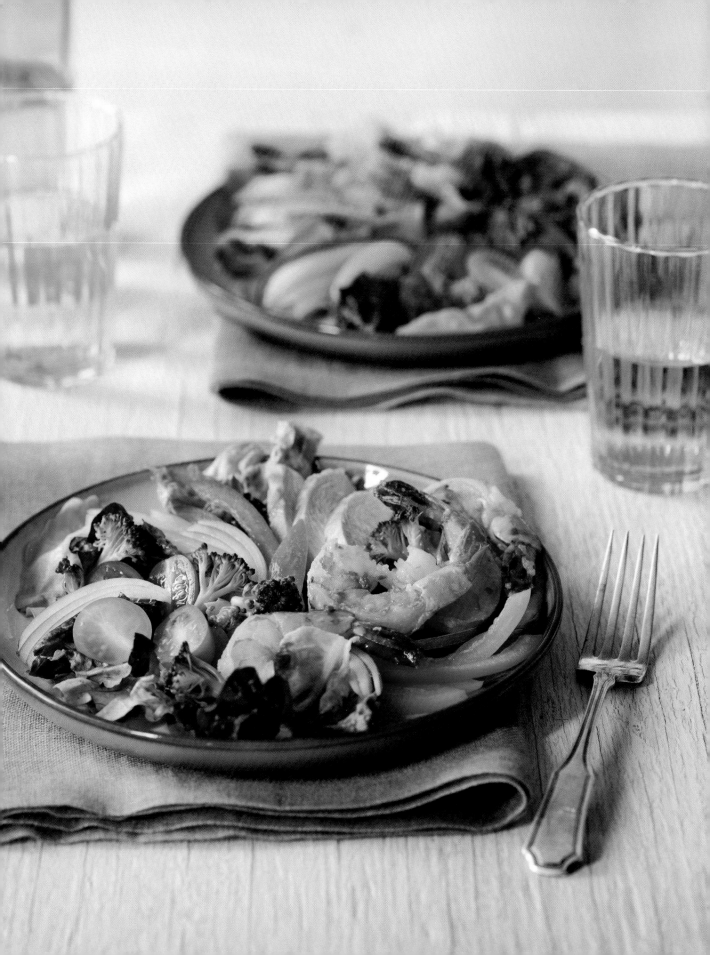

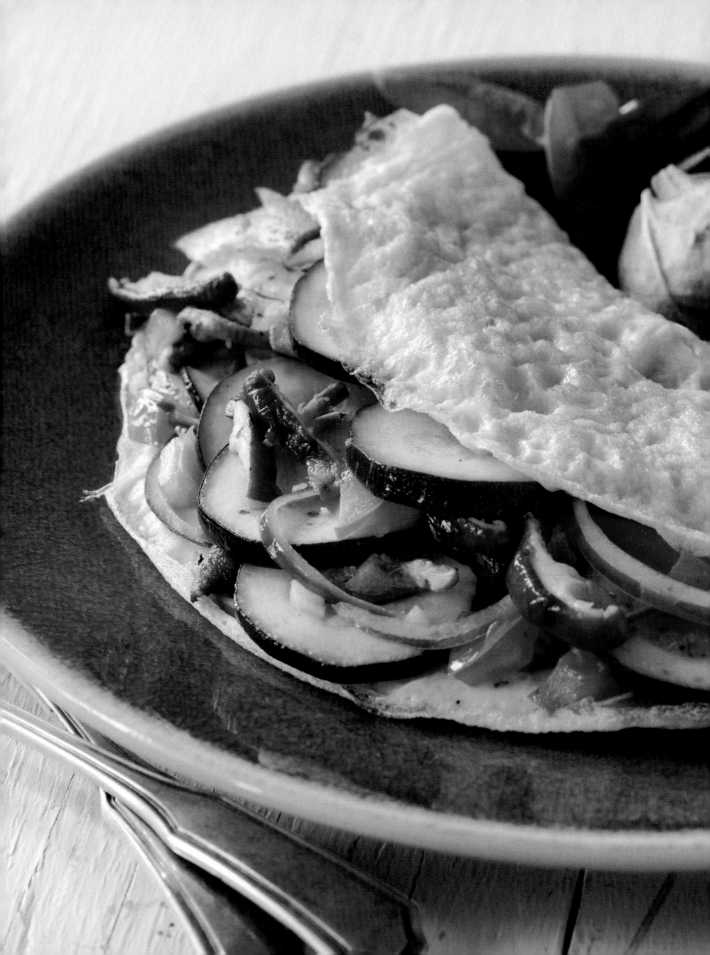

# Egg-White Veggie Omelet

**Prep time:** 10 minutes
**Cooking time:** 20 minutes
**Yield:** 2 servings

Egg-whites are essential sources of lean protein. They're a healthy alternative to meat, without losing the amino acids that help aid in muscle repair. This meal is simple and quick to make, which is great for those early mornings before your busy day.

## Ingredients

- Cooking spray
- ½ **red onion**, thinly sliced
- ½ **red pepper**, sliced into strips
- 1 cup **shiitake mushrooms**, sliced
- 1 **zucchini**, sliced into ¼-inch coins
- 1 tsp minced **garlic**
- 1 **tomato**, chopped
- ¼ tsp **oregano**
- 6 **egg whites** (separated eggs or prepared egg whites)
- **Black pepper**, to taste

## Method

1 Spray nonstick skillet with cooking spray. Heat on medium-high. Add onion and red pepper and sauté for 5 minutes. Add mushrooms and zucchini and sauté for another 5 minutes. Stir in garlic, tomato and oregano. Cover and simmer on low for about 4 minutes.

2 Meanwhile, separate eggs. Discard yolks. Whisk egg whites until frothy.

3 Spray second nonstick skillet with cooking spray and heat over medium-high. Once pan is hot, add egg whites.

4 Turn heat to medium. Allow eggs to cook for 1 minute. With a rubber spatula, separate the egg in the middle, allowing uncooked egg to seep through to cook. Conversely, you can lift the side of the egg and tilt the pan, allowing the uncooked egg to flow to the bottom.

5 Once the egg is nearly cooked through, flip it over so the remaining uncooked section can cook. Turn the heat off immediately.

6 Add the vegetables to one half of the egg, crack black pepper overtop and then fold the other half over. The omelet should resemble a half-moon at this point. Cut in half to serve.

**TIP:** You can customize this omelet by switching the type of mushrooms, throwing in some fresh herbs or heating things up with some sliced jalapeño.

**Nutritional value per serving:**
Calories: 148 | Calories from Fat: 11 | Protein: 15 g | Carbs: 22 g | Total Fat: 0.4 g | Saturated Fat: 0 g | Trans Fat: 0 g | Fiber: 3 g | Sodium: 349 mg | Cholesterol: 0 mg

# Lemon Dill Whitefish
## with Broiled Asparagus

**Prep time:** 20 minutes
**Cooking time:** 13 minutes
**Yield:** 4 x 1 fillet with ½ pound asparagus

White fish contain lean proteins that provide essential omega-3 fatty acids to your body. Asparagus is full of vitamins and makes a gourmet-tasting side dish. When doused with dill, this meal benefits stomach digestion and simply tastes divine!

## Ingredients

- ¼ cup chopped fresh dill
- Juice of 1 lemon
- 2 Tbsp grainy Dijon mustard
- White wine vinegar
- Olive oil spray
- 2 pounds fresh asparagus
- 4 x 6 oz white fish fillets
- One Vidalia onion, thinly sliced
- 1 lemon, sliced

## Method

1  Set broiler to low.

2  Mix first four ingredients together well in a small bowl. Allow to sit for 30 minutes to combine flavors.

3  Meanwhile, cut or break off the toughest part of the asparagus stems and discard. Prepare a baking sheet by spraying it with olive oil. Lay the asparagus in a single layer on the sheet and place in oven, six inches from the flame. Broil, keeping a close watch to make sure the asparagus doesn't brown too much, for about 5 minutes.

4  While the asparagus cooks, rub the fish with the lemon-dill mixture. Spray a baking sheet with cooking spray. Lay the onion slices on the baking sheet and lay the fillets on the onions.

5  Remove the pan from the oven and turn the asparagus. When you return the asparagus to the oven, put the white fish pan into the oven as well, both six inches from the flame if possible. If not, place the asparagus one rack lower, and the fish on the top rack.

6  Cook the asparagus and fish together for 8 minutes. To serve, divide asparagus evenly among four plates and place a fillet of fish on top.

**TIP:** If you don't have fresh dill handy, you can substitute it with 1 Tbsp dried dill instead.

**Nutritional value per serving:**
Calories: 336 | Calories from Fat: 117 | Protein: 44 g | Carbs: 11 g | Total Fat: 13 g | Saturated Fat: 2 g | Trans Fat: 0 g | Fiber: 3 g | Sodium: 294 mg | Cholesterol: 131 mg

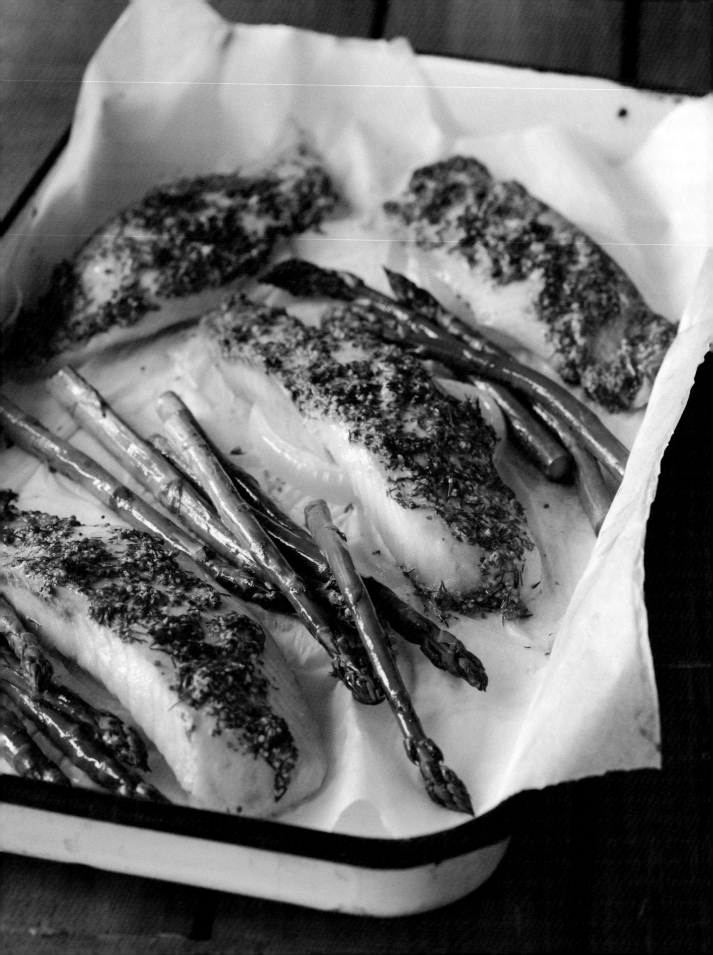

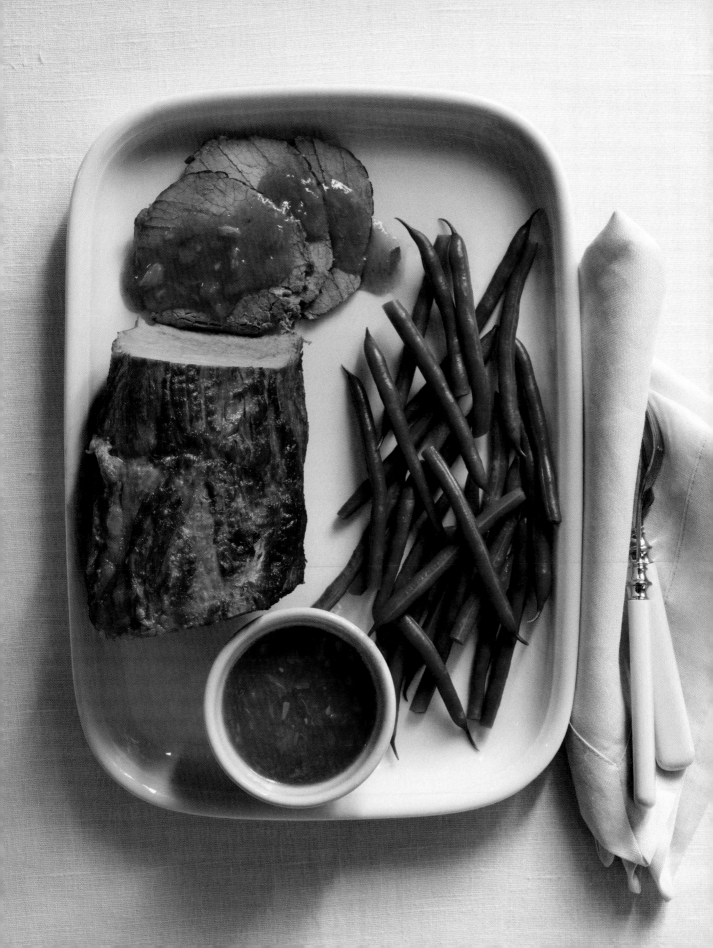

# Pot Roast
## with Green Beans

**Prep time:** 15 minutes
**Cooking time:** 3 hours
**Yield:** 6 x 4 oz beef
with 1 cup green beans

There's nothing like a big roast to complete a Sunday dinner. Trimming the fat off the meat makes this meal extra lean, and the green beans provide another dose of protein for an added bonus. It's a healthy meal the whole family will devour!

## Ingredients

- 1 Tbsp extra virgin olive oil
- 2 lb eye of round roast, visible fat removed
- 2 oz beef broth, more if necessary
- 3 cooking onions, sliced
- 3 bay leaves
- 1 bulb garlic, peeled
- 6 cups green beans, topped and tailed
- 1 Tbsp whole wheat flour

## Method

**1** In a large heavy pot or Dutch oven, heat the olive oil to medium-high. Add the roast and leave for about 45 seconds to brown that side. Turn to another side and continue this process until roast is completely browned. Remove from pot momentarily.

**2** Deglaze pot with 2 oz broth. Add the onions and bay leaves to the pot and cook for 5 minutes. Add roast back to pot, cover and turn to low. Cook for 30 minutes.

**3** After 30 minutes, open pot and place bulbs of garlic down the sides of the roast. Add another ounce or more of broth only if necessary. Cover pot again and cook for 2 hours.

**4** Again, remove meat from the pot just long enough to add green beans. Place the roast on top of the beans, close pot again and cook for 15 minutes further.

**5** Remove meat from pot to slice. Mix flour in with 6 oz cold water or broth. Mix together well, and add to the pot. Increase heat to high until boiling. Reduce heat to low and simmer until sauce thickens.

**6** To serve, place slices of pot roast on plate and spoon saucy onion/garlic/bean mixture on top.

**TIP:** For a lean alternative to beef, try roasting up some bison, venison or elk. Opt for low-fat, high-protein, grass-fed game meats for the best nutritional profile.

**Nutritional value per serving:**
Calories: 367 | Calories from Fat: 121 | Protein: 37 g | Carbs: 26 g | Total Fat: 13 g | Saturated Fat: 4 g | Trans Fat: 0 g | Fiber: 6 g | Sodium: 129 mg | Cholesterol: 69 mg

# Protein Shake

**Prep time:** 5 minutes
**Cooking time:** 0 minutes
**Yield:** 1 x 1 ½ cups

Simple, yet full of a sweet, fresh flavor, this protein shake makes for a great breakfast or post-workout drink. The protein will help with muscle repair while the carbs from the strawberries will boost your energy.

## Ingredients

- 1 cup water
- 1 tsp flaxseed oil
- 6 frozen strawberries
- Sugar-free vanilla whey protein powder
  (1 scoop for females, 2 scoops for males)

## Method

Blend first three ingredients, then add whey and blend again until smooth.

### Options:

Instead of strawberries you can use ¾ cup blackberries, blueberries or raspberries.

**TIP:** Whey protein powder is great for burning fat and building muscle. Check out page 152 for more info on this key ingredient.

**Nutritional value per serving (1 scoop protein):**
Calories: 164 | Calories from Fat: 40 | Protein: 24 g |
Carbs: 6 g | Total Fat: 5 g | Saturated Fat: 0.4 g | Trans Fat: 0 g |
Fiber: 0 g | Sodium: 47 mg | Cholesterol: 5 mg

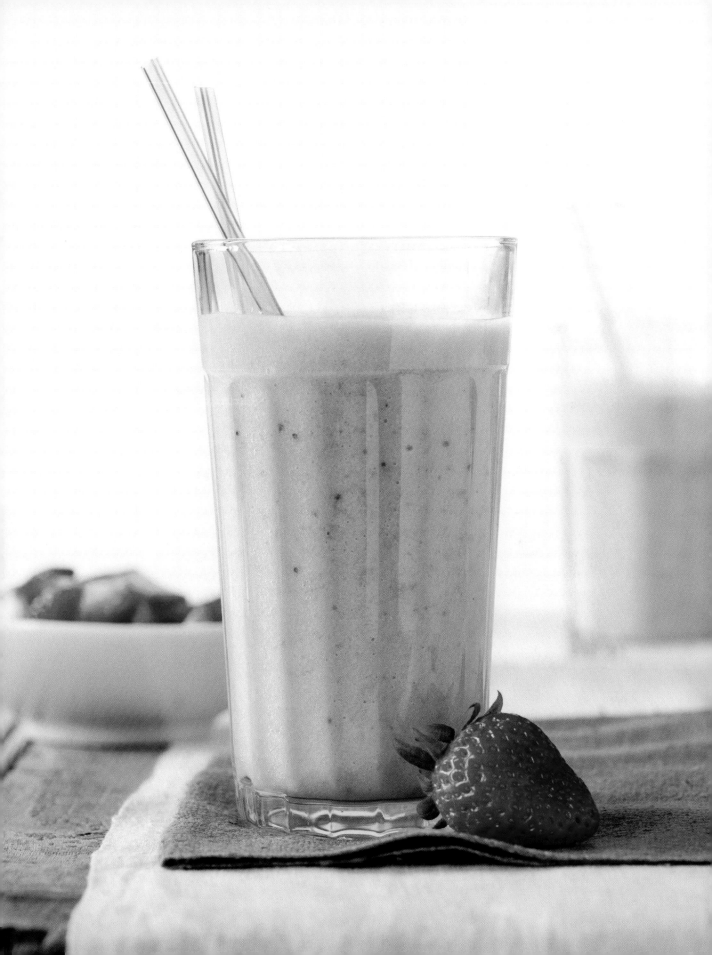

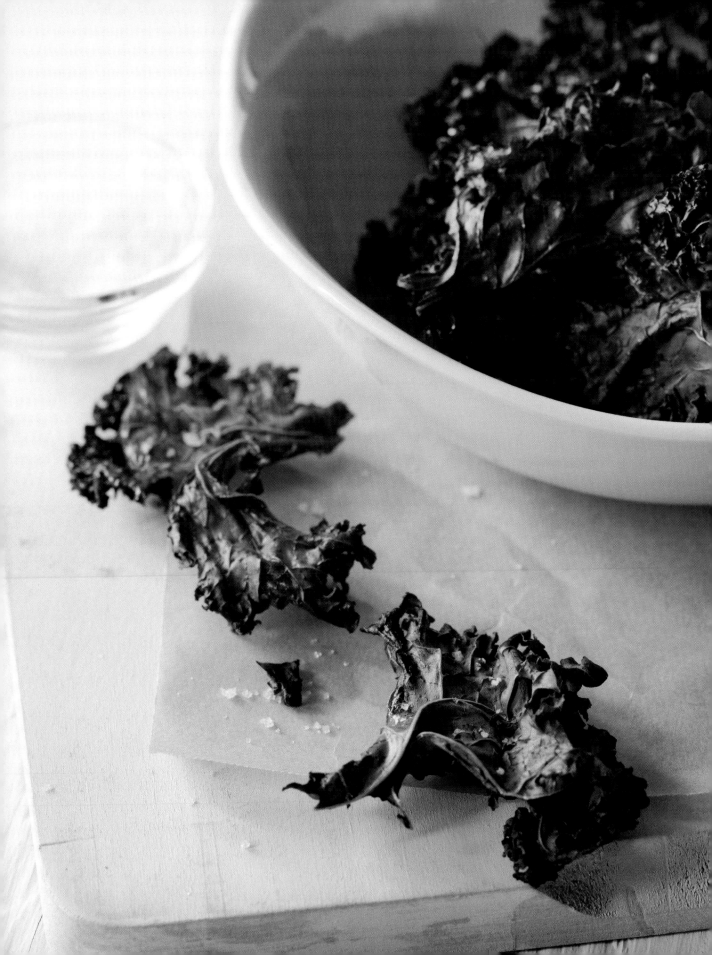

# Kale Chips

**Prep time:** 10 minutes
**Cooking time:** 30-35 minutes
**Yield:** 2-4 servings

Instead of trans-fatty potato chips and chip dip, here's a healthy snack you can dip into some all-natural hummus. Not only does it satisfy your salty-crunch craving, but the kale helps to lower cholesterol and offers disease-fighting minerals. A bag of store-bought chips can't do all that!

## Ingredients

- 1 bunch kale (flat-leaf kale is best if you can find it)
- 1 Tbsp extra virgin olive oil
- 1 Tbsp balsamic vinegar (optional)
- 2 pinches salt (sea salt is best)

## Method

1  Preheat oven to 300°F.

2  Wash kale well. Remove stalks and ribs, and rip into bite-sized pieces. Place in salad spinner and spin until very dry.

3  Place kale in a food-grade plastic bag. Add the olive oil and vinegar (if using), and massage into the kale through the bag.

4  Spray a large baking sheet with cooking spray. Lay the kale in a single layer on the sheet, sprinkle with salt and place on the middle rack in the oven.

5  Bake for approximately 30 to 35 minutes, or until crispy. Cooking time will likely be 30 minutes if using flat leaf, 35 if curly.

**TIP:** As an excellent source of dietary fiber, kale will keep you feeling full and help you maintain a slim waistline. These "chips" will satisfy your craving for a crunchy snack.

**Nutritional value per serving:**
Calories: 66 | Calories from Fat: 34 | Protein: 2 g |
Carbs: 4 g | Total Fat: 4 g | Saturated Fat: 1 g | Trans Fat: 0 g |
Fiber: 1 g | Sodium: 31 mg | Cholesterol: 0 mg

# Oven-Steamed Greens

**Prep time:** 20 minutes
**Cooking time:** 13-18 minutes
**Yield:** 4 x 1½ cups

Here's to greens, greens and more greens! Overloaded with vitamins and minerals, this dish makes a powerful sidekick to any meat- or protein-filled main course.

## Ingredients

- 1 bunch kale
- 1 bunch Swiss chard, preferably red
- 1 bunch collard greens
- 2 Tbsp balsamic vinegar
- 1 red onion, chopped
- Cooking spray
- 1 bulb garlic, each clove peeled
- 1 tsp smoked paprika
- Black pepper

## Method

1 Preheat oven to 400°F.

2 Wash greens thoroughly. Remove the toughest stems. Chop the rest of the leaves and stems and mix together in a large bowl. Sprinkle with vinegar and toss with clean hands or tongs. Add red onion, and mix again.

3 On a baking sheet, lay one or two sheets of aluminum foil or parchment paper, large enough that you will be able to wrap it around the pile of greens and still fold it together.

4 Spray the bottom of the foil/parchment with cooking spray. Scatter the cloves of garlic over the foil/parchment. Scoop all the greens/onion mixture on top. Sprinkle with smoked paprika and black pepper.

5 Wrap the foil/parchment over the greens, folding all along the center seam to seal. Fold each side closed so the whole bundle is sealed.

6 Place the baking sheet on the middle rack in the oven. Cook for 10 to 15 minutes. Be careful when opening the packet – very hot steam will rush out.

**TIP:** It's better to steam vegetables than to boil them, since fewer nutrients are leached out. Steaming provides the best retention of flavor, color and texture.

**Nutritional value per serving:**
Calories: 59 | Calories from Fat: 4 | Protein: 3 g |
Carbs: 12 g | Total Fat: 0.4 g | Saturated Fat: 0 g | Trans Fat: 0 g |
Fiber: 2 g | Sodium: 60 mg | Cholesterol: 0 mg

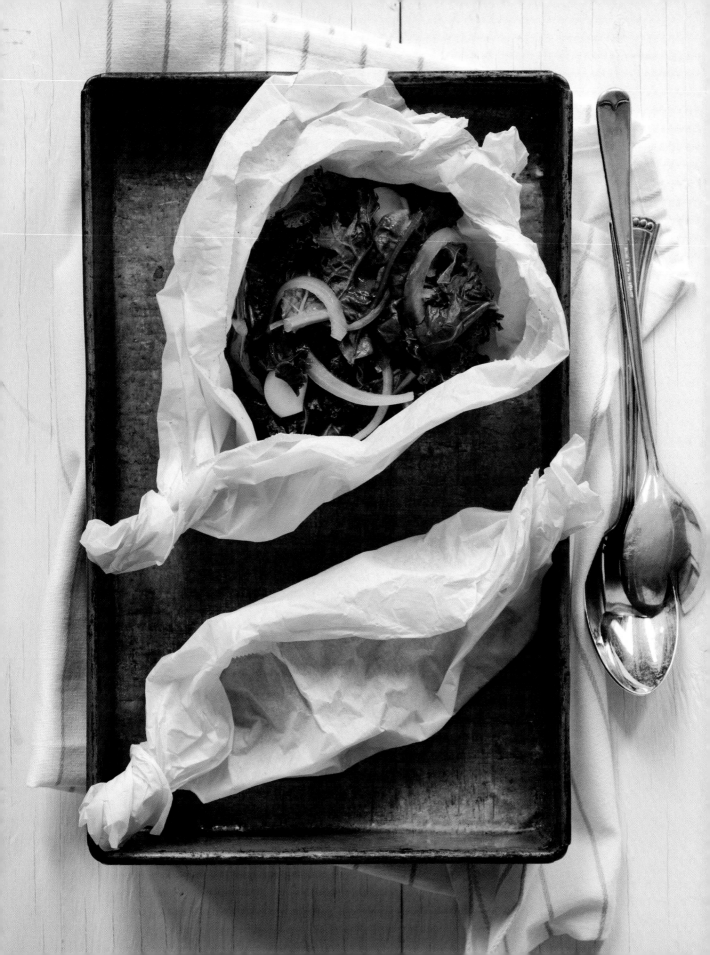

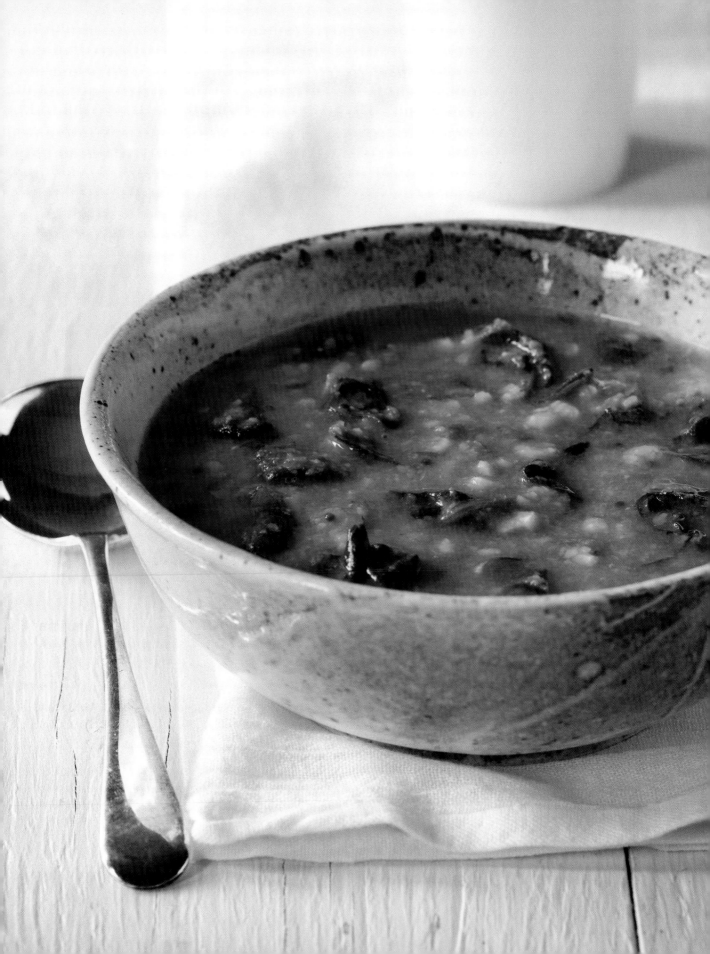

# Spicy Split Pea Soup

**Prep time:** 10 minutes
**Cooking time:** 45 minutes + 20 minutes
**Yield:** 4 x 1½ cups

This hearty, vegetable-laden soup will boost your metabolism with a kick of hot pepper and spices. The comforting, creamy texture will definitely leave you feeling satisfied after every bowl.

## Ingredients

- 1 cup split yellow peas
- 1 Tbsp extra virgin olive oil
- ½ tsp mustard seeds
- ½ tsp cumin seeds
- 2 cloves
- 1 hot pepper
- 3 medium tomatoes, blended
- 1 tsp minced fresh ginger
- 1 Tbsp minced fresh garlic
- 1 tsp ground cumin
- ½ tsp turmeric
- 4 cups fresh baby spinach or one package frozen chopped spinach
- 3 Tbsp chopped cilantro
- 3 Tbsp freshly squeezed lemon juice

## Method

1 Wash and rinse split peas, discarding any stones. Place in a medium-large pot with 3 cups water. Bring to a rolling boil and then turn down to simmer until soft – about 45 minutes. Scoop off any foam and discard. Blend with an immersion blender or mash until smooth. This step can be performed up to a day before, if desired.

2 In a large pot, heat oil on medium. Add mustard seeds, cumin seeds and cloves. Cook for 2 minutes or until you hear the mustard seeds pop.

3 Add the rest of the ingredients except spinach, cilantro and lemon juice. Cook for 6 minutes. Add blended split peas, stir well and cook for 10 minutes longer.

4 Stir in spinach, cilantro and lemon juice.

**TIP:** Make a big pot of this hearty soup and save some for leftovers. It's a quick dinner after a long day or a warm lunch on a cold afternoon.

**Nutritional value per serving:**
Calories: 117 | Calories from Fat: 42 | Protein: 6 g |
Carbs: 15 g | Total Fat: 4 g | Saturated Fat: 1 g | Trans Fat: 0 g |
Fiber: 5 g | Sodium: 43 mg | Cholesterol: 0 mg

# Lemon Garlic Spinach

**Prep time:** 5 minutes
**Cooking time:** 5 minutes
**Yield:** 4 x ½ cup

Spinach is a high-protein vegetable that's packed with disease-fighting phytonutrients. Throwing in some garlic makes this dish your immune system's best friend, and fresh lemon juice adds a zesty flavor!

## Ingredients

- 1 Tbsp extra virgin olive oil
- 3 cloves garlic, minced
- 20 oz baby spinach
- Juice of ½ lemon
- Black pepper, to taste

## Method

1  In a large skillet, heat oil on medium high. Add minced garlic and cook, stirring, for 1 minute.

2  Add spinach and cover skillet. Cook for 1 minute, then open and stir so uncooked spinach touches skillet surface. Cover and cook 1 minute more. Remove lid and squeeze lemon over entire skillet. Stir again and cook for 1 to 2 minutes more, or until all spinach is wilted but not overcooked.

3  Grind black pepper over entire skillet, and serve.

**TIP:** If you want to know why Popeye was so strong, check back to page 146 for the low-down on the health benefits of spinach.

**Nutritional value per serving:**
Calories: 66 | Calories from Fat: 35 | Protein: 5 g |
Carbs: 7 g | Total Fat: 4 g | Saturated Fat: 1 g | Trans Fat: 0 g |
Fiber: 5 g | Sodium: 111 mg | Cholesterol: 0 mg

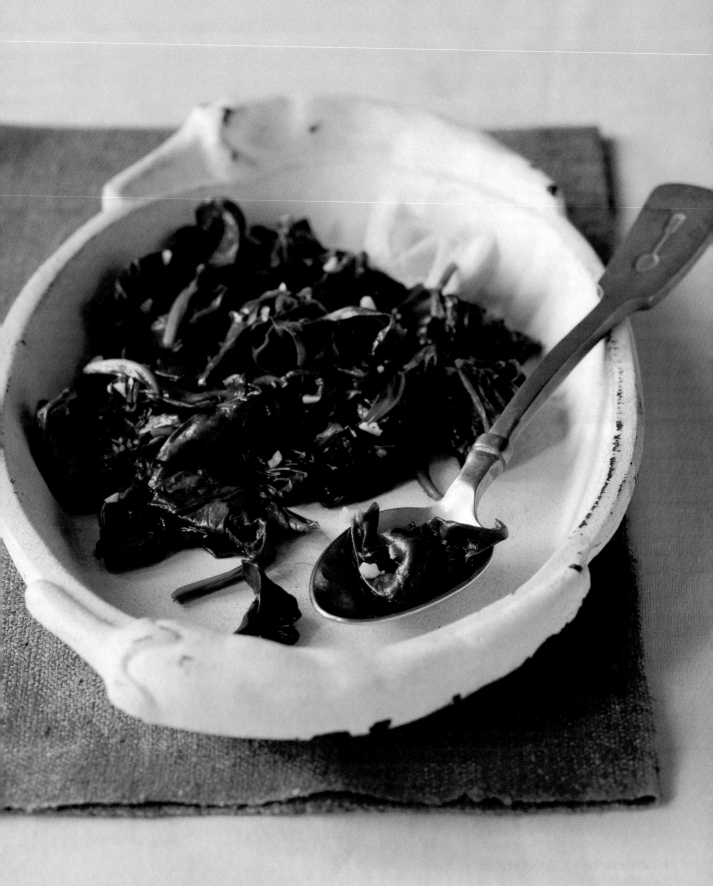

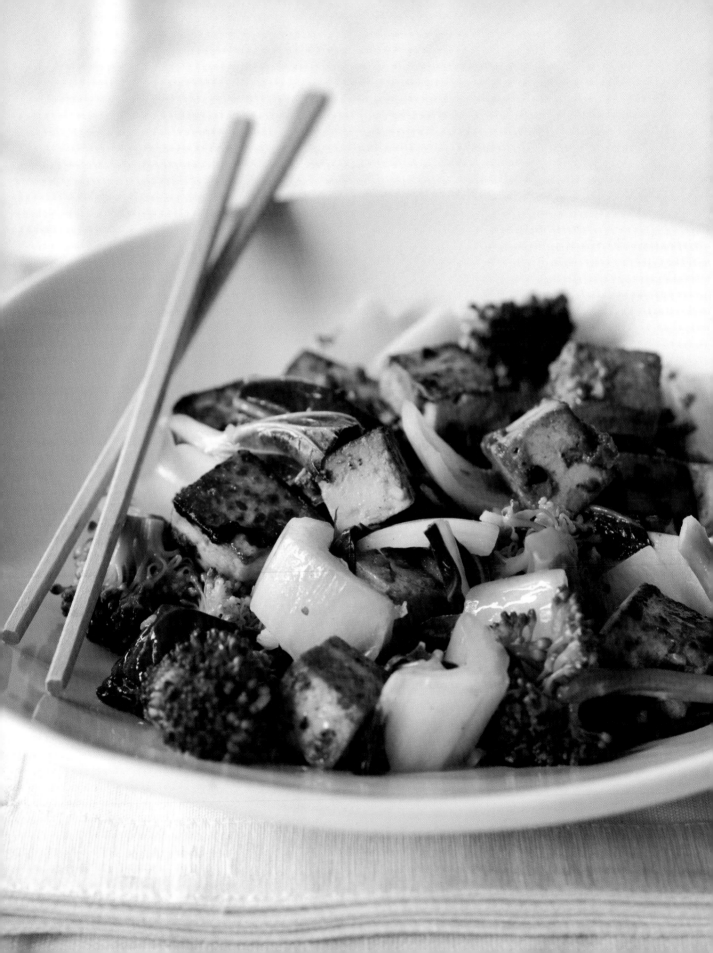

# Marinated Tofu Stir-Fry

**Prep time:** 25 minutes
**Cooking time:** 35 minutes
**Yield:** 4 x 2 cups

Tofu contains enough protein and minerals to power you through your workouts. This lean meal is the perfect meatless dish for vegetarians or for those taking a break from eating red meats and poultry.

## Ingredients

- ¼ cup low-sodium tamari
- ¼ cup rice vinegar
- ¼ cup Worcestershire sauce
- 2 Tbsp Dijon mustard
- 3 cloves garlic, minced, divided
- 2 inches fresh ginger, finely chopped, divided
- 1 lb extra firm tofu
- 2 tsp sesame oil
- 1 medium onion, chopped
- 1 large bunch broccoli, peeled and cut into small florets and stem pieces
- 1 head Chinese cabbage or bok choy, chopped roughly

## Method

1 To make marinade, place tamari, vinegar, Worcestershire sauce and mustard in a medium-sized flat-bottomed container. Add one minced clove of garlic and one inch of finely chopped ginger. Mix together well.

2 Take tofu from package and cut into ½- to ¾-inch cubes. Place cubes in marinade and stir to ensure marinade touches all surfaces. Refrigerate for one hour.

3 Meanwhile, prepare vegetables.

4 Heat oil in large skillet or wok on high. Add onion. Sauté for about 3 minutes. Add the rest of the garlic and the rest of the ginger. Sauté for another 3 minutes.

5 Add broccoli a bit at a time, stir-frying. Remove some of the cooked broccoli as you go along to make more room to stir-fry the next batch. Once the broccoli is done, remove to a plate and add Chinese cabbage or bok choy, again a bit at a time. Remove cabbage or bok choy and set aside.

6 Get tofu from fridge and add to pan with about ¼ to ½ cup of the marinade. Cook just until heated through. Add vegetables back in and stir gently to combine. Once everything is heated through, you may serve.

**TIP:** Since tofu is flavorless, it will absorb the marinade nicely. You can even leave it overnight so it bursts with tang and spice for your stir fry the next day!

**Nutritional value per serving:**
Calories: 262 | Calories from Fat: 96 | Protein: 22 g |
Carbs: 26 g | Total Fat: 11 g | Saturated Fat: 2 g | Trans Fat: 0 g |
Fiber: 8 g | Sodium: 1248 mg | Cholesterol: 0 mg

# Beef Fajita Wraps

**Prep time:** 12 minutes
**Cooking time:** 30 minutes
**Yield:** 4 fajitas

These fajitas let you savor Mexican flavors without the bad fats from sour cream and cheese. Jalapeños give your metabolism a kick, while the avocado throws in a dose of healthy fat.

## Ingredients

- 1 Tbsp extra virgin olive oil
- 1 lb flank steak, visible fat removed
- 4 pinches salt
- Pepper, to taste
- Garlic powder, to taste
- 2 oz beef broth
- 1 onion, sliced
- 1 green bell pepper, sliced
- 1 or 2 jalapeño peppers, chopped
- 2 cloves garlic, minced
- 1 tsp chili powder
- 1 tsp ground cumin
- 1 tsp ground coriander
- Juice of ½ lime
- 4 x 7-inch whole wheat tortillas
- ½ cup Greek yogurt
- ½ avocado, cut into 8 slices
- 4 tsp chopped cilantro
- Salsa, optional

## Method

1 Heat olive oil in a large skillet on high. Season steak with salt, pepper and garlic powder. Sear 4 minutes each side. Remove from heat, let rest 5 minutes and then cut into thin strips.

2 Add beef broth to pan and deglaze. Reduce heat to medium-high and add onion to skillet. Sauté for about 5 minutes. Add the green pepper and jalapeño peppers. Sauté for 3 minutes. Add the garlic.

3 Immediately return the beef to the pan and stir to combine with onions and peppers. Sprinkle with spices and then stir to blend flavors throughout the dish. Cook for about 4 to 5 minutes. Add lime juice and stir in, then remove from heat.

4 To make fajitas, spread each tortilla with 2 Tbsp Greek yogurt. Lay two slices of avocado on top. Spoon ¼ of the beef mixture on top of the avocado, and top with 1 tsp cilantro. Add salsa if desired, then roll up tightly, closing the bottom of the tortilla as you go. You will need a toothpick to keep this closed.

**TIP:** Flank steak can be a tougher cut of meat because of its low fat content. Slicing the meat thinly against the grain will help.

**Nutritional value per serving:**
Calories: 381 | Calories from Fat: 146 | Protein: 32 g |
Carbs: 25 g | Total Fat: 16 g | Saturated Fat: 4 g | Trans Fat: 0 g |
Fiber: 4 g | Sodium: 1384 mg | Cholesterol: 48 mg

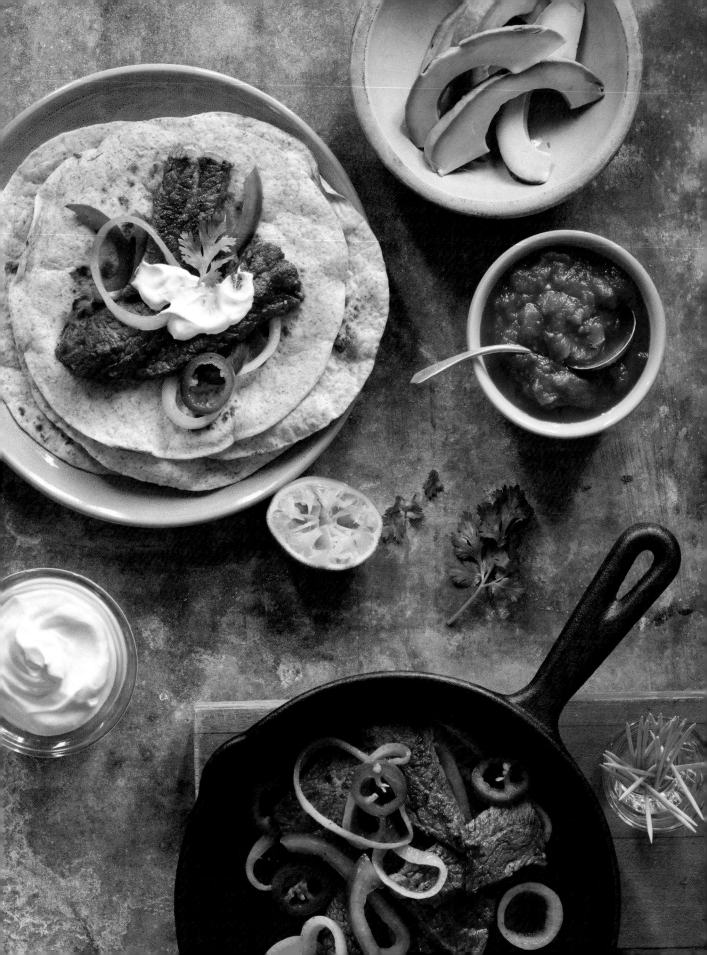

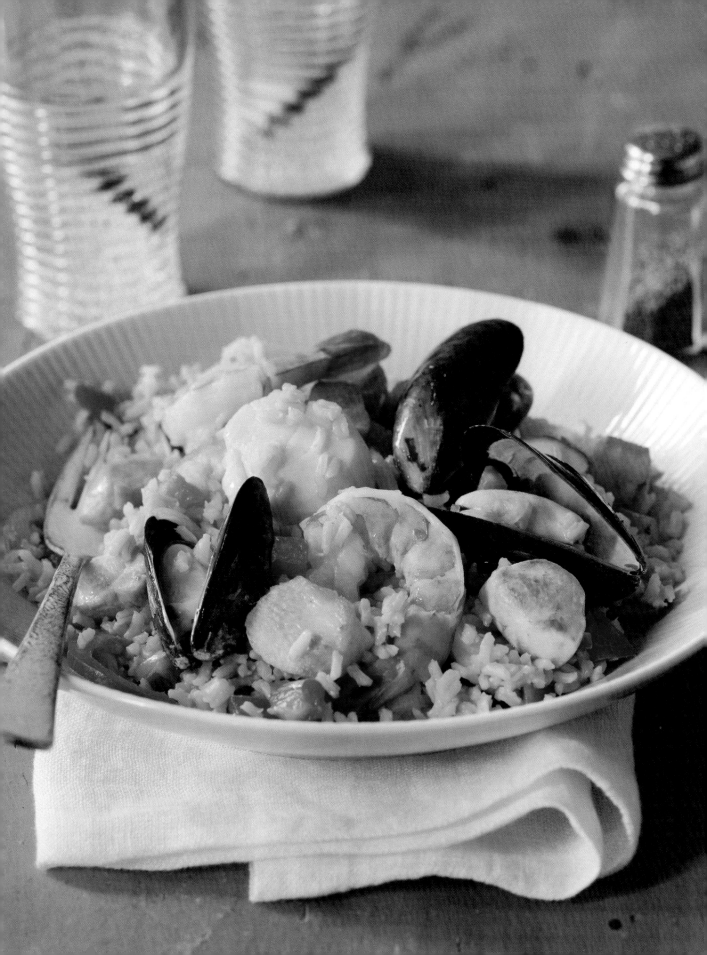

# Paella

**Prep time:** 25 minutes
**Cooking time:** 1 hour
**Yield:** 4 x 2 cups

Paella is a traditional rice dish that originates from Spain. You can whip up your own Spanish flavor with this nutrient-rich and satisfying recipe. Using brown rice instead of the traditional white rice adds an extra dose of antioxidants and manganese for energy. *Olé!*

## Ingredients

- 1 Tbsp olive oil
- 4 x 4-oz chicken breasts, cut into 1-inch cubes
- 1 cooking onion, sliced
- 1 Tbsp garlic, chopped
- 2 cups diced tomatoes
- 1 cup sliced red pepper
- 1 cup sliced green pepper
- 1 cup sliced zucchini
- 4 large scallops
- 8 medium shrimp
- 8 mussels
- Pinch saffron
- 2 Tbsp chopped fresh basil
- 1 cup brown rice
- Salt and pepper to taste
- 2 cups chicken broth
- Juice of ½ lemon

## Method

1 Heat olive oil in a large skillet on medium high. Add chicken and brown. Remove from pan and reserve.

2 Add onion to pan and sauté for 3 minutes. Add garlic and tomatoes and simmer for 4 to 5 minutes. Add peppers and zucchini. Cook for 5 minutes.

3 Stir in the seafood, then saffron, basil and rice. Mix well and add broth. Bring to a boil.

4 Reduce heat and let simmer until rice is cooked – about 45 minutes. Squeeze lemon juice on top and season with salt and pepper.

**TIP:** Shrimp have gotten a bad rap because of their cholesterol content, but they also contain healthy omega-3 fatty acids and cancer-fighting selenium.

**Nutritional value per serving:**
Calories: 535 | Calories from Fat: 114 | Protein: 50 g |
Carbs: 32 g | Total Fat: 12 g | Saturated Fat: 3 g | Trans Fat: 0 g |
Fiber: 5 g | Sodium: 488 mg | Cholesterol: 187 mg

# Seafood Frittata

**Prep time:** 20 minutes
**Cooking time:** 30 minutes
**Yield:** 4 x 2 slices

Here's one recipe that will supply you with a healthy dose of omega-3 fatty acids! Combining eggs, seafood and veggies not only tantalizes the taste buds, but infuses your body with essential nutrients – a great morning meal to give you energy throughout the day!

## Ingredients

- 1 Tbsp coconut oil
- 1 cup thinly sliced red onion
- 1 zucchini, thinly sliced
- 1 cup thinly sliced red peppers
- 2 tsp minced garlic
- ½ cup Greek yogurt
- 2 Tbsp fresh thyme

- 8 egg whites + 2 whole eggs
- 8 oz fresh shrimp
- 8 oz fresh salmon, preferably wild caught
- 2 cups thinly sliced shiitake mushrooms
- Salt and pepper, to taste

## Method

1 Preheat broiler to low.

2 In a deep ovenproof frying pan, heat oil on medium high and sauté onions until soft – about 5 minutes. Add zucchini, mushrooms, peppers and garlic. Cook until vegetables soften, another 5 to 6 minutes.

3 Meanwhile, in a small bowl, whip thyme into Greek yogurt until yogurt is smooth and creamy.

4 In a large bowl, beat the eggs until frothy. Season with salt and pepper. Stir in salmon and shrimp. Add herbed yogurt. Combine well.

5 Add this mixture to the vegetable mixture and cook for 5 minutes. Place pan under broiler until eggs are set and top is browned.

6 Cut into 8 slices and serve.

**TIP:** Alaska wild-caught salmon offers the most health benefits with the lowest risk of contaminants such as mercury.

**Nutritional value per serving:**
Calories: 333 | Calories from Fat: 102 | Protein: 37 g | Carbs: 21 g | Total Fat: 12 g | Saturated Fat: 4 g | Trans Fat: 0 g | Fiber: 3 g | Sodium: 372 mg | Cholesterol: 181 mg

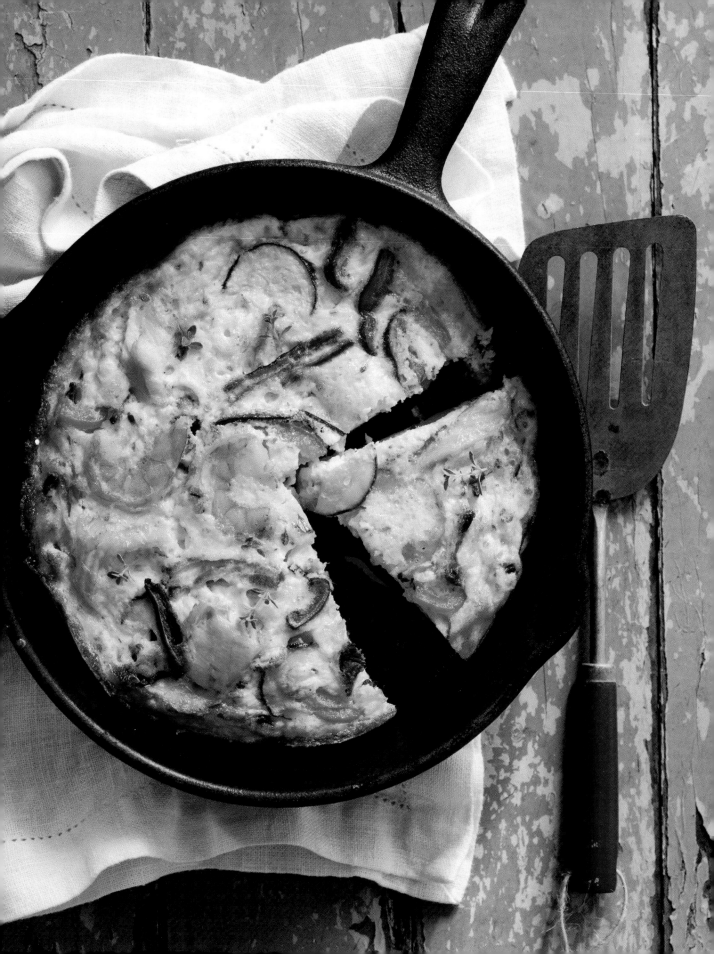

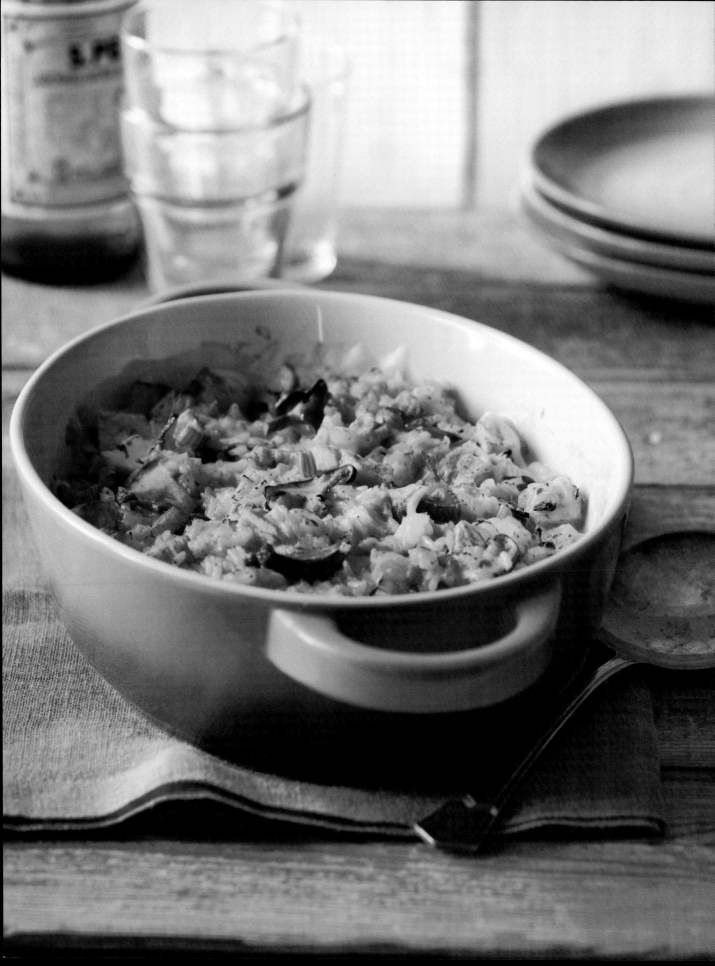

# Turkey Rice Casserole

**Prep time:** 15 minutes
**Cooking time:** 50 minutes
**Yield:** 4 x 2 cups

This recipe is great with fresh turkey or even festive turkey leftovers. The poultry itself contains lean protein and will increase your metabolic rate. This meal will leave you feeling relaxed, since turkey supplies you with tryptophan that keeps your stress levels down.

## Ingredients

- 1 Tbsp coconut oil or butter
- 2 cooking onions, chopped
- 3 stalks celery, chopped
- 2 cloves garlic, minced
- 1 cup sliced shiitake mushrooms
- 4 cups diced cooked turkey
- 4 cups cooked brown rice
- 2 Tbsp whole wheat flour
- 1 cup cold skim or 1% milk
- 1 cup cold chicken or vegetable stock

## Method

1 Preheat oven to 350°F.

2 In a skillet, heat the coconut oil on medium high. Add onions and celery and cook for about 3 to 4 minutes, stirring. Add the garlic and mushrooms and cook for 1 minute more.

3 Place turkey and rice in a 2-quart casserole dish. Spoon onion mixture overtop and mix in thoroughly.

4 Place flour in a small bowl. Add cold milk and stock, and mix until smooth with no lumps. Pour over the turkey mixture in the casserole dish. Mix gently so liquid is evenly dispersed.

5 Place casserole, uncovered, on middle rack in oven. Cook for 45 minutes. Allow to sit for 5 minutes before serving.

**TIP:** In the United States alone, turkey consumption has increased 108% since 1970. Not surprising, given its nutrient profile!

**Nutritional value per serving:**
Calories: 602 | Calories from Fat: 93 | Protein: 53 g |
Carbs: 73 g | Total Fat: 11 g | Saturated Fat: 5 g | Trans Fat: 0 g |
Fiber: 8 g | Sodium: 291 mg | Cholesterol: 141 mg

# Cabbage Rolls

**Prep time:** 25 minutes
**Cooking time:** 40 minutes
**Yield:** 6 servings of 2 cabbage rolls

These bundles of protein and fiber are the perfect champion's snack or meal! Cabbage is packed with glutamine to help maintain muscle mass and benefit the digestive tract. There's also an abundance of vitamins C and A to amp up the immune system and help keep skin and eyes healthy.

## Ingredients

- 12 cabbage leaves
- 1 lb ground chicken
- ¾ cup cooked brown rice or quinoa
- 1 cup finely chopped red onion
- 1 egg
- ½ cup skim or 1% milk
- 1 tsp black pepper
- 2 Tbsp cornstarch

## Sauce

- 2 cups diced tomatoes
- 1 cup good-quality low-sodium tomato sauce
- 1 Tbsp basil
- 2 Tbsp vinegar
- ½ cup chicken broth

## Method

1 Preheat oven to 400°F.

2 Boil at least 8 cups of water in a large pot. Boil or steam cabbage leaves for 3 minutes. You can do this in batches if you like. Remove from heat immediately.

## Sauce

1 Combine all sauce ingredients in a medium-sized bowl. Set aside.

## Filling

1 In a large bowl, combine chicken, rice or quinoa, onion, egg, milk and pepper. Mix well and divide into 12 equal portions.

2 Place each portion in a cabbage leaf. Roll up and secure with a toothpick.

3 Place cabbage rolls side by side in a baking dish at least two inches deep and with a cover. Pour sauce over top.

4 Bake, covered, for 40 minutes.

5 When cooked, remove cabbage rolls from baking dish. Transfer juices to saucepan. Mix cornstarch with ¼ cup cold water and stir into juices. Bring to a boil and then reduce heat. Simmer until this mix thickens. Pour over cabbage rolls when serving.

**TIP:** Steaming cabbage instead of boiling it causes the fiber to bind together better with acids in your digestive tract, resulting in lower cholesterol for you!

**Nutritional value per serving:**
Calories: 274 | Calories from Fat: 93 | Protein: 22 g | Carbs: 23 g | Total Fat: 11 g | Saturated Fat: 3 g | Trans Fat: 0 g | Fiber: 5 g | Sodium: 140 mg | Cholesterol: 112 mg

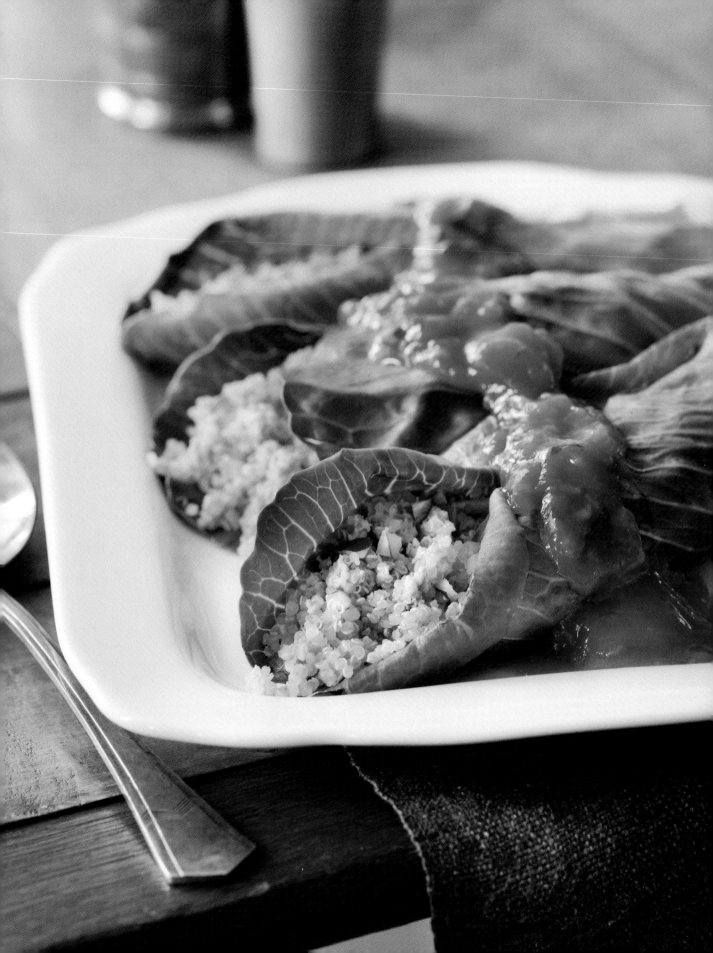

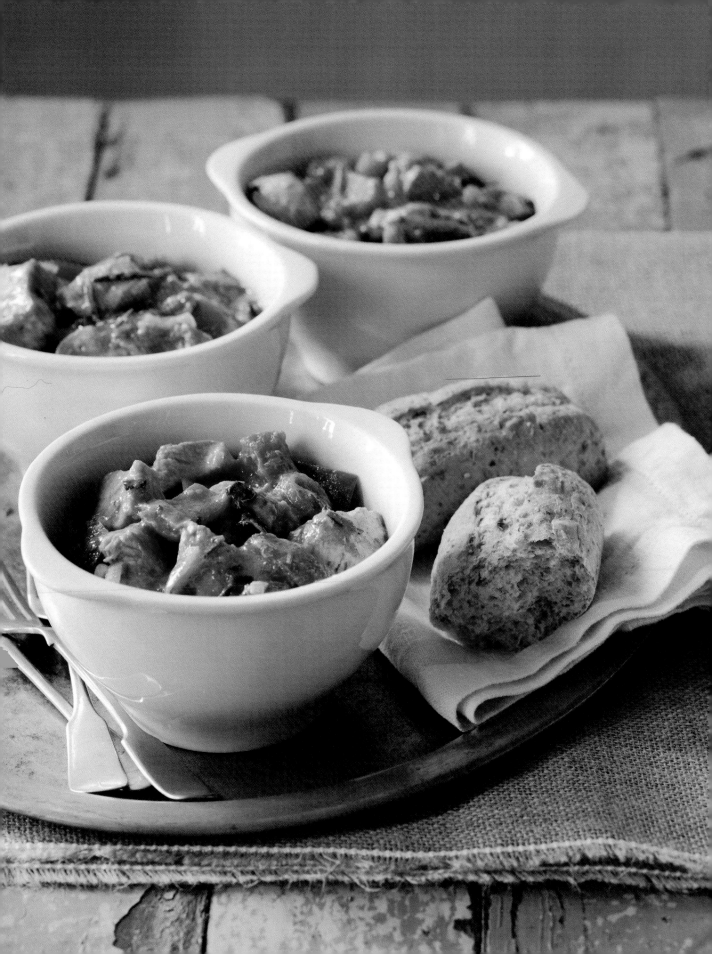

# Hungarian Turkey Stew

**Prep time:** 20 minutes
**Cooking time:** 1 hour
**Yield:** 4 x 2 cups

Low-fat, high-protein turkey paired with metabolism-boosting spices and bunches of vitamin-rich veggies makes this a nutrient powerhouse-in-a-pot! Not to mention, leftover stew is great during the week when you need something quick.

## Ingredients

- 2 lbs turkey breast, cut into 1-inch cubes
- Pinch each sea salt and black pepper
- ½ tsp garlic powder
- 2 Tbsp coconut oil or
- 1 cup sliced leeks
- 2 cups sliced shallots

- 2 cups sliced red peppers
- 2 cups sliced green peppers
- 1 Tbsp chopped garlic
- 1 cup cremini mushrooms, sliced
- 1½ Tbsp paprika
- or to taste

- 2 cups canned plum tomatoes, chopped
- 1 Tbsp lemon juice
- 1 Tbsp Worcestershire sauce
- 1 tsp fresh rosemary, chopped
- Sea salt and black pepper, to taste

## Method

**1** Spray a large pan with cooking spray. Add turkey breast and sprinkle with salt, pepper and garlic powder. Sauté until golden brown. Remove from pan.

**2** In same pan, heat 1 Tbsp coconut oil and sauté leeks, shallots and peppers until caramelized – about 10 minutes. Add garlic. Cook 2 minutes. Remove onion mixture from pan and set aside.

**3** Add remaining coconut oil to pan and sauté mushrooms until browned. Once mushrooms are browned, mix in the onion and pepper mixture along with turkey. Add the paprika and cayenne pepper.

**4** Mix in tomatoes, lemon juice, Worcestershire sauce, rosemary, salt and pepper. Bring to a boil. Reduce heat and simmer for 20 minutes. Turn off heat.

**5** Mix together yogurt and cornstarch. Add this mixture to the pan and stir until sauce thickens.

**TIP:** Feel the heat! The capsaicin found in cayenne pepper causes thermogenesis (heat production) in the body when consumed. Your body burns energy – and calories! – to create all that heat.

**Nutritional value per serving:**
Calories: 609 | Calories from Fat: 135 | Protein: 77 g |
Carbs: 38 g | Total Fat: 15 g | Saturated Fat: 8 g | Trans Fat: 0 g |
Fiber: 5 g | Sodium: 782 mg | Cholesterol: 158 mg

# INDEX

# BIOGRAPHY

Although it might be hard to believe that someone not yet 30 could earn national acclaim for helping hundreds of people take control of their health and habits, Charles D'Angelo has done exactly that.

A decade ago, the idea of such a bright and promising future would have been incomprehensible to Charles. He was morbidly obese, miserable and had resigned himself to lifetime of lonely nights spent gorging on junk food in front of the TV.

It took one sudden, terrifying experience to help Charles make the decision that saved his life. In a matter of years, he was able to change not only his body – going from wearing a size-50 pant to having an enviably lean, muscular physique – but also his entire world. Through his own transformation, which included extensive studies of the masters of psychology, Charles learned that success starts in the mind. Armed with this newfound knowledge, determination and an arsenal of valuable strategies, he set out on a mission to improve as many lives as possible.

With each new success story, Charles became known for creating remarkable transformations in the minds, bodies, and spirits of all those he coached.

While he's not a doctor, personal trainer, dietician, or nutritionist, his success in helping people transform surpasses that of many of the nation's most respected professionals in these fields.

In fact, many doctors, therapists, dieticians and personal trainers have sought his personal counsel and even recommended his approach to healthy living. His secret? Fitness success is not found in the science of nutrition, it's found in the mastering of your own thoughts!

Many of Charles' clients, including CEOs and nationally recognized politicians, have traveled thousands of miles to seek his help as their personal coach. Although he regrets that he can't counsel the country's more than 200 million overweight citizens personally, he knows that by sharing the strategies that have helped so many in *Think and Grow Thin,* he will be well on his way to creating a healthier, happier world.

Are you ready to let Charles D'Angelo "The Weight-Loss Coach" help you transform your life?

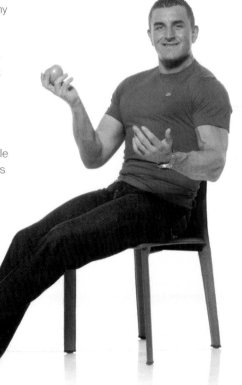

# ACKNOWLEDGMENTS

Think of your favorite film, one that really moved you and changed the way you look at life. Got one? Now, I bet you can name the lead actor, maybe one or two supporting actors, right? Can you tell me who engineered the lighting? Do you know who built the sets? Probably not. Although we don't often stay glued to our seats as the credits roll, we are aware that countless folks are working tirelessly behind the scenes to ensure everything comes out just right. They all believe wholeheartedly in the message of the movie, and they all want the audience to leave the theater changed for the better. Writing a book works much in the same way, and I'm blessed to have a team behind me that believes as much in my message as I do.

It's with tremendous humility that I extend my appreciation to all those who have helped bring me to this point in life, a point where I'm making my dream of helping millions to change their lives a reality. Nothing is accomplished alone. With this in mind, you can imagine just how difficult it is to name all those who've been such a positive part of my life.

- I want to express my gratitude to God, our Creator. His direction led me to those who've been so instrumental in bringing my message of Hope to the world. I am simply a conduit. It's because of Him that you're reading this!

- I want to express my infinite love and appreciation to my mother and father, Laura and Charles, my sister Lauren and brother Vince. My parents made many sacrifices for their children and worked hard to instill the conviction that through absolute faith and hard work, any challenge could be overcome.

- To my adopted grandmother, Mrs. Valerie White, whose tremendous faith in God and in the innate goodness that exists in all humans changed my life. Coming to personally know God helped me realize that truly lasting change would come only through mental transformation. I owe much to this saint-like woman. I can't think of anyone who's influenced me more deeply.

- To my grandparents, Rose, Charlie and Marie, who are smiling down from heaven. Their lives and influence serve as a constant reminder to work hard and serve others.

- To Joyce, a magnificent spirit, great friend and tremendous help in my mission of spreading the message of Hope to the world through my book.

- To all the countless clients who've worked so hard in achieving their goals. You've spread my message everywhere from local parties all the way to the White House! It's because of all of you that I've been able to reach – and help – so many, and for that I'm extremely grateful.

- To President Bill Clinton. Your passion for doing what's right, your tireless efforts in improving our global society and serving others less fortunate means more to me than you'll ever know, and this has helped me make critical life decisions fueling my fire to do what's right and serve others with my gifts. I look up to you so much. I hope to one day have as positive an impact on our world as you have. Thank you for the wonderful influence you and your life has provided me.

- To a man I will forever treasure, and who radically changed me along with my worldview, Mr. David Steward. He is a walking, talking testament to our Lord's message. I'm blessed to call him my mentor and dear friend. I'm indebted to him for all of his support, wisdom and guidance. His commitment to bettering the lives of others is unparalleled and serves as an inspiration to me.

- To Wendy Morley, director at Robert Kennedy Publishing. Her unwavering support and faith literally brought my book to Bob Kennedy's attention and masterfully carried it though every step of the editorial process, resulting in the high-quality product that you are holding right now. If it wasn't for Wendy listening to God's call and her gift in editing and publishing, this book couldn't have been so magnificent.

- To my mentor, Mr. Ray Bahr, who's been supportive, loving and willing to listen to all my creative impulses. His example of the value of honesty, structure, discipline and commitment affected me deeply.

- To all of my teachers, friends and other staff members at Christian Brothers College High School, you helped mold me into the man I am today.

- To all the great educators, staff and friends I made at St. Louis University, my alma mater. Your example of God's love in an environment that nurtured intellectual, emotional and spiritual development helped foster much of the creativity that is found in my book.

- In particular, to my SLU psychology professor, mentor and dear friend, Dr. Frank Gilner. Thank you for your wisdom and your insights into truly serving others. Your course introduced me to some new ways of thinking and helped shape my skills in helping others overcome psychological challenges encountered in transformation.

- To Dr. Edward Sabin, also a great professor, mentor and friend. Thanks for being so tremendously supportive of my business vision from the start, and for giving me one of my first speaking opportunities. It ignited a fire that continues to blaze. Thanks for your ideas on reaching out and helping others as well.

- To Roger Semsch, owner of the first gym I joined, who recognized God's spark in me, helped me begin to understand the basics of fitness, appreciated my passion and desire to serve others, and gave me a chance early on to do just that in his wonderful fitness center.

- To Mr. Valeriy Fradkin, who not only made primary school bearable for me, but also taught me that I had something of value, a talent that could bring joy to both myself and others.

- To all the staff members at Robert Kennedy Publishing, especially Gabby and Amy, who helped package my material in such an entertaining and comprehensible way. (They made this process fun!)

- To all of the great teachers, visionaries and leaders of the past and present whose work influences and continues to inspire me. I hope one day my work joins the ranks of yours and serves to change and positively influence as many lives.

And to all of you whom I haven't mentioned specifically, thank you for your undying faith and support in my efforts to help others. Please continue to spread my message of Hope, making this book the answer so many people have been searching for. If we work together, I know we can end the strife so many Americans now believe they're facing.